NUTRITION

NUTRITION: CHEMISTRY AND BIOLOGY

JULIAN E. SPALLHOLZ, Ph.D.

Professor of Nutrition and Director
Institute for Nutritional Sciences
Texas Tech University and
Texas Tech University Health Sciences Center

PRENTICE HALL, Englewood Cliffs, New Jersey 07632

LIBRARY OF CONGRESS
Library of Congress Cataloging-in-Publication Data

Spallholz, Julian E.
    Nutrition, chemistry and biology / Julian E. Spallholz.
        p.   cm.
    Bibliography.
    Includes index.
    ISBN 0-13-627241-X
    1. Nutrition. 2. Metabolism.   I. Title.
QP141.S59 1988
    574.1'3--dc19   88-1028
                                                              CIP

Editorial/production supervision and
    interior design: Mary A. Bardoni
Cover design: Photo Plus Art
Manufacturing buyer: Margaret Rizzi and Peter Havens

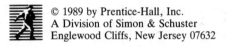 © 1989 by Prentice-Hall, Inc.
A Division of Simon & Schuster
Englewood Cliffs, New Jersey 07632

Printed in the United States of America

10 9 8 7 6 5 4 3 2 1

ISBN   0-13-627241-X

Prentice-Hall International (UK) Limited, *London*
Prentice-Hall of Australia Pty. Limited, *Sydney*
Prentice-Hall Canada Inc., *Toronto*
Prentice-Hall Hispanoamericana, S.A., *Mexico*
Prentice-Hall of India Private Limited, *New Delhi*
Prentice-Hall of Japan, Inc., *Tokyo*
Simon & Schuster Asia Pte. Ltd., *Singapore*
Editora Prentice-Hall do Brasil, Ltda., *Rio de Janeiro*

To Students of All Ages

Contents

Preface

The manuscript for *Nutrition: Chemistry and Biology* originated with a collection of teaching notes and is presented in the order of instruction that I have used to teach Advanced Nutrition. The material accompanying the text fulfilled my perceived need of students at Texas Tech University for the one semester course with prerequisites of introductory nutrition, anatomy, and one semester of biochemistry.

Chapter 1, *Concepts in Chemistry and Biology,* beginning with the periodic table, is a review of some basic principles of inorganic, organic, and biochemistry with inclusion of some thermodynamic principles relating to nutrition. I have found this review useful for some students. *The Elements of Life,* Chapter 2, sets the scene for the origin and use of the organic and inorganic nutrients by all living species of plants, animals, and man.

Chapter 3, *The Nutrients,* outlines the chemical and functional attributes of the nutrients beginning with what were probably the first macromolecules, the proteins, and ending with the most important nutrient of life, water. Where possible and where it contributes to the understanding of the function of the nutrients, some physical, biochemical, nutritional, and metabolic information is provided. The vitamins are presented in the order of their historical discovery and the minerals in descending order of their abundance in the human body.

Assuming the presence of all nutrients in a typical meal, each nutrient or nutrient class is taken through digestion and absorption, Chapter 4. Chapter 5 provides a comparison of the microanatomy of a typical mammalian and plant cell. *Photosynthesis,* Chapter 6, not always found in textbooks on nutrition, is included to show the requirement of plants as primary producers of energy for agricultural food chains: carbohydrates, proteins, and oils. ATP synthesis from solar energy and carbon dioxide fixation is followed through the light and dark reactions of plants. Energy stored by plants as carbohydrates, oils, and proteins is followed through the catabolic and anabolic pathways of heterotrophs, Chapters 7 and 8.

Chapter 9 describes the chemistry of dietary fiber and briefly touches upon the physiology and some of the attributes and health implications associated with it. The essential fatty acids and their nutritional role as precursors to the prostaglandins and related compounds is covered in Chapter 10. Oxygen toxicity, free radicals, and lipid peroxidation is covered in Chapter 11, followed by the function of the dietary and other antioxidant molecules and enzymes in preventing peroxidation reactions *in vivo,* Chapter 12. The text concludes with an overview of drug–nutrient interactions as they may affect the utilization of nutrients and the metabolism of xenobiotics, Chapter 13.

The study of nutrition draws from many sciences and is a diverse and evolving science. If the text appears to be preoccupied with the chemical–biochemical aspects of this science, it is because I am a captive of my own interests and because it is the foundation of nutrition. As Levoisier once stated, "La vie est une fonction chemique."

In conclusion, I would like to thank the students in FN 4320 who helped inspire me to want to take on the task of preparing a textbook; colleagues, friends, and family who provided encouragement during the writing; and finally my editor at Prentice Hall, Susan B. Willig, who asked, believed, and trusted that I could accomplish such an undertaking. A special thank you goes to Mrs. Dunree Norris who patiently and skillfully assisted me in the preparation of the manuscript. With all of the advice, suggestions, and encouragement received, the shortcomings of the book are mine. If you receive any nutritional insights not previously held, then it will all have been worthwhile.

Julian E. Spallholz

NUTRITION

1

Concepts in Chemistry and Biology

THE PERIODIC TABLE

It has been said that we are what we eat. More correctly, we are the atoms we eat. The periodic table, first established by the Russian chemist Dmitri Mendeleev (1834–1907) in 1869 and independently, by the German chemist Julius Meyer (1830–1895) in 1870, now contains more than 100 elements (atoms), of which 90 occur naturally. Beginning with the smallest element, hydrogen (element 1), and progressing through the periodic table, the elements become increasingly larger by the addition of protons, neutrons, and electrons. As the elements get physically larger, they increase in mass correspondingly. For the experimental nutritionist, the periodic table contains and retains fascinating information. On the practical side, the periodic table provides information on atomic numbers and atomic weights. As we explore in more detail in Chapter 2, life's elements have been selected, often in groups and clusters, with great specificity. On the basis of physical and chemical properties alone, the elements of the periodic table have been grouped into light metals, transition metals, heavy metals, and nonmetals.

MOLECULAR WEIGHTS

Weights of the elements are obtained from the periodic table and are standardized against the atomic weight of the element carbon (C) equal to 12. The atomic weight of the smallest element, hydrogen, is 1. The heaviest element is the man-made element lawrencium, of atomic weight 103. All other elements have atomic weights between hydrogen and lawrencium. In determining the molecular weights of molecules of two or more atoms, the sum of the atomic weights of the atoms equals its molecular weight. Thus the molecular weight of oxygen (O_2) is 32, water (H_2O), 18; and ethane (C_2H_6), 30. The molecular weight of any molecule, regardless of size, can be calculated by addition of the atomic weights of the constituent atoms.

BONDING

In the biological world, as in the more inanimate chemical world, few elements exist entirely by themselves. Almost all elements are found in association with other elements as molecules. Elements are composed of neutrons and protons which comprise the nucleus. Surrounding the nucleus of each element are ordered layers of orbiting electrons. It is electrons (e^-), small negatively charged particles orbiting the nucleus with its positively charged protons (p^+) and uncharged neutrons (n^0), which permit the bonding of elements into molecules. There are many possible combinations of elements that make up molecules and there are then additional interactions between molecules involving bonding forces related to orbiting electrons.

The Covalent Bond

The most important bond in the biological world is the covalent bond. In the simplest case, two atoms of hydrogen share their single orbiting electron to form a single covalent bond (Figure 1.1).

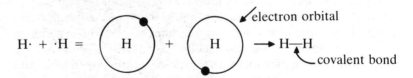

Figure 1.1 Covalent bond of hydrogen.

Most biological molecules exit by sharing a pair of outer orbital electrons which comprise the covalent bond, designated by —. Whereas the covalent bond of hydrogen is relatively simple, more complex and important covalent bonds exist in the bioorganic molecules, including the carbon–carbon bond (—C—C—), the carbon-hydrogen bond (—C—H), and the carbon–oxygen double bond (—C═O) as well as other carbon bonds. Every covalent bond of every molecule represents a small amount of stored energy (Table 7.4). In the chapters that follow, we explore how this small amount of energy is stored, transferred and utilized by living systems.

The Ionic Bond

The ionic bond is commonly found in inorganic compounds, such as salts. Examples of this class of compounds include NaCl, KI, and $FeSO_4$. Like the covalent bond, outer orbiting electrons of atoms enter into ionic bonds that also exist in pairs. Unlike the covalent bond, in which each atom donates and shares an electron pair, in the ionic bond a single electron in the shared pair of electrons is donated by only one of the paired atoms. For this reason NaCl can also be written Na^+Cl^-. In this example of an ionic bond, the sodium (Na^+) cation's outermost electron shell is deficient by one electron. In contrast, the chloride (Cl^-) anion has an extra electron (e^-) in its outer electron shell. In NaCl the sodium atom donates a single electron to the chloride atom forming the ionic bond. When dissolved in water, many salts undergo either partial or total dissociation. Dissociated salts in solution separate, with the electrons that formed the ionic bond being retained by the donor atom. For example, NaCl in solution

Equation 1.1
Dissociation of sodium chloride.

$$NaCl \rightarrow Na^+ + Cl^-$$

dissociates, producing the sodium cation (Na^+) and the chloride anion (Cl^-). In Equation 1.1 Na^+ has donated its electron, forming anionic Cl^-. The ionic bond and principles of dissociation are of more importance to the inorganic chemist and biochemist than to the nutritionist.

The Coordinate Covalent Bond

The coordinate covalent bond possesses properties of both the covalent bond and the ionic bond. In the coordinate covalent bond, two electrons are donated from one atom to another atom, forming the bond. In many instances, coordinate covalent bonds are formed between nitrogen ($\ddot{N}$) atoms and metal ions. Molecules called chelates (meaning "claw") form coordinate covalent bonds between two or more nitrogens and a metal ($\ddot{N} \longrightarrow Fe^{2+}$). Molecules derived from pyrroles form tetrapyrroles, which form coordinate covalent bonds with iron (Fe), cobalt (Co), and magnesium (Mg). These molecules are of particular interest, for they form the biologically important molecules hemoglobin, myoglobin, cytochromes, vitamin B_{12}, and the chlorophyll family of molecules. Each of these molecules and its important biological functions are discussed separately in later chapters.

Other Bonding

The covalent, ionic, and coordinate covalent bonds are forms of intramolecular associations of atoms in the assembly of molecules. There are other forms of intramolecular and intermolecular bonding which are probably of less interest but are no less important in biological systems. These bonding associations include hydrophobic bonding, hydrogen bonding, electrostatic bonding, and van der Waals forces. An appreciation of hydrophobic interactions (bonding) and hydrogen bonding is essential, for such interactions are important in lipids (hydrophobic bonds) and contribute to water's special properties (hydrogen bonding). The hydrogen bond and the dipole moment are unique properties of the most important nutrient, water. Hydrophobic interactions are discussed in the section "Lipids" Chapter 3. Hydrogen bonding is defined in the section "Water" (Chapter 3). Electrostatic forces and van der Waals forces occur as a result of charged separation in molecules (bond dipoles) and may exist as either intermolecular or intramolecular partitioning of polar molecular species.

FUNCTIONAL ORGANIC GROUPS OF NUTRITIONALLY IMPORTANT COMPOUNDS

While the study of the chemistry of carbon and its compounds is the purview of organic chemistry, it is useful to review and again become familiar with those functional organic groups that are important to the nutrients and their metabolic intermediates. Table 1.1 lists the names of these functional groups.

THERMODYNAMICS

Thermodynamics is often viewed as being an esoteric concept of the chemist, biochemist, or physicist. Not so! Thermodynamic principles are easily understandable and should be familiar to all advanced students who study nutrition. Understanding nutrition—why animals and people eat—as well as understanding photosynthesis and energy flow, is to have an understanding of thermodynamics. The principles of thermodynamics are embodied in the three laws of thermodynamics.

1. The first law of thermodynamics is a statement of the conservation of matter and energy: Matter and energy can be neither created nor destroyed, but their form can be changed. In nutritional terminology, matter consists of carbohydrates, lipids, and protein, which is converted into physical movement (work) and heat or is stored as body fat. The first law of thermodynamics is embodied in Einstein's equation, $E = mc^2$ (E = energy, m = mass, c = speed of light). Although this equation is not directly applicable to nutrition, both obesity and starvation are realities of the first law.

2. The second law of thermodynamics is only slightly more esoteric than the first law but is no less important to the understanding of the biological world. The second law is embodied in the idea of structural order within any system: molecule, machine, man, or universe. The law states that the entropy (S) of the universe tends toward maximum disorder. In different words, the

TABLE 1.1 FUNCTIONAL ORGANIC GROUPS IN NUTRIENTS

Functional group name	Formula	Found in these nutrients
Hydroxyl	R—OH (primary)	Carbohydrates, proteins, lipids, vitamins
Amino	R—NH$_2$ (primary)	Proteins
Carboxylic acid	R—COOH	Proteins, lipids
Ester	$\begin{matrix} & O \\ & \parallel \\ R-O-&C-R \end{matrix}$	Lipids
Ether	R—O—R	Carbohydrates
Amide	$\begin{matrix} & O \\ & \parallel \\ R-N-&C-R \\ H \end{matrix}$	Proteins, vitamins
Phosphate esters	$\begin{matrix} & O \\ & \parallel \\ R-O-&P-O-R \\ & \mid \\ & OH \end{matrix}$	Lipids, vitamins
Methylene	R—CH$_2$—R	Proteins, lipids, vitamins
Alkyl	R—CH$_2$—CH$_2$—CH$_3$	Lipids, proteins
α-Keto acid	$\begin{matrix} & O \\ & \parallel \\ R-&C-COOH \end{matrix}$	Important metabolic intermediates
Imine	R—NH (secondary)	Proteins, heterocyclics
Methyl	R—CH$_3$	Lipids, vitamins, proteins
Aldehyde	R—CHO	Carbohydrates, vitamins
Keto	$\begin{matrix} R \\ \\ R \end{matrix}\!\!\!>C=O$	Carbohydrates, proteins
Thiol	R—SH	Proteins
Aryl	R—⬡	Proteins
Phosphate	$\begin{matrix} & OH \\ & \mid \\ R-O-&P-OH \\ & \parallel \\ & O \end{matrix}$	Energy intermediates, phospholipids
Halide	R—I	Thyroid hormones (minerals)

second law says that all order of the universe generally progresses in a unilateral direction toward ever-increasing disorder. Entropy, then, is a quantitative measure of how much order exists in the universe or in any other defined system at any time.

3. The third law of thermodynamics states that the entropy (S) of a perfect crystal, like a perfect diamond with perfect order, is equal to zero [at absolute temperature ($0°K$)]. In a state of perfect order, $S = 0$. Combining the second and third laws of thermodynamics provides the limits for entropy where S exists within theroretical values of $S = 0$ (perfect order) to $S = \infty$ (maximum or infinite disorder). In the real world, S never equals zero or infinity in any system, but possesses intermediate values. We shall learn that the amount of entropy of any system can be either increased or decreased, but that any decrease in entropy of one system is at the expense of increased entropy of another system. Students may be surprised to find that this is what happens when people eat.

ENZYMOLOGY

The study and understanding of enzymes—enzymology—and their functions are described by biochemical specialists called enzymologists. General concepts of enzymology are important aspects of an understanding of the biological world. It is within the study of enzymes that we discover the nutritional need and functions of the vitamins and many minerals. The vitamins, minerals, and their functions are described in Chapter 3. Here, a general presentation is made of the action of enzymes, simple enzyme kinetics, and the thermodynamic concepts of "free" or biologically useful energy, G. (G stands for Gibbs, who was the first person to describe useful energy).

Structurally, enzymes are proteins of varied molecular weights and differing amino acid composition. Functionally, enzymes are organic catalysts often possessing extraordinary specificity. Enzymes exist because the reactions in which they participate normally would not proceed at the human body temperature or at the subzero temperatures often encountered by fish. As catalysts, enzymes enter into reactions that would not ordinarily occur by lowering the energy of activation, which results in a reaction proceeding at a faster (sometimes very fast) rate without itself being consumed in the reaction.

In the simplest cases, an enzyme acts on a substrate or substrates to produce one or more products. The enzyme is often named for the function it performs, and/or for the substrate on which it acts, by adding the suffix *ase*. Examples are shown in Equation 1.2.

Equation 1.2
Enzyme–substrate terminology.

$$(1) \quad \text{sucrose} \xrightarrow{\text{sucrase}} \text{fructose} + \text{glucose}$$

$$(2) \quad \text{fructose} + \text{glucose} \xrightarrow[\text{synthetase}]{\text{sucrose}} \text{sucrose}$$

In example (1), sucrose, the substrate, is hydrolyzed to yield the products fructose and glucose by the enzyme sucrase. In example (2), fructose and glucose, the substrates for the reaction, are combined by the enzyme, a synthetase, to yield the product, sucrose. The substrate in reaction (1) becomes the product in reaction (2). In the reactions above, the enzymes are shown to react without the requirement for cofactors or coenzymes. Many reactions require organic coenzymes, vitamins, to complete the structural requirements of the active site of an enzyme. This aspect of enzymology is described in the section on "vitamins" in Chapter 3.

Enzymes acting on substrates have physical and chemical limits to their catalytic activity. This notion is demonstrated in Figure 1.2.

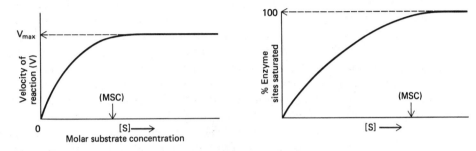

Figure 1.2 Enzyme–substrate kinetics.

In this example, the rate of the enzymatic reaction or velocity is seen to increase with substrate concentration until further increases in substrate concentration beyond the maximum substrate concentration (MSC) result in no increase in reaction velocity. At [S] equal to the (MSC), the enzyme is said to be saturated and it is operating at V_{max}, maximum velocity. V_{max} is also a measure of how fast an enzyme is able to convert substrate(s) to products, and V_{max} is different for each enzyme.

Enzymes acting on substrates in cooperation with coenzymes (vitamins) often exhibit different kinetics. The kinetics exhibited with the cooperative binding of coenzymes in completing the active site is sigmoidal, as shown in Figure 1.3.

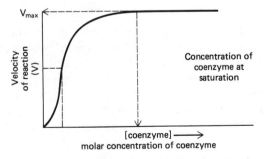

Figure 1.3 Enzyme–coenzyme–substrate kinetics.

In this example of enzyme kinetics, the concentration of coenzyme in the presence of excess substrate [S] is the limiting factor in attaining maximum enzyme catalytic activity (V_{max}) when the concentration of enzyme is held constant. Each enzyme molecule in this situation is not able to function catalytically until there is enough coenzyme present to fulfill the binding requirements to structurally complete all the active sites on the enzymes for substrate attachment. Such limiting conditions of coenzyme saturation are paramount to the induction of a vitamin deficiency, and if the deficiency is severe enough, the onset of disease.

Energy Requirements of Enzymatic Reactions

Many enzymatic reactions proceed with either a requirement for energy or the liberation of energy. When enzyme reactions proceed without any energy requirement, they often, but not always, liberate internal energy contained within the substrate. The difference in internal energy—the difference in energy contained within the substrate and the energy contained within the products—is called the "free energy" of the enzymatic reaction and is designated (G), Gibbs' free energy. G, or more appropriately ΔG, the change in free energy, is a thermodynamic property of the reaction. In addition to the change in the thermodynamic property of the enzymatic reaction (ΔG), there will be an associated change in the overall state of order of the reaction: the entropy (ΔS) of the reaction. The relationship between the free energy of the enzymatic reaction and the change in the entropy, the internal order of the reaction, is shown in Equation 1.3.

Equation 1.3
Free energy, entropy, and total energy within enzyme reactions.

			$\Delta G^{\circ\prime}$	ΔS	E_{total}
(1)	substrate $\xrightarrow{\text{enzyme}}$ product(s)		reaction ($-$) exothermic and spontaneous	increased ($+$) disorder	($-$) declines
(2)	substrate(s) $\xrightarrow{\text{enzyme}}$ product(s)		reaction ($+$) endothermic and nonspontaneous	increased ($-$) order	($+$) increases

In example (1), the enzyme reaction proceeds spontaneously and may be exothermic, releasing energy, $-\Delta G$. The net result within the reaction at completion is an increase in the entropy of the substrate and a decrease in the total energy of the reaction. In example (2), the enzyme reaction cannot proceed without an input of energy, $+\Delta G$, and is therefore a reaction that will not proceed spontaneously. If this reaction is completed to yield a product, energy, often supplied to the enzymatic reaction as adenosine triphosphate (ATP), will be consumed during catalysis. Entropy in this reaction will decline; there will be increased order within the reaction products and the total energy within the product will increase. The relationships in enzyme reaction (2) between ΔG, ΔS, and E_{total} is an example of the thermodynamic state of nutrition, which relates free energy, entropy, and total energy to growth, food (energy source), maintenance, and aging.

OXIDATION–REDUCTION (Redox) REACTIONS

Oxidation–reduction reactions, redox reactions, are important in nutrition because the release of "energy" from food is a basic oxidative process. Reduction reactions are also important, as these processes are paramount in the synthesis of carbohydrates by plants, the synthesis of fatty acids and the subsequent storage of body fat, and the synthesis of other essential organic compounds by animals and humans. No oxidation reaction will take place without a concurrent reduction reaction taking place. Conversely, no reduction reaction will take place without an oxidation reaction also taking place. Therefore, oxidation and reduction reactions occur simultaneously in close contact and are referred to as redox reactions. Redox reactions are most easily understood by example and the application of three rules.

1. No oxidation reaction takes place without something being reduced, and no reduction reaction takes place without something being oxidized.
2. In inorganic chemistry, oxidation is the loss of electrons (e^-), and in organic chemistry oxidation is the loss of hydrogen (H).
3. In inorganic chemistry, reduction is the gain of electrons (e^-), and in organic chemistry reduction is the gain of hydrogen (H).

These rules are almost absolute and should be retained as a guide to recognizing redox reactions. In Equation 1.4 a simple redox reaction is shown for iron (Fe). This reaction can be viewed as an example of an inorganic redox reaction. *In vivo*, such reactions are carried out biologically by a group of iron-containing proteins, the cytochromes.

Equation 1.4
Inorganic redox reaction.

$$\text{(reduced) } Fe^{2+} \underset{-\ e^-}{\overset{+\ e^-}{\rightleftharpoons}} Fe^{3+} \text{ (oxidized)}$$

Iron(II)   Iron(III)
Ferrous ion   Ferric ion
[Fe(II) has been   [Fe(III) has been
oxidized to produce   reduced to produce
Fe(III)]   Fe(II)]

In biological systems, instead of transferring electrons (e^-), redox reactions transfer hydrogen (H), as shown in Equation 1.5. In this reaction, FAD, flavin adenine dinucleotide, is a coenzyme in which the vitamin riboflavin participates in the redox reaction.

Equation 1.5
Organic redox reaction.

$$\text{FAD} \underset{-\ 2H}{\overset{+\ 2H}{\rightleftharpoons}} \text{FADH}_2$$
(oxidized form)   (reduced form)

Examples of several vitamin redox reactions are presented in Chapter 3.

Additional redox reactions of nonvitamin coenzymes and minerals will also be encountered in metabolism.

ENERGY, WORK, AND ATP

As defined by physics, energy is the capacity for doing work and overcoming resistance. Work, for example physical movement, is movement through a measured distance. There are, in the biological world, several types of work and various forms of energy. The various types of work that require energy include mechanical work, chemical work, and osmotic and electrical work. All are different types of biological work. In animals and humans, the energy that sustains the various forms of biological work is derived from the carbohydrates, lipids, and proteins of the diet. Animals and humans, which derive their energy from a variety of food sources, are called heterochemotropes. Plants, on the other hand, derive their primary energy from photosynthesis from the sun and are called phototropes. In an indirect way, mediated by plants, people are solar powered.

All forms of energy may be described as consisting of either potential or kinetic energy. Gasoline (hydrocarbons) in the tank of an automobile is potential energy. A gasoline engine transforms the fuel into the kinetic energy of a flywheel or momentum for work to be accomplished. For people, food is a source of potential energy. A second source of potential energy for people is represented by the body's own store of its carbohydrates, lipids, and protein, which can be called upon in the absence of an intake of food to provide the body with energy.

Whereas potential energy sources—the sun, food, and plant and body stores of carbohydrates, lipids, and protein—are rather extensive for biological processes, most chemical, mechanical, osmotic, and electrical work (kinetic energy) is mediated by a single energy-bearing molecule, adenosine triphosphate (ATP). When energy requiring processes of the body do not use ATP directly, they are mediated by ATP in a preexisting or subsequent step in metabolism. Energy flows through great biological systems from the sun to people. This energy transfer is shown in Figure 1.4.

Energy flow and energy requirements are measured in calories, kilocalories, or joules. By definition, the energy content of 1 calorie (cal) is the amount of heat needed to raise the temperature of 1 gram (g) of water 1°C. The amount of heat needed to raise the temperature of 1 kilogram (1000 g) of water 1°C is the kilocalorie (kcal). Thus 1000 calories equals 1 kcal. A normal human diet containing 2000 kcal contains 2,000,000 calories. It is technically correct to define energy units as either calories or joules (1 J = 0.239 kcal). Whereas the use of the joule for quantitating energy is now preferred by convention, the continuing widespread acceptance and usage of the calorie as a measure of energy, including its use in the Table of Recommended Intakes of the Food and Agricultural Organization and the World Health Organization of the United Nations, prompt its use herein.

The caloric values of the major energy nutrients are: proteins and carbohy-

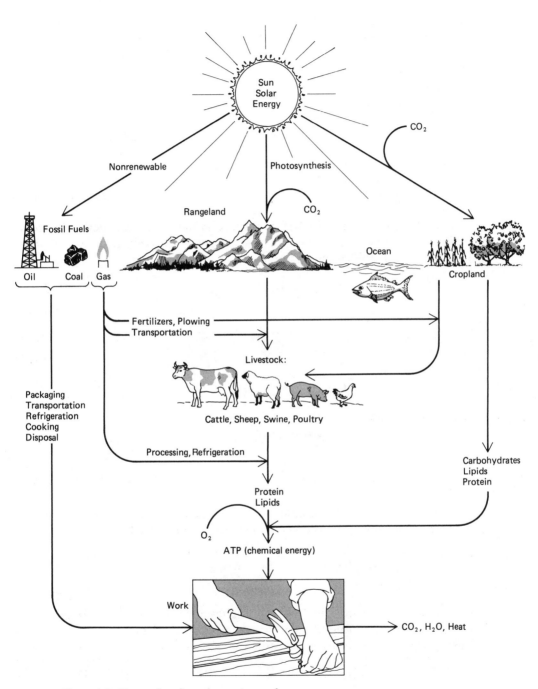

Figure 1.4 Energy flow from the sun to people.

drates, 4 kcal/g, and lipids, 9 kcal/g. Through the metabolic processes, the potential energy of food is converted into the universal carrier of potential chemical energy, ATP. The potential energy stored in ATP is released upon hydrolysis according to Equation 1.6.

Equation 1.6
Hydrolysis of ATP.

$$\text{ATP} \xrightarrow[\text{H2O}]{\text{ATPase}} \text{ADP} + \text{P}_i + (\Delta G^{\circ\prime} = -7.3 \text{ kcal/mol})$$

In the equation, hydrolysis of ATP is shown to liberate (yield) free energy in the amount -7.3 kcal/mol (1 mol of ATP $= 6.02 \times 10^{23}$ molecules). It is evident that each individual molecule of ATP contains only $6/10^{23}$ kcal, a very small amount of energy.

The energy "stored" in ATP is retained in the structural, chemical, electrostatic, and resonant properties of the molecule and is released only upon hydrolysis. The structure of ATP is shown in Figure 1.5.

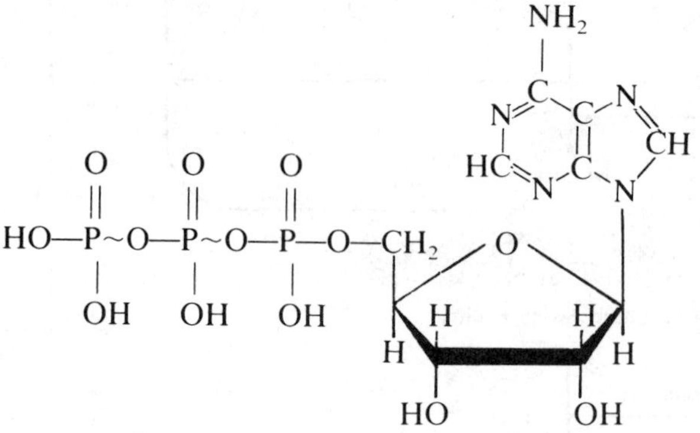

Adenosine triphosphate (ATP)   **Figure 1.5**   Chemical structure of ATP.

Upon hydrolysis, the -7.3 kcal/mol of released energy that has been "stored" in the terminal phosphate of ATP is summarized in Equation 1.7.

Equation 1.7
Energy stored within ATP.

	kcal/mol
Energy contribution from hydrolysis of the terminal phosphate	$\Delta G^{\circ\prime} = -3.0$
Energy contribution from phosphoric acid electrostatic repulsion	$\Delta G^{\circ\prime} = -2.0$
Energy from change in resonance structure of π electrons	$\Delta G^{\circ\prime} = -2.3$
Summary: ATP $\rightarrow$ ADP + P$_i$	$\Delta G^{\circ\prime} = -7.3$

Under biological conditions, the hydrolysis of ATP may yield somewhat greater amounts of free energy. There also exist compounds other than ATP that can yield free energy (some more free energy and some less free energy than ATP), and we will encounter some of these compounds in subsequent chapters.

pH AND pOH

Although pH and pOH are not a primary focus of attention in nutrition, it is important to recall that the pH of the stomach may approach pH 1 and the pH of the duodenum, 7 to 8, with the remaining small intestine being approximately neutral, pH 7. The letter p in pH stands for "$-\log$ of"; thus pH is a measurement, $-\log [H^+]$, the molar hydrogen ion concentration. The pH scale runs from 0 to 14. The pH value and the pOH ($-\log$ of the $[OH^-]$, the molar hydroxyl ion concentration) value are always equal to 14.

Pure water is only weakly dissociated; $HOH \rightleftharpoons H^+ + OH^-$, with a concentration of $[H^+] =$ to $10^{-7} M$ and $[OH^-] =$ to $10^{-7} M$. This condition is commonly referred to as neutral pH, pH 7. pH values below 7 are acidic and pH values greater than 7 are basic or alkaline. The [pH–pOH] scale is shown in Figure 1.6. The pH scale is logarithmic, so that the difference between pH 7 and 8 is a factor of 10 in the $[H^+]$, whereas between pH 7 and 9 the $[H^+]$ is decreased by a factor of 100; and so on.

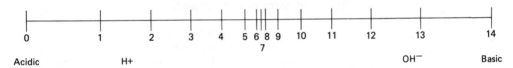

0	1	2	3	4	5 6 8 9	10	11	12	13				14
					7								
Acidic		H+								OH⁻		Basic	

Figure 1.6 pH scale (not to proper log scale).

POLARITY AND SOLUBILITY

Wherever life exists as we know it, water is necessary as the primary sustenance of that life. The property of water that allows it to sustain life is its fluidity and versatility as a solvent. Water's most unique property in these respects is its polarity. Water possesses a dipole moment (Figure 1.7) that is considerably larger than that of other liquid solvents.

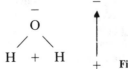

Figure 1.7 Dipole moment of water.

This property, the large dipole moment, permits solvation of inorganic salts; solvation of carbohydrates and proteins; and in the presence of certain amphipathic molecules, such as soaps and detergents, the solubilization of lipids that are hydrophobic. Most organic solvents are generally poor biological solvents because of their smaller dipole moment (Table 1.2).

TABLE 1.2 DIELECTRIC CONSTANTS

Solvent		Dielectric constant (measure of polarity, Debye units)	
Water	HOH	80	
Methanol	CH_3OH	33	
Ethanol	CH_3CH_2OH	24	
Butanol	$CH_3CH_2CH_2OH$	18	
Acetone	CH_3—C—CH_3 $\underset{}{\overset{\|}{}}$ O	21	increasing polarity
Benzene	(ring) or (ring)	2.3	
N-Hexane	$CH_3CH_2CH_2CH_2CH_2CH_3$	1.9	

WEIGHTS AND MEASURES

Commonly used weights and measures are listed in Table 1.3.

TABLE 1.3 COMMONLY USED
WEIGHTS AND MEASURES

(m) 1 meter	= 3.2808 feet
(cm) 1 centimeter	= 0.3937 inch
(g) 1 gram	= 0.035274 ounce
(kg) 1 kilogram	= 2.2046 pounds
1 liter	= 1.05671 quarts
1 mm	= 10^7 Å
100 mm	= 1 centimeter
100 cm	= 1 meter
1000 ng	= 1 µg
1000 µg	= 1 mg
1000 mg	= 1 g
1000 g	= 1 kg
1000 µl	= 1 ml
1000 ml	= 1 L
1 dl	= 100 ml
1000 ppb	= 1 ppm
1 ppm	= 1 µg/mg = 1 mg/kg
1 ppm	= 1 µg/ml = 1 mg/L
1000 calories	= 1 Calorie (1 kilocalorie)
1 mole	= 1 gram-molecular weight
temperature: °C	= $\frac{5}{9}$ (°F − 32)
212°F	= 100°C
32°F	= 0°C
1 Cal (1 kcal)	= 4.184 kilojoules (kJ)

2

The Elements of Life

PERIODIC ARRANGEMENT OF ELEMENTS AND THE ORGANIC CLUSTER

The periodic table contains 103 elements. Only 90 of these elements occur naturally in the environment, and still fewer elements comprise the living world. Scientists have long sought means to predict, interpret, detect, and measure quantitatively the elements necessary for life. The discovery of life's elements, contained by the totality of present knowledge, suggests that life has evolved from the less complex to the more complex. From bacteria to higher vertebrates and humans, nature has repeatedly selected for all life forms a basic group of only six elements. These six elements, the organic cluster (Figure 2.1), include the first element of the periodic table (Figure 2.2), hydrogen, then carbon, nitrogen, oxygen, phosphorus, and sulfur. These six relatively small elements comprise most of the structural organization of the nutrients: proteins, carbohydrates, lipids, and vitamins. In addition, they make up most of the structural forms of the nucleic acids, deoxyribonucleic and ribonucleic acids, and all the metabolic intermediates of metabolism.

The primordial selection of these six elements, which comprise the total bulk of all living matter, appears to have been made on the basis not only of physical size but also on chemical reactivity and the requirement to form intramolecular covalent bonds. Proteins, lipids, and carbohydrates are composed principally of monomers, small molecular units of carbon, oxygen, hydrogen, and nitrogen. The ability of carbon to form —C—C— bonds, extended carbon chains, and cyclic compounds permitted the formation of the myriad of organic compounds. Silicon,

15

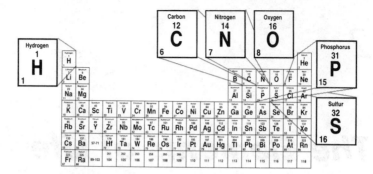

Figure 2.1   Organic cluster.

located just below carbon in the periodic table, is also capable of forming extended chains.   Chains of silicon, however, alternate with oxygen (—O—Si—O—Si—O—), forming silicones.   Such molecules were not biologically selected over carbon, for what would have been a much different type of macromolecular world.

The elements of the organic cluster appear also to have been selected because of their abundance in the primordial atmosphere at the time the first molecules, probably amino acids, were found in the primordial soup.   Evidence does suggest that the composition of the primordial atmosphere was probably much different from our present atmosphere in that it contained no oxygen but was comprised mostly of methane, ammonia, and smaller amounts of carbon monoxide.   Such gaseous mixtures saturated with water vapor, when subjected to electric discharge in the laboratory, result in the synthesis of organic molecules.   The primordial atmosphere, as it is believed to have existed, together with the addition of sulfur as hydrogen sulfide (H_2S) and driven by intense ultraviolet radiation through an ozone-free atmosphere, provided conditions suitable for the synthesis of the first biological organic molecules.

DISTRIBUTION OF ELEMENTS IN THE UNIVERSE, ON EARTH, AND IN THE HUMAN BODY

While the true origin of the organic molecules remains open to conjecture, the association of the elemental composition of the human body to that of the universe, the primordial atmosphere, the earth's crust, and seawater remains fascinating to contemplate.   The universe is composed of 91% of hydrogen and 8.7% of helium. All of the other 88 naturally occurring elements make up the remaining 0.3% of the universe and can be viewed in the periodic table as being derived from hydrogen and helium.   There is within the periodic table a general inverse relationship between elemental abundance and atomic number.   In different words, the larger the atomic number, generally, the rarer the element is in the universe, land and sea.   After H and He, we find four elements of the organic cluster, C, N, O, and

Periodic Table of The Elements

In the periodic table the elements are arranged in order of increasing atomic number. Vertical columns are headed by Roman numerals and are called *groups*. A horizontal sequence of elements is called a *period*. The most active elements are at the top right and bottom left of the table. The staggered line (groups IIIA-VIIA) roughly separates metallic from non metallic elements.

Groups—Elements within a group have similar properties and contain the same number of electrons in their outside energy shell.
— The first group (IA) includes hydrogen and the alkali metals.
— The last (VIIIA) contains the *inert gases.*
— Group VIIA includes the *halogens.*
— The elements intervening between groups IIA and IIIA are called *transition elements.*
— Short vertical columns without Roman numeral headings are called *subgroups.*

Periods—in a given period the properties of the elements gradually pass from a strong metallic to a strong non-metallic nature, with the last number of a period being an inert gas.

LIGHT METALS

NON METALS

Key

Name of element — small type
Atomic wt. — under name
Atomic symbol — bold set
Atomic number — bottom left corner

The organic cluster

The macrominerals

The microminerals

Not proven to be essential for humans; may be essential for other animals and/or plants.

Figure 2.2

17

TABLE 2.1 APPROXIMATE ELEMENTAL COMPOSITION (PERCENT TOTAL NUMBER ATOMS)[a]

Human	Universe	Today's atmosphere	Primordial atmosphere	Earth's crust	Seawater	Seawater (ppm)	
H 63	H 91	N 78.1	H $\quad$ CH$_4$(?)	O 47	H 66	Br 65	La 0.0003
O 25.5	He 8.7	O 20.9	C $\quad$ NH$_4$(?)	Si[b] 28	O 33	Sr 13	Ye 0.0003
C 9.5	O 0.057	Ar 0.934	N $\quad$ CO(?)	Al 7.9	Cl[b] 0.33	B[b] 4.6	Ni[b] 0.0001
N 1.4	N 0.042	C 0.009	O $\quad$ H$_2$S(?)	Fe[b] 4.5	Na[b] 0.28	Si[b] 4.0	Sc 0.00004
Ca[b] 0.31	C 0.021		S	Ca[b] 3.5	Mg[b] 0.33	F[b] 1.4	Hg 0.00003
P 0.22	Si[b] 0.003			Na[b] 2.5	S 0.17	N 0.7	Au 0.000006
Cl[b] 0.03	Ne 0.003			K[b] 2.5	Ca[b] 0.006	Al 0.5	Ra
K[b] 0.06	Mg[b] 0.002		Exclusive of water vapor	Mg[b] 2.2	K[b] 0.006	Ru 0.2	Cd
S 0.05	Fe[b] 0.002			Ti 0.46	C[b] 0.0014	Li 0.1	Cr[b] ⎫
Na[b] 0.03	S 0.001	Exclusive of water vapor		H 0.22	Br 0.0005	P 0.1	Co[b] ⎬ Trace
Mg[b] 0.01				C 0.19		Ba 0.05	Sn ⎭
<0.01[c]	<0.01[c]	<0.10[c]		<0.10[c]	<0.10[c]	I[b] 0.05	and others
						As 0.02	
						Fe[b] 0.02	
						Mn[b] 0.01	
						Cu[b] 0.01	
						Zn[b] 0.005	
						Pb 0.004	
						Se[b] 0.004	
						Cs 0.002	
						U 0.002	
						Mo[b] 0.0005	
						Th 0.0005	
						Ce 0.0004	
						Ag 0.0003	
						V[b] 0.0003	

[a] Boxed elements are of the organic cluster.
[b] Essential mineral.
[c] All other elements.

TABLE 2.2 ELEMENTS REQUIRED BY BACTERIA, PLANTS, AND HUMANS[a]

Bacteria	Source of elements	Plants	Source of elements	Humans	Source of elements
H	H_2O	H	H_2O	H	H_2O, protein
O	HCO_3^-, glucose, citrate	O	CO_2	O	Carbohydrates, lipids
C		C		C	Carbohydrates, lipids, protein
N	NH_3, NH_4^+	N	NH_3, NH_4^+	N	Protein
Ca		Ca		Ca	
P	PO_4^{-2}	P	PO_4^{-2}	P	PO_4^{-2}
S	SO_4^{-2}	S	SO_4^{-2}	S	Amino acids, vitamins
K		K		K	
Cl		Cl		Cl	
Na		—		Na	
Mg		Mg		Mg	
Fe	Salts	Fe	Salts	Fe	Salts
Zn		Zn		Zn	
Cu		Cu		Cu	
Se[b]		—		Se	Se-amino acids
Mn		Mn		Mn	
—		—		I	
Mo		Mo		Mo	
—		—		Cr[b]	
—		—		Co	Vitamin B_{12}
—		B[b]		B[b]	
—		Ni[b]		Ni[b]	
—				F[b]	
—		Si[b]		Si[b]	?
—				Sn[b]	
—		V[b]		V[b]	
—		As[b]		As[b]	
W[b]		—		—	

[a] Listed by decreasing amounts in humans. Details on the functions of most elements are given in Chapter 3. The requirements for elements by bacteria, plants, animals, and humans are similar, but the nutritional source of the elements becomes increasingly more complex for animals and humans than for bacteria and plants.

[b] May or may not have a biological function in all species within each class heading.

S, to be relatively abundant in the universe. In the earth's crust and atmosphere we also find H, C, N, and O to be abundant. The composition of seawater closely approximates the elemental composition of the human body. People are composed of approximately 88.5% H and O, salt water is 99% H and O, and only 1% of seawater includes all the other elements listed in Table 2.1.

ELEMENT REQUIREMENTS OF MICROORGANISMS, PLANTS, ANIMALS, AND HUMANS

Plants, animals, and humans require, in addition to the organic elements, various amounts and types of other elements, collectively referred to as minerals. Reexamination of Table 2.1 reveals that all major elements of the universe, with the exception of the inert gases He and Ne, are included in plant and/or animal life. With the exception of Al, Ti, and Br, all major elements of the earth's crust and seawater include those elements needed by bacteria, plants, animals, and humans.

As life forms increase in complexity from the simplest single cells of the amoeba and bacteria to the more complex plants and animals, there is a general increase in the requirements for those elements that comprise less than 0.1% and often less than 0.01% of our environment. The latter elements are the micro- and ultramicro-(trace) elements, elements required by life forms in minute amounts. The element requirements of many bacteria, plants, and humans are given in Table 2.2. The required elements for bacteria, plants, and humans as representative of the vertebrates shows 15 elements in common to all life forms. With some exceptions, bacteria and plants have similar known element requirements, with the element requirements of humans the most extensive.

The biological complexity of life changes the requirements and the ways in which the need for the elements of the organic cluster can be met. Bacterial requirements for the elements of the organic cluster are met by simple common salts and an inorganic or organic carbon source. Plants fulfill their need for the elements of the organic cluster from atmospheric CO_2 and the remaining elements from soils. Animals and humans rely solely on the organic molecules—carbohydrates, lipids, proteins, and vitamins produced by bacteria and plants—to fulfill their needs for the elements of the organic cluster. Macro-, micro-, and ultramicro-(trace) elements are provided to humans by foods from both plant and animal origin.

3

The Nutrients

PROTEINS

Proteins, from the Greek work *proteus*, meaning "first," are assembled from their basic units, the amino acids. Amino acids or organic compounds of similar nature were probably first formed in that primordial soup at the beginning of biological time. There are many present-day amino acids, but only 20 amino acids are commonly found in proteins. With the exception of glycine, all amino acids assembled into protein in animals and humans are L-amino acids (Figure 3.1). Glycine does not exist as either the D- or L-isomer because it does not possess an (asymmetric) chiral carbon center as do all other amino acids found in protein and in biological fluids. Amino acids of the D-isomer are found in bacteria and racemic mixtures of synthetically made amino acids, but they are not incorporated into animal or human protein. The D-amino acids must undergo isomerization and be converted to the L-isomer of the amino acid before being incorporated into protein.

Amino acids can be and have been classified in several ways. The classifi-

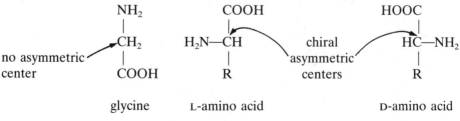

Figure 3.1 Asymmetry in amino acids.

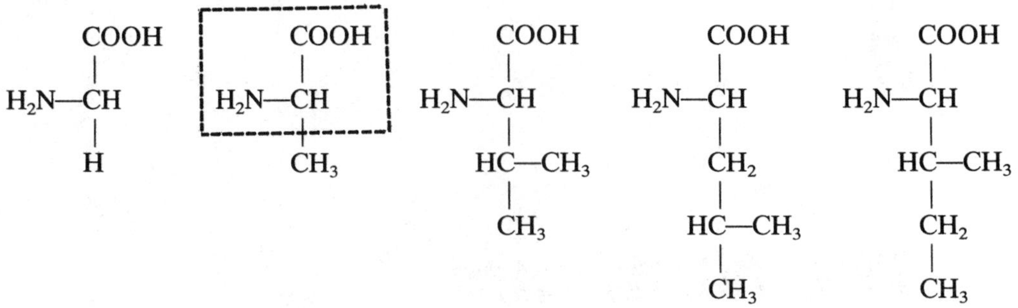

COOH   COOH   COOH   COOH   COOH
 | | | | |
H₂N—CH   H₂N—CH   H₂N—CH   H₂N—CH   H₂N—CH
 | | | | |
 H   CH₃   HC—CH₃   CH₂   HC—CH₃
                             | | |
                            CH₃   HC—CH₃   CH₂
                                           | |
                                          CH₃   CH₃

glycine   alanine   valine   leucine   isoleucine
Gly   Ala   Val   Leu   Ile
1820   1881   1901   1820   1903

Figure 3.2 Aliphatic amino acids.

cation used here is one based on the structural similarities of amino acids. The structural divisions include the aliphatic, acidic, basic, aromatic, sulfur-containing, and secondary amino acids. The structures of 22 amino acids are presented with names, abbreviations, and dates of discovery (Figures 3.2 to 3.8).

Each of the aliphatic amino acids possesses a common structural component, shown within the boxed area of alanine (Figure 3.2). Among the branched-chain aliphatic amino acids, valine, leucine, and isoleucine, metabolism is sometimes prevented, owing to the lack in newborns, of an enzyme, a branched-chain α-keto acid dehydrogenase, resulting in an inborn error of metabolism called MSUD, maple syrup urine disease. This disease cannot be corrected but is controllable by limiting these amino acids in the diets of children. Serine and threonine differ in structure by a methyl group and are the hydroxyl-containing amino acids (Figure 3.3).

Aspartic acid and glutamic acid (Figure 3.4) are acidic amino acids because each possesses two carboxylic acids and only one amino group. These two amino acids differ by only a single methylene, which when added to aspartic acid becomes glutamic acid. The monosodium salt of glutamic acid is commonly used as a flavor

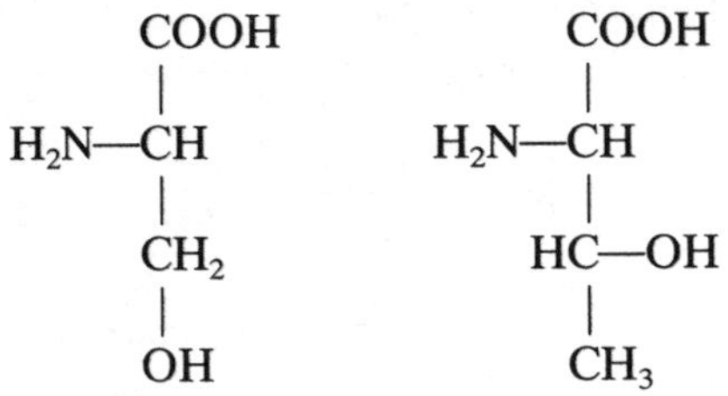

COOH   COOH
 | |
H₂N—CH   H₂N—CH
 | |
CH₂   HC—OH
 | |
OH   CH₃

serine   threonine
Ser   Thr
1865   1935   **Figure 3.3** Hydroxyl amino acids.

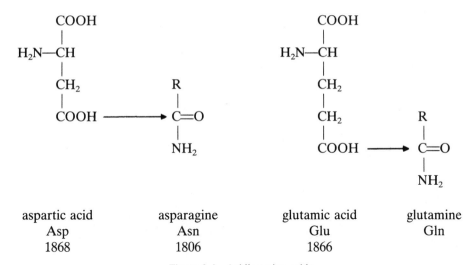

Figure 3.4 Acidic amino acids.

enhancer in foods and is known as MSG, monosodium glutamate. Sometimes, protein contains the amide derivatives of aspartic acid, asparagine, and glutamic acid, glutamine. Ammonia (NH_3) from the degradation of protein and amino acids is commonly carried in body fluids as glutamine, the ammonia having been fixed to glutamic acid (see Equation 7.15).

Lysine, arginine, and histidine (Figure 3.5) are the basic amino acids because

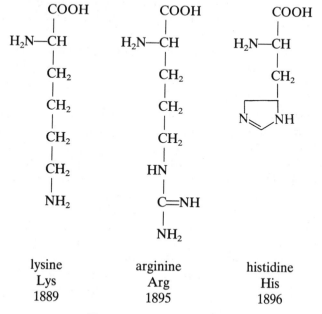

Figure 3.5 Basic amino acids.

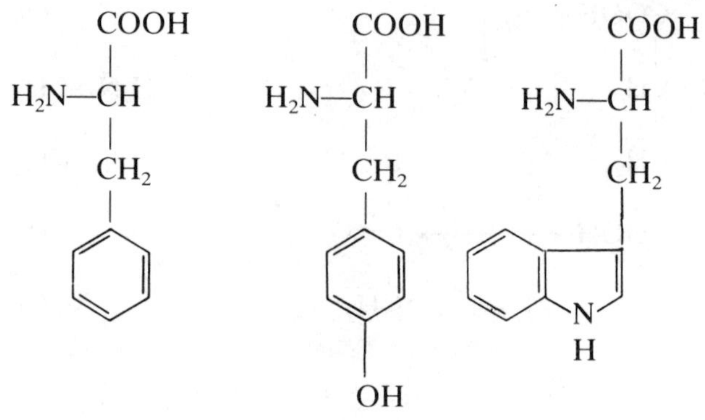

phenylalanine Phe 1881 | tyrosine Tyr 1849 | tryptophan Try 1901

Figure 3.6 Aromatic amino acids.

they each possess at least two amino groups or amine equivalents and only one carboxylic acid. Lysine is nutritionally one of the most important amino acids, as it is often the limiting dietary essential amino acid of plant protein.

The aromatic acids (Figure 3.6) contribute to the ultraviolet-absorbing property that most proteins possess. The methyl ester of phenylalanine and the acidic amino acid aspartic acid are combined as a dipeptide forming the sweetener aspartame, one trade name for which is NutraSweet®. Children born without the enzyme phenylalanine hydroxylase, which converts phenylalanine to tyrosine, have the inborn metabolic disease PKU, phenylketoneuria. This disease, like MSUD, is managed by controlling the quantity of phenylalanine in the diet. Persons with this disease are cautioned to limit or not use products with NutraSweet® because of its phenylalanine content.

The sulfur amino acids methionine and cysteine (Figure 3.7) are two predominant sulfur-containing compounds in many cells. Only methionine need be included in the diet, as cysteine is derived from *S*-adenylsylmethionine, the principal methylating agent of cells. When incorporated into protein, cysteine can undergo oxidation and combine with another oxidized cysteine residue, forming cystine. Cystine is commonly referred to as a disulfide and functions as both an interchain and intrachain cross-linking amino acid in protein structure (see also Figure 3.9). Cysteine is a component of another important thiol compound, glutathione, the tripeptide γ-glutamylcysteinylglycine. This abundant intracellular thiol, common to all cells and functions to prevent harmful oxidation reactions in cells (see Chapter 12). Glutathione also detoxifies carcinogens and xenobiotics by forming glutathione derivatives with these compounds, which are then excreted (see Chapter 13).

methionine Met 1922 | cysteine ½Cys 1899 | cystine* Cys 1899

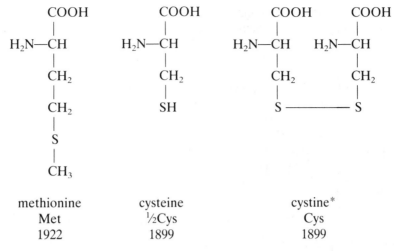

Figure 3.7 Sulfur amino acids.

*Dimer of cysteine formed post-translationally.

Sulfur (S) has chemical properties similar to those of its sister element selenium (Se), located just below S in the periodic table. From simple selenium salts and organic selenium compounds, selenium can replace the sulfur atom in cysteine, forming the uncommon amino acid selenocysteine. This seleno-amino acid is found in some proteins and enzymes of bacteria, animals, and humans but is not known in plants. Plants, cereal grains, and yeasts synthesize another selenoamino acid, selenomethionine, which is a major dietary source of selenium. Selenocystine is not formed in protein from selenocysteine as cystine is formed from oxidized cysteine.

Proline and hydroxyproline are not primary amino acids but are the only two secondary amino (imino) acids (Figure 3.8). Proline interrupts α-helical formations in protein. Hydroxyproline is extensively found in collagen, a protein of connective tissue. Hydroxylation of proline, forming hydroxyproline, occurs with the participation of ascorbic acid (see Figure 3.29).

Proteins are assembled from their constituent amino acids, one by one and

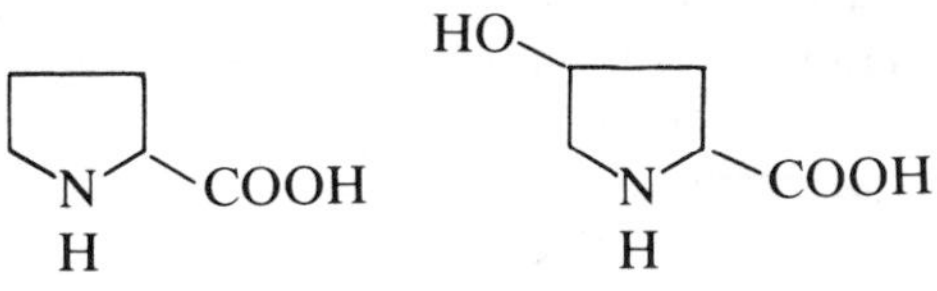

proline Pro 1901 | hydroxyproline Hyp 1902

Figure 3.8 Secondary amino (imino) acids.

one at a time.   Two amino acids are initially combined, forming a dipeptide by the exclusion of a molecule of water from the carboxylic acid (R_1) and the amino group of the second amino acid (R_2), as shown in Equation 3.1.

Equation 3.1
Peptide bond formation: synthesis of a dipeptide.

```
          O      [H]
      H   ||      |      H
H₂N—C—C—|OH|+ N—C—COOH  ⟶
      |          |   H  |
      R₁         |      R₂
               H₂O
```

```
          O
      H  |||      H
H₂N—C+C—N+C—COOH          peptide bond
      |   |H|   |
      R₁        R₂
```

The result is formation of a dipeptide with its amide, "peptide bond."   Addition of a third amino acid to the dipeptide results in the formation of a second peptide bond and a tripeptide (Equation 3.2).

To the tripeptide is added, in similar fashion, another amino acid, forming a tetrapeptide, and so, one by one, polypeptides are assembled from amino acids.

Equation 3.2
Peptide bond formation: synthesis of a tripeptide.

```
          O       O      [H]
      H   ||   H  ||      |      H
H₂N—C—C—N—C—C—|OH+|N—C—COOH  ⟶
      |    H  |          H  |
      R₁      R₂         |   R₃
                       H₂O
```

```
          O       O
      H  |||   H  |||      H
H₂N—C+C—N+C+C—N+C—COOH      second peptide
      |   |H|  |   |H|  |          bond
      R₁       R₂       R₃
```

When polypeptides begin approaching 50 amino acids in length they are called proteins. Hormones of the pituitary gland, thyroid-stimulating hormone (MW 30,000) and follicle-stimulating hormone (MW 26,000), are moderately large proteins. Other hormones of the pituitary gland, vasopressin, oxytosin (nine amino acid residues), and human β-melanocyte-stimulating hormone with 22 amino acid residues, are polypeptides. Insulin (Figure 3.9), a pancreatic hormone with its 51 amino acids, is a small protein. Proteins vary extensively in size and function and are physically described by their amino composition (primary structure), which determines their molecular weight. Proteins are further described by their α-helical content stabilized by hydrogen-bonding between amino acid residues (secondary structure), and the spatial arrangement of secondary structure contributed by —S—S— bonding (tertiary structure). Some proteins will assemble themselves by the association of individual subunits (quaternary structure). They are the principal components of muscle, connective tissues, hair and nails, serum, antibodies, and enzymes. It is the catalytic function of proteins that makes all life processes possible. Proteins are believed to have been the first molecules, for it is their catalytic activity that permits the assembly of the nucleic acids and all the other bioorganic molecules. Proteins do not always exist singularly but are often associated with other compounds. Such complex proteins in association with nucleic acids, lipids, carbohydrates, and minerals are often classified according to the molecule with which the protein associates. Such protein complexes are named in Table 3.1.

Amino acids and their specific order in the primary protein structure provides the chemical specificity that dictates their function. No *de novo* synthesis of protein can be sustained without a continuous dietary intake of the essential amino acids. The essential amino acids cannot be synthesized *in vivo* from nonprotein sources in sufficient quantity to meet the body's needs, and so must be supplied to humans

TABLE 3.1 COMPLEX PROTEINS

Complex	Example	Non-peptide moiety
Glyproteins	Blood antigens A, B, AB, O	Carbohydrates
Lipoproteins	HDLs, LDLs, VLDLs	Triglycerides, cholesterol
Nucleoproteins	Chromosomes, ribosomes	Nucleic acids
Metalloproteins	Metallothionine	Zinc
	Dehydrogenases	Zinc
	Cytochromes	Iron
Chromoproteins	Hemoglobin	Heme iron
	Myoglobin	Heme iron
	Cytochromes	Heme iron

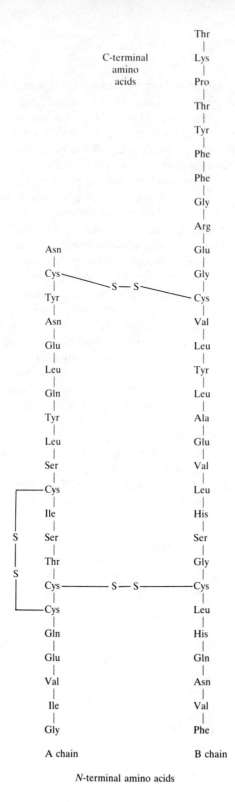

Figure 3.9 Amino acid sequences of A and B chains of human insulin. The amino acid sequence of human insulin and the positions of the —S—S— cross-linkages; 51 amino acids.

28

TABLE 3.2 ESSENTIAL AMINO ACIDS

Amino acids required by the human infant and adult		Amino acids synthesized in vivo (nonessential amino acids)	
Valine	Leucine	Hydroxyproline	Tyrosine
Threonine	Lysine	Glycine	Alanine
Tryptophan	Phenylalanine	Serine	Glutamine
Isoleucine		Glutamic acid	Asparagine
Methionine		Aspartic acid	Proline
Histidine[a]		Cysteine	
Arginine[a]		Cystine	

[a]May not be required by the human adult.

from either plant or animal proteins. There are 10 essential amino acids required in the diet of the human infant and eight amino acids required by the human adult. These essential amino acids are given in Table 3.2. Our understanding of the nutritional needs for the essential amino acids was mostly determined by W. C. Rose of the University of Illinois over a period of several years during the 1930s. The last of the essential amino acids, threonine, was isolated by Rose in 1935.

In addition to supplying the essential amino acids, dietary protein supplies the nitrogen for the synthesis of the nucleic acids. Aspartic acid is incorporated into pyrimidines, and glycine becomes a part of the purines (Chapter 8). Proteins in the diet also supply energy. Proteins contain approximately 4 kcal/g, and 12% of the caloric requirements of an average American is supplied by protein. Nearly 45 g of protein, representing 180 kcal, is recommended as a daily dietary intake for adults. It is estimated that 450 million people, about 10% of the world's population, continuously suffer from hunger. Much prolonged hunger, as recently occurred in people in the Sahara Desert of Africa, results in protein-calorie malnutrition, protracted starvation, and even death. In Western countries, people generally consume excessive amounts of high-quality protein, such as meat. Third-world peoples more often than not consume inadequate amounts of protein, which is often of the lower-quality protein provided by vegetables and cereal grains containing limited amounts of the essential amino acids lysine and methionine. With world population continuing to grow at disconcerting rates, future droughts, floods, and political disruptions will probably lead to increasing incidences of protein-calorie malnutrition in the world.

CARBOHYDRATES

The word *carbohydrate* has been compounded from the description of this group of organic molecules, the "carbon hydrates," whose carbon compounds are extensively hydrated. The carbohydrates are either polyhydroxyaldehydes or polyhydroxyketones. Dietarily, carbohydrates provide approximately 48% of the caloric needs of Americans.   Being derived from plants, vegetables, and cereal grains, a greater proportion of the caloric needs of third-world people are met by carbohydrates.   Carbohydrates are grouped according to the number of carbon atoms per molecule, such as the trioses (three-carbon unit), the pentoses (five-carbon unit), and the hexoses (six-carbon unit).   Nutritionally, the most important carbohydrates are the hexoses.   The most important hexose metabolically is a monosaccharide, D-Glucose.   D-glucose is commonly referred to as blood glucose or blood sugar.   Glucose comes in two epimeric forms, α-D-glucose and β-D-glucose (Figure 3.10).

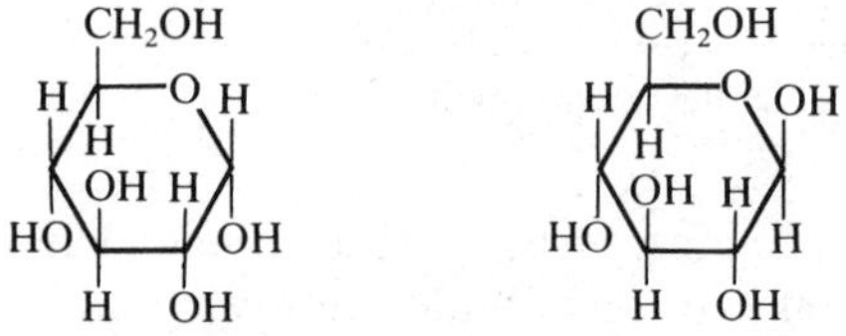

α-D-glucose   β-D-glucose   **Figure 3.10**   Structure of glucose.

While it is the most important metabolic carbohydrate, glucose, galactose, fructose, sorbose, and other monosaccharides are infrequent dietary carbohydrate constituents.   Insignificant amounts of glucose are naturally consumed in diets.   Far more important as dietary constituents are the disaccharides lactose and sucrose (Figure 3.11).

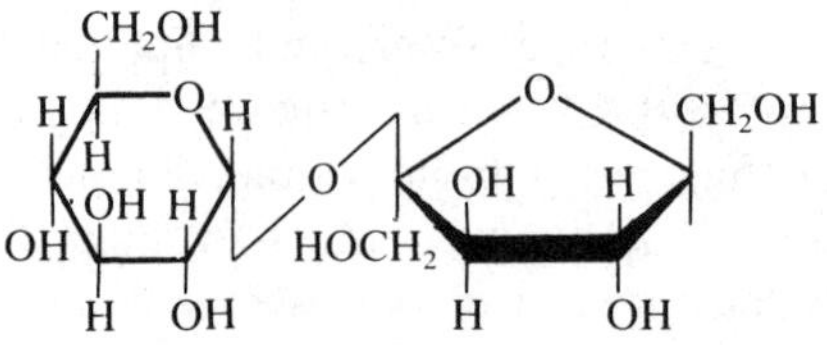

sucrose

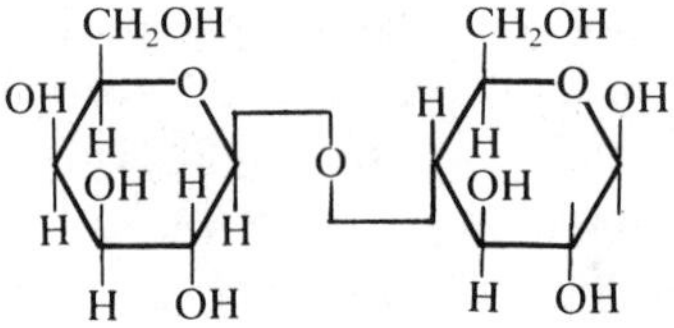

lactose

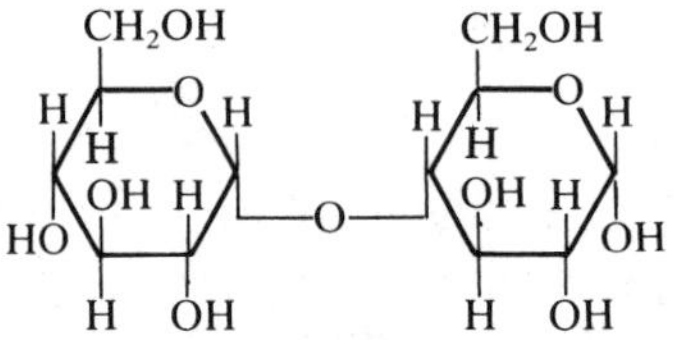

maltose   **Figure 3.11** Predominant dietary disaccharides.

Lactose, known also as milk sugar, is a major dietary carbohydrate of nursing infants. Upon hydrolysis, lactose yields the monosaccharides glucose and galactose. Infants and adults lacking the intestinal enzyme lactase are often confronted with an intolerance to lactose and may need to avoid milk and dairy products.

A major dietary carbohydrate, providing as much as 20 to 30% of total dietary calories, is the disaccharide sucrose (Figure 3.11). Although found primarily as an extensively used food additive in the American diet, smaller amounts of sucrose are naturally found in a few foods. Because sucrose is sweet and inexpensive, processed foods often contain proportionately large amounts of sucrose. Upon hydrolysis of sucrose by sucrase, the monosaccharides glucose and fructose are liberated. The hexose fructose can be a major dietary carbohydrate when fruits, honey, and preserves are eaten. Maltose, a disaccharide consisting of two molecules of glucose, is not naturally found to any great extent in the diet. It is found as a hydrolysis product of starch, in the malting process of fermentation, and is present in corn syrups, another major food additive.

Polysaccharides

Three homopolysaccharides of glucose comprise the major dietary carbohydrates and the major carbohydrate store of liver and muscle. These three homopolysaccharides are starch, cellulose, and glycogen. All are synthesized from glucose, made either by the photosynthetic activity of plants, or in animal and human tissues. All three polysaccharides are substantially different as determined by the composition of their glycosidic (R—O—R) linkage between glucose subunits. The polysaccharide providing the largest proportion of dietary calories is starch. Starch is assembled from glucose by plants as a principal energy store of the cereal grains (wheat) and tuberous (potato) vegetables. Starch contains two types of glucose–glucose bonding (Figure 3.12). The bond providing the extended glucose polymer

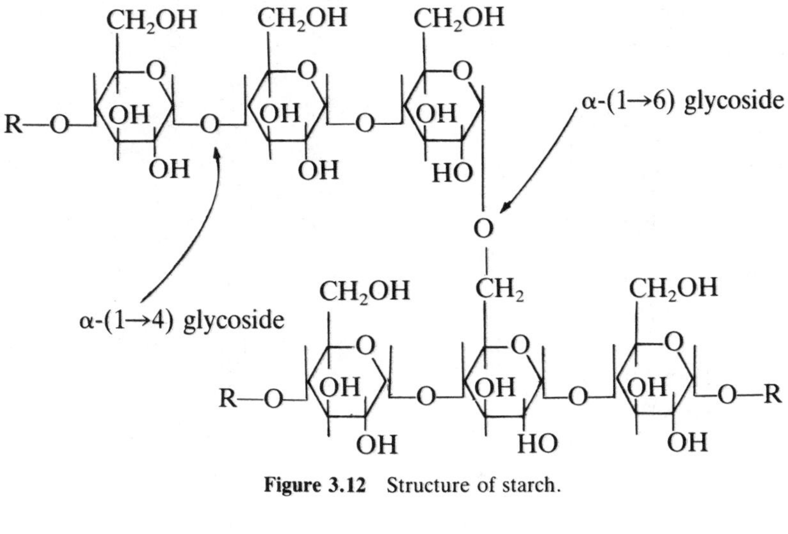

Figure 3.12 Structure of starch.

in the starch molecule is the α-(1→4) glycoside. A second glycoside, the α-(1→6) glycoside, provides for branching and termination of the linear arrays of α-(1→4) glycoside chains of glucose. Polymers of glucose in α-(1→4) linear chains is amylose. Amylose with α-(1→6) glycosidic branching is amylopectin. Digestive enzymes specific for α-(1→4) glycosides and α-(1→6) glycosides in the mouth and small intestine rapidly degrade the starch polymer to polysaccarides, fragments of starch containing terminal α-(1→6) glycoside residues that cannot be degraded further by the α-(1→4) maltoglycosidase, to dextrins, maltose, and ultimately to the monosaccharide glucose. Limit dextrins are further degraded to maltose, isomaltose, and glucose by the enzyme α-(1→6) isomaltoglycosidase, isomaltase; and α-(1→4) glycosidase, maltase.

Polysaccharides stored in liver and muscle are glycogen. Glycogen (Figure 3.13) is structurally very similar to starch, containing both the α-(1→4) and α-(1→6) glycosides linking the glucose units. The difference between starch and glycogen is that glycogen is more highly branched, as it contains a proportionately higher amount of α-(1→6) glycosides than does starch. The larger amount of branching, ( ), provides for the rapid hydrolysis of glycogen to glucose to provide energy for muscular contraction and for the elevation of blood glucose from liver.

The third polysaccharide of glucose is the most abundant of all organic molecules in the biosphere. It is cellulose (Figure 3.14). One need only view a pristine forest to contemplate the vast amounts of cellulose present in wood fiber. The cell walls of trees and other plants are composed mainly of cellulose. This polysaccharide is similar in composition to amylose, but instead of the α-(1→4) glycosidic bond, cellulose possesses a β-(1→4) glycoside between glucose units. Equal quantities of starch and cellulose contain the same caloric value, but the

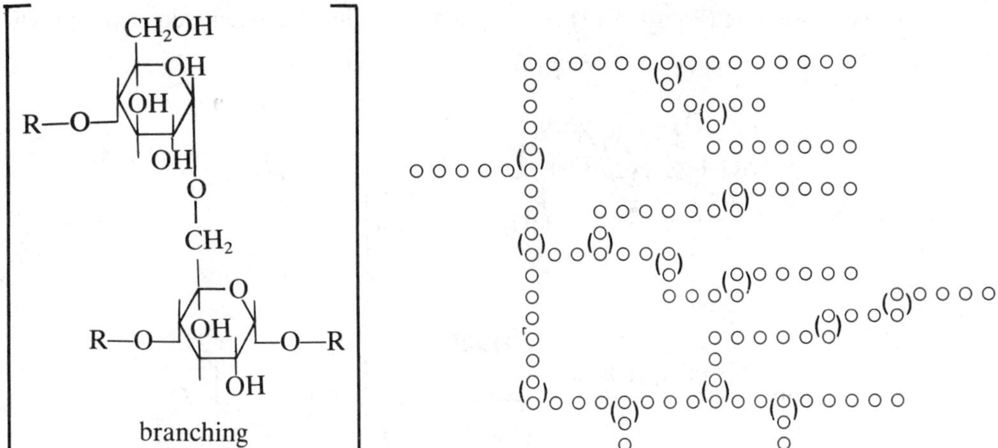

Figure 3.13 Structure of glycogen.

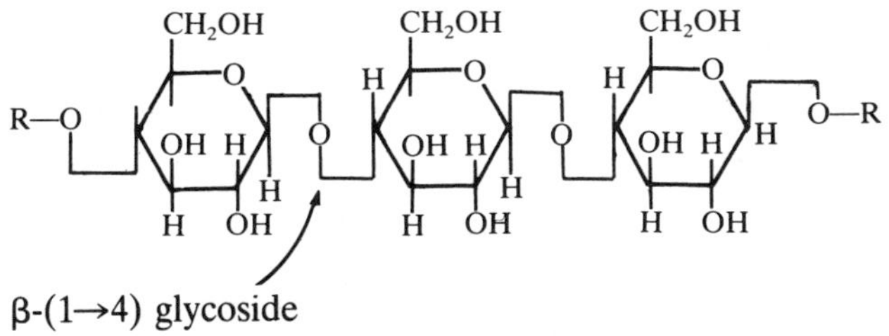

β-(1→4) glycoside

Figure 3.14 Structure of cellulose.

calories within cellulose are largely unavailable to monogastric animals and humans because they do not possess a β-(1→4) glycosidase and consequently the glucose cannot be released from its polymer structure. β-(1→4) glycosidases are synthesized by many bacteria, and in the human gastrointestinal tract some small amount of glucose may be released from cellulose to the extent that β-(1→4) glycosidases are present. Ruminants (cattle, sheep) derive calories from cellulose because of the extensive hydrolytic action of the β-(1→4) glycosides produced by bacteria and other microflora of the rumen.

Fiber

Hemicelluloses, pectins, gums, and mucilages are heteropolysaccharides: polysaccharides composed of monosaccharides—glucose, galactose, pentoses, uronic acid, and so on. These carbohydrates, present in plants together with cellulose (Figure 3.14) and lignin, constitute what is called dietary fiber (see Chapter 9). Dietary fiber is not subject to a universally accepted definition. Different types of fiber have been defined, classified by the solubility of the fiber in acid or alkali solutions or as the carbohydrate not subject to human digestive enzymes. The author's preferred definition of dietary fiber is: that portion of dietary carbohydrate and lignin unabsorbed following digestion by human or bacterial enzyme activity. Glucose and similar monosaccharides from starch, cellulose,* and most other components of dietary fiber possess the same caloric values following intestinal absorption, irrespective of the source of hydrolytic enzymes.

LIPIDS

Lipid is a generic word for a diverse group of organic compounds. Chemically, the lipids are defined as those organic compounds that are insoluble in water, but are generally soluble in one or a mixture of several organic solvents. Many organic solvents are able to dissolve lipid compounds because both are non-polar. Table

---

*Cellulose, lignin, and other components of dietary fiber do not provide dietary calories to humans, but do supply significant calories to ruminants (cattle, sheep) and horses, which have a cecum.

TABLE 3.3 PROPERTIES OF SOME SOLVENTS

Solvent	Polarity, E	Boiling point (°C)
Nonlipid		
Water, H_2O	80	100
Ethanol, CH_3CH_2OH	24	79
Acetone, CH_3CCH_3	21	57
O		
Lipid		
Chloroform, $CHCl_3$	4.8	61
Ether, $(CH_3CH_2)_2O$	4.3	35
n-Hexane, $CH_3(CH_2)_4CH_3$	1.9	37

3.3 lists the polarity and boiling points of some commonly used organic solvents that can be compared to water, which is extensively hydrogen bonded (Table 3.3).

Lipid Classifications

Lipids, as heterogeneous as they are, are usually classified as being either simple or compound lipids (Table 3.4). That classification is maintained here with only a few modifications. The primary emphasis for the lipids, as it was for the carbohydrates, is to focus attention on the most important dietary lipids. Dietary lipids of significant importance include the fatty acids, the triglycerides, cholesterol and esters of cholesterol, and the fat-soluble vitamins. Discussion of the fat-soluble vitamins is deferred to the nutrient section, "Vitamins."

The extreme diversity of lipid compounds, both in structure and function, makes any classification of these molecules almost unsatisfactory. As a collection of molecular diversity, however, most of the lipids are formed from a small number of identifiable biological molecules which comprise the building blocks of this group of compounds.

Fatty acids and glycerol. All of the important lipid nutrients that yield either calories or are essential are comprised of fatty acids or fatty acids esterified to glycerol. If phosphatidic acid is included, all phosphatidyl derivatives are then included as derivatives of fatty acids and glycerol.

Isoprene derivatives. Isoprene,

$$CH_2{=}C{-}CH{=}CH_2$$
$$\overset{\displaystyle |}{\underset{}{CH_3}}$$

is a five-carbon compound derived from acetylcoenzyme A (see Chapter 7). Isoprene molecules can be thought of as the "glucose" or "amino acid" of the lipid

TABLE 3.4 CLASSIFICATION OF THE LIPIDS

Simple lipids
    Fatty acids: C_2 to C_{24}, saturated and unsaturated
    Monoglycerides: monoacylglycerol
    Diglycerides: diacylglcerol
    Triglycerides: triacylglycerol
    Cholesterol: cholesterol esters
    Bile acids: cholic acid, taurocholic acid, glycocholic acid, etc.
    Vitamin A: vitamin A esters
    Waxes: esters of alcohols
    Prostaglandins: hormones of the essential fatty acids
Compound lipids: derivatives of phosphatidic acid
    Phosphatidylcholine (lecithin)
    Phosphatidylethanolamine
    Phosphatidylserine
    Phosphatidylinositol
    Sphingolipids
    Plasmologens
Other lipids
    Glycolipids
    Liproproteins
    Adrenocorticotropins
    Androgens
    Estrogens
    Chylomicrons, HDLs, LDLs, VLDLs

compounds. From isoprene, "polylipids" are synthesized by plants, animals, and humans, giving rise to β-carotene and vitamin A, plant sterols, cholesterol and bile acids, all the adrenocorticosteroids, sex hormones, vitamins D, E, and K, and related compounds such as ubiquinone. Classifying the lipids or viewing them as a heterogeneous group of molecules formed from primarily fatty acids, glycerol, or units of isoprene simplifies one's perspective of this large array of diverse molecules. As nature fashioned, its simple units continue to unfold biological diversity.

Fatty Acids

Much can be learned about the nutritionally important lipids—their metabolism, structure, and function—by understanding the properties of the saturated and unsaturated fatty acids. Saturated fatty acids of dietary importance are composed of straight-chain monocarboxylic acids, $CH_3CH_2CH_2(CH_2)_nCOOH$. The simplest fatty acid of dietary importance is acetic acid, CH_3COOH. A dilute solution of acetic acid is known as vinegar. Fatty acids are extended by the addition of methylene ($-CH_2-$) groups between the terminal methyl and carboxylic acid moieties. The carbon range of saturated fatty acids is from C_2 to C_{24}, with the predominant nutritional fatty acids being of even carbon numbers, C_{14}, C_{16}, C_{18}.

    Examination of the properties of the saturated monocarboxylic fatty acids

TABLE 3.5 SATURATED FATTY ACIDS

Name	Carbon atoms	Molecular weight	Solubility (g/100 ml H_2O)[a]	Melting point (°C)
Acetic (ethanoic)	$C_2:0$	60	∞	16.6
Proprionic	$C_3:0$	74	∞	−22.0
Butyric	$C_4:0$	88	5.6	−7.9
Pentanoic	$C_5:0$	102	3.7	−59.0
Caproic	$C_6:0$	116	0.4	−9.5
Heptanoic	$C_7:0$	130	0.24	−10.0
Caprylic	$C_8:0$	144	0.25	16.0
Pelargonic	$C_9:0$	158	vsl	12.0
Capric	$C_{10}:0$	172	sl	31.5
Undecylic	$C_{11}:0$	186	i	29.3
Lauric	$C_{12}:0$	200	i	40.0
Tridecylic	$C_{13}:0$	214	i	51.0
Myristic	$C_{14}:0$	228	i	58.0
Pentadecylic	$C_{15}:0$	232	i	—
Palmitic	$C_{16}:0$	256	i	64.0
Margaric	$C_{17}:0$	270	i	61.0
Stearic	$C_{18}:0$	284	i	69.0
Nondecylic	$C_{19}:0$	298	i	—
Arachilic	$C_{20}:0$	312	i	76.3
Behenic	$C_{22}:0$	340	i	80.7
Lignoceric	$C_{24}:0$	369	i	81.0

[a]vsl, very slightly soluble; sl, slightly soluble; i, insoluble.

(Table 3.5) reveals that the smaller (C_2 to C_5) fatty acids have appreciable solubility in water and do not strictly adhere to the definition given for lipids. In these few fatty acids, the carboxylic acid moiety dominates chemically over the hydrocarbon portion of the molecule. Intermediate-sized fatty acids (C_6 to C_{11}) are oils, and higher-molecular-weight fatty acids are solids at room temperature. In these larger fatty acids, the hydrocarbon portion of the molecule chemically dominates the carboxylic acid moiety. This dominance by the hydrocarbon portion of the molecule in these higher-molecular-weight fatty acids is measurable as increasing melting points. Even-numbered fatty acids have higher melting points than those of the preceding odd-numbered fatty acids. Nutritionally, the even-numbered fatty acids, beginning with acetic acid, predominate in the diet. The majority of saturated monocarboxylic fatty acids in the diet are the C_{14}, C_{16}, and C_{18} even-numbered fatty acids. These three fatty acids—myristic, palmitic, and stearic, respectively—comprise a large proportion of the saturated fatty acids found in plant oils and animal fats (Table 3.7).

A second type of fatty acid, the monocarboxylic monounsaturated and mono-carboxylic polyunsaturated fatty acids, contain one or more carbon–carbon

$$(-C{=}C-)$$
$$|\quad\ |$$
$$H\quad H$$

double bonds. Double bonds in fatty acids are distinguished by a suffix in the abbreviated formula. Steric acid is a fully saturated fatty acid with a full complement of hydrogen atoms. Its formula is $C_{18}:0$ (Table 3.5) and no double bonds are in its structure. Oleic acid is a common C_{18} monounsaturated fatty acid. Its formula is $C_{18}:1$, designating that one double bond exists in the molecule. Since the double bond could occur in any one of 16 different positions in the aliphatic carbon chain, the position of the double bond in the molecule is usually parenthetically noted in some manner in the formula, as, for example, $C_{18}:1(9)$ and $C_{18}:1^{\Delta 9}$. These formulas tells us that the double bond exists in oleic acid between the number 9 and 10 carbon atoms of the fatty acid counting from the C_1, the carboxylic acid carbon atom. This same nomenclature is followed for the polyunsaturated fatty acids, with the number and position of each double bond explicitly noted.

Table 3.6 reveals that the addition of a single double bond to an otherwise identical saturated fatty acid lowers the melting point. The addition of more double bonds (more unsaturation) results in still further lowering of the melting point of fatty acids of comparable or larger carbon chain length. The addition of double bonds not only results in lower melting points but in unsaturated fatty acids becoming oils as compared to similar saturated fatty acids being solids at room temperature.

Monounsaturated fatty acids may exist in two different isomeric forms, as determined by the orientation of the hydrogen atoms about the carbon–carbon double bond. If both hydrogen atoms are positioned on one side of the carbon–carbon bond, a monounsaturated fatty acid would be in the *cis* configuration (Figure 3.15). If one H is positioned on one side of the carbon–carbon double bond and the other H is positioned on the opposite side, a monocarboxylic unsaturated fatty acid would be in the *trans* configuration (Figure 3.15). With few exceptions, naturally occurring mono- and polyunsaturated fatty acids are found to exist in the cis configuration. When heated to high temperatures, mono- and polyunsaturated fatty acids of triglycerides are partially hydrogenated by the addition of hydrogen to the carbon–carbon double bonds to form some trans fatty acids. The American

TABLE 3.6 SOME UNSATURATED FATTY ACIDS

Name	Carbon atoms	Molecular weight	Solubility[a]	Melting point (°C)
Acrylic[1]	$C_3:1$	72	∞	12.3
Methacrylic[1]	$C_4:1$	86	s	16.0
Oleic	$C_{18}:1^{\Delta 9}$	282	i	14.0
Eleomargaric	$C_{17}:2^{\Delta 9,13}$	280	i	48.0
Linoleic	$C_{18}:2^{\Delta 9,12}$	280	i	−5.0
Linolenic	$C_{18}:3^{\Delta 9,12,15}$	278	i	−11.0
Arachidonic	$C_{20}:4^{\Delta 5,8,11,14}$	304	i	−49.5

[a]g/100 ml H_2O; s, soluble; i, insoluble.
[1]not dietary fatty acids

$$\begin{matrix} H & H \\ ----C=C---- \end{matrix}$$

$$\begin{matrix} H \\ ---C=C--- \\ H \end{matrix}$$

cis configuration   trans configuration

Figure 3.15 Cis and trans configurations of unsaturated fatty acids.

diet therefore contains trans fatty acids formed in corn oil and other margarines and in foods cooked at high temperatures in fats and oils.

It is estimated that stick margarines formed of partially hydrogenated vegetable oils may contain up to 36% of the total fatty acids in the trans isomeric form. It follows that processed and snack foods using margarine or cooked in partially hydrogenated vegetable oils will also contain trans fatty acids. The average per capita consumption of trans fatty acids in the American diet is estimated to be 12 g per day: 5 g per day from animal fats and 7 g per day from margarine and shortenings. Trans fatty acids appear to be absorbed and metabolized similar to cis fatty acids (Figure 7.5) and yield energy, although their metabolism may be slightly slowed. The trans fatty acids appear in all lipid fractions of the body, and concern has been expressed about the long-term safety of trans fatty acid consumption. There are presently no strongly correlated associations between trans fatty acid consumption and cancer of the colon or breast, atherosclerosis, or heart disease.

The chemical and physical characteristics of the fatty acids can be summarized as follows:

1. Fatty acids are weak organic monocarboxylic acids with hydrocarbon chains which are most often acyclic and unbranched.
2. Fatty acids contain a polar (hydrophylic) carboxylic acid and a nonpolar (hydrophobic) hydrocarbon whose carbon chain length determines some of the physical properties of the fatty acid.
3. Dietary fatty acids are most often even carbon chain lengths, C_{12}, C_{14}, C_{16}, C_{18}, C_{20}.
4. Fatty acids may be saturated or unsaturated and the unsaturated fatty acids may exist in either the cis or trans isomeric forms, with the cis form predominant in nature. Carbon–carbon double bonds are usually not found between the carboxylic moiety C_1 and C_9 of the hydrocarbon chain.

Mono-, Di-, and Triglycerides

Human and animal diets contain very few "free" unbound fatty acids. With the exceptions of acetic acid from bacterial fermentation and the presence of other short-chain fatty acids in milk, dietary fatty acids exist bound to a water-soluble

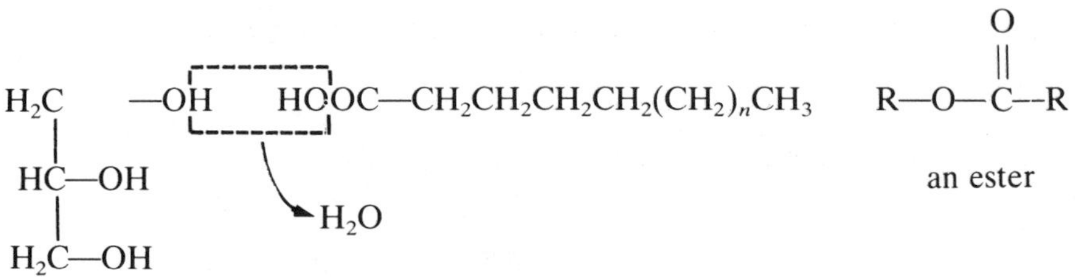

$$H_2C \quad\ \ —OH \qquad HOOC—CH_2CH_2CH_2CH_2(CH_2)_nCH_3 \qquad R—O—\overset{\overset{\displaystyle O}{\|}}{C}\text{--}R$$

$$HC—OH$$

$$H_2C—OH \qquad\qquad\qquad \searrow H_2O \qquad\qquad\qquad\qquad\qquad \text{an ester}$$

Figure 3.16 Structure of a monoglyceride.

triose, glycerol. Fatty acids combine with glycerol, forming the neutral lipids. The linkage between glycerol and the fatty acid is an ester bond formed by the elimination of a molecule of water from the hydroxyl of glycerol and the carboxylic acid moiety of the fatty acid forming a monoglyceride shown in Figure 3.16.

Esterification of additional fatty acids to the monoglyceride results in the formation of a diglyceride and triglyceride (Figure 3.17). The triglyceride is a neutral lipid. It is the major caloric lipid of the diet and is commonly referred to as animal fat and plant oil. Fats and oils are the major storage forms of lipids (depot fat) and energy in the body.

Triglycerides, fats and oils, contain fatty acids of variable carbon chain length (e.g., mixed triglycerides) and degree of saturation or unsaturation. The glycerol portion of the triglyceride contributes little to the physical characteristics of the glycerides. It is, rather, the characteristics of the individual fatty acids that determine whether the triglyceride will be a fat or oil. Fats are triglycerides which are primarily of animal origin and contain a greater proportion of long-chain saturated fatty acids esterified to glycerol. The major saturated fatty acids found in animal fats is palmitic (C_{16}:0) acid, followed by lesser amounts of stearic (C_{18}:0) acid. Fats contain more oleic (C_{18}:1) acid than palmitic acid or stearic acid, but contain much less polyunsaturated fatty acids than do most oils. At room temperature, most animal fats are solids. Oils are extracted from plant seeds and are usually liquids at room temperature because of their greater content of the mono-

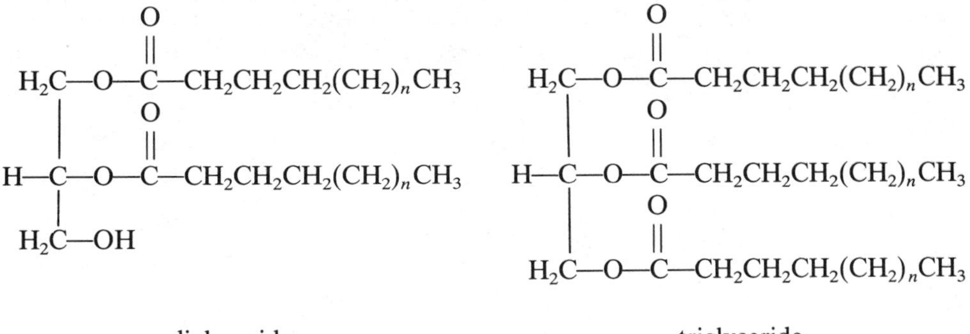

diglyceride   triglyceride

Figure 3.17 Structure of a diglyceride and triglyceride.

TABLE 3.7 FATTY ACID COMPOSITION OF FATS AND OILS (PERCENT FATTY ACIDS)[a]

| Name | Saturated FA | | | PUFA | Melt. Pt. °C |
	$(C_4:0–C_{14}:0)$	$(C_{16}:0–C_{18}:0)$	$(C_{18}:1)$		
Fats					
Butter	21.6	38.4	25.1	3.7	25
Tallow	4.7	43.5	36.0	4.3	40
Lard	2.0	36.7	40.9	11.4	30
Poultry	2.4	30.2	39.2	17.6	25
Menhaden (fish)	9.0	22.8	15.5	28.5	−5
Oils					
Coconut	74.2	11.2	5.7	1.8	25
Olive	0	13.8	71.5	8.9	−6
Peanut	0.1	11.8	45.6	31.0	3
Soybean	0.3	14.0	22.8	57.6	−16
Corn	0	12.4	24.6	58.1	−20
Sunflower	0.1	9.9	21.7	66.7	−17

Adapted from G. J. Brisson, *Lipids in Human Nutrition* (Englewood, N.J.: Jack K. Burgess, Inc., 1981).

[a]The higher content of saturated fatty acids in animal fats and much higher content of unsaturated and PUFA in oils are very apparent and contrast sharply with one another. Coconut oil is the exception among the plant oils in having a high proportion of saturated shorter-chain fatty acids. At room temperature coconut oil is a solid.

unsaturated fatty acid oleic ($C_{18}:1$) acid and the polyunsaturated fatty acids linoleic ($C_{18}:2$) acid and linolenic ($C_{18}:3$) acid. Linoleic and linolenic are two of the polyunsaturated fatty acids (PUFA). The composition of some common fats and oils is shown in Table 3.7.

Among mammals, the fatty acid content of depot fat is subject to slight variation and is influenced only slightly by diet. The fatty acid content of milk is

TABLE 3.8 APPROXIMATE COMPOSITION OF DEPOT AND MILK FATS (PERCENT FATTY ACIDS)[a]

	Human depot fat[b]		Human milk fat[a]	Beef depot fat[b]	Beef milk fat[a]
$C_4:0$	—		—	—	17
$C_6:0$	—		—	—	6
$C_8:0$	—		—	—	2
$C_{10}:0$	—		1	—	4
$C_{12}:0$	—	1	3	—	4
$C_{14}:0$	3	5	6	7	13
$C_{16}:0$	23	26	30	29	27
$C_{18}:0$	6	5	7	21	8
$C_{16}:1$	5		—	—	—
$C_{18}:1$	50		41	41	17
$C_{18}:2$	10		12	3	2

[a]Adapted from G. J. Brisson, *Lipids in Human Nutrition* (Englewood, N.J.: Jack K. Burgess, Inc., 1981).
[b]Compiled from other sources.

under genetic control and contains a higher proportion of the shorter-chain fatty acids. A comparison of human depot fat and milk fat with beef depot and milk fat is given in Table 3.8. The data reveals similarity between the fatty acid composition between human and beef depot fat and greater diversity in the fatty acids of milk. Beef milk fat has a higher proportion of short-chain fatty acids than does human milk and a lower content of oleic acid, exhibiting an overall tendency toward greater lipid saturation.

Cholesterol and Derivatives

Usually classified as a simple lipid, cholesterol (Figure 3.18) is the most widely distributed sterol in animal and human tissues. Present in the diet from the ingestion of only animal foods, cholesterol esters (Figure 4.6) are hydrolyzed and absorbed as chylomicrons and circulate with the lipoproteins (Table 4.3). Cholesterol is also actively synthesized from acetyl-CoA and isoprene (Figure 7.11) by the liver, intestinal epithelium, adrenal glands, and skin. Cholesterol is present in tissues as cholesterol esters in plasma, adrenals, intestinal epithelium, and liver and as free cholesterol in the central and peripheral nervous systems.

From cholesterol, specialized body tissues and intestinal bacteria synthesize many derivatives of cholesterol—sterols and steroids—some of which are metabolically active as hormones or hormone-like compounds (Figure 3.19). From the adrenal are synthesized the adrenocorticoids; from the ovaries and testes, the estrogens and androgens; and from the skin, 7-dehydrocholesterol and vitamin D. The liver synthesizes the bile acids, which are converted in the gastrointestinal tract into bile salts which assist with lipid digestion and absorption (Figure 4.7). The microflora of the intestinal tract convert cholesterol into unabsorbed excretory products, the neutral sterols (Figure 4.13).

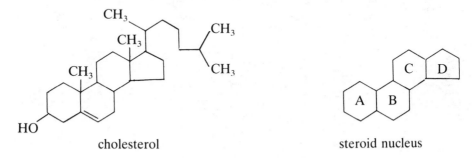

cholesterol   steroid nucleus

Figure 3.18 Structure of cholesterol and the steroid nucleus.

Phosphatidic Acid and Derivatives

Addition of phosphoric acid forming a phosphoester of any α,β-diglyceride provides the principle nucleus, phosphatidic acid (Figure 3.20), precursor to a large variety of compound lipids collectively named phospholipids.

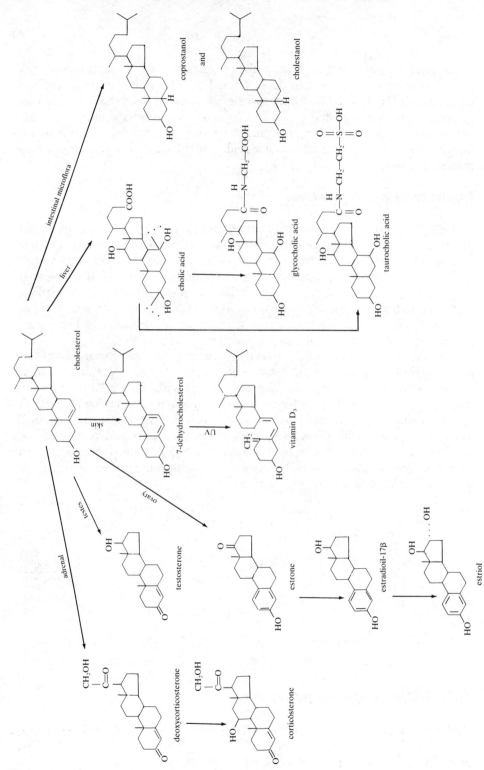

Figure 3.19 Derivatives of cholesterol.

42

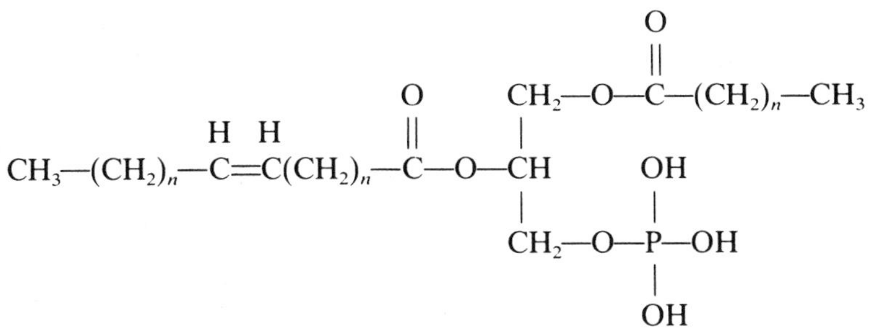

$$CH_3-(CH_2)_n-\overset{H}{\underset{}{C}}=\overset{H}{\underset{}{C}}(CH_2)_n-\overset{O}{\overset{\|}{C}}-O-CH \quad \begin{array}{c} CH_2-O-\overset{O}{\overset{\|}{C}}-(CH_2)_n-CH_3 \\ | \\ OH \\ | \\ CH_2-O-\overset{}{\underset{\underset{OH}{|}}{\overset{|}{P}}}-OH \end{array}$$

L-phosphatidic acid
(diacylglycerolphosphate)

Figure 3.20 Structure of phosphatidic acid.

Phospholipids

Dietary compound lipids are essential in the diet only to the extent that they provide calories, the mineral phosphorus, and possibly esterified essential fatty acids. Phospholipid derivatives are cellularly synthesized *de novo* from α-glycerol phosphate, fatty acids, and some other molecule which, when esterified to phosphatidic acid, gives the phospholipid their name and special chemical characteristics. Generally, phospholipids comprise the major structural component of membranes (65 to 85%) where, because of their amphipathic (hydrophobic-hydrophilic) property, they chemically mediate the transition between the more lipid characteristics of the membrane and its aqueous environment. Table 3.9 lists some of the charac-

TABLE 3.9 CHARACTERISTICS OF THE PHOSPHOLIPIDS AND GLYCOLIPIDS

Lipid	Major function
Phospholipids	
Phosphatidylcholine (lecithin)	Major membrane lipid of most cells
Phosphatidylethanolamine (cephalin)	Major membrane lipid of most cells
Phospatidylserine (cephalin-like)	Bacterial phospholipid
Phosphatidylinositol (inositide)	Major brain phospholipid
Phosphatidylglycerol	Bacterial phospholipid
Diphosphatidylglycerol (cardiolipin)	Heart lipid, concentrated in mitochondria
Plasmalogens	Membrane components of heart, brain, liver, and muscles
Sphingomyelin	Insulates nerve axon
Glycolipids	
Ceramide	Major brain glycolipid
Cerebroside	Provides the different blood types; brain and nerve glycolipids
Ganglioside (hexosamine)	Cell surface glycolipids, found in nerve endings

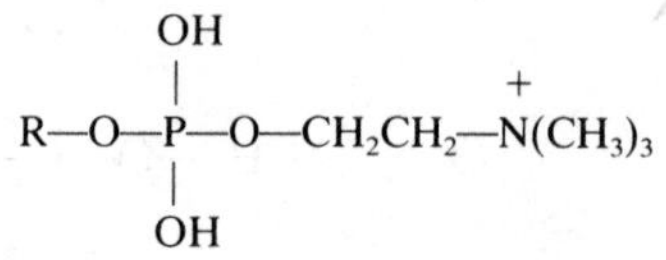

$$
\begin{array}{c}
OH \\
| \\
R-O-P-O-CH_2CH_2-\overset{+}{N}(CH_3)_3 \\
| \\
OH
\end{array}
$$

phosphatidylcholine (lecithin)

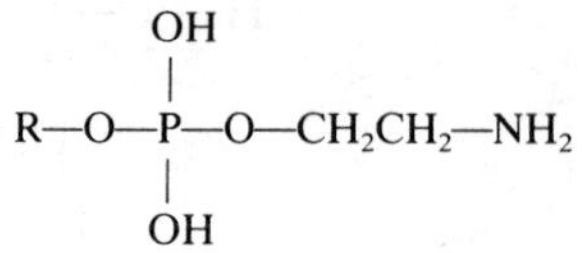

$$
\begin{array}{c}
OH \\
| \\
R-O-P-O-CH_2CH_2-NH_2 \\
| \\
OH
\end{array}
$$

phosphatidylethanolamine (cephalin)

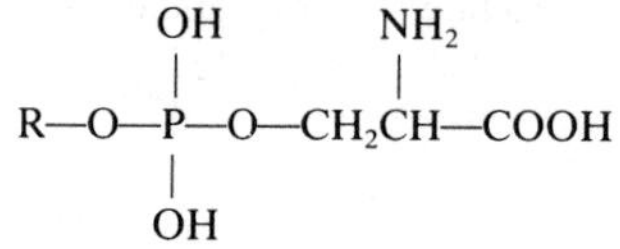

$$
\begin{array}{c}
OH \qquad\quad NH_2 \\
| \qquad\quad\ | \\
R-O-P-O-CH_2CH-COOH \\
| \\
OH
\end{array}
$$

phosphatidylserine (cephalin-like)

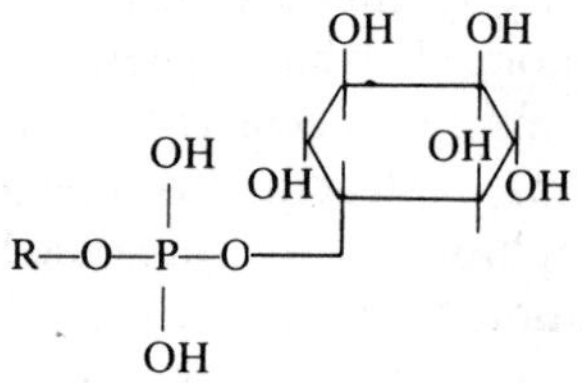

phosphatidylinositol

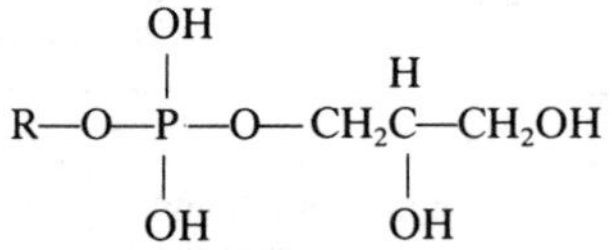

$$
\begin{array}{c}
OH \qquad\qquad H \\
| \qquad\qquad | \\
R-O-P-O-CH_2C-CH_2OH \\
| \qquad\qquad | \\
OH \qquad\quad\ OH
\end{array}
$$

phosphatidylglycerol

$$
\begin{array}{c}
OH \qquad\qquad\qquad\qquad OH \\
| \qquad\quad H \qquad\qquad | \\
R-O-P-O-CH_2C-CH_2-O-P-OH \\
| \qquad\quad | \qquad\qquad | \\
OH \qquad\ OH \qquad\qquad OH
\end{array}
$$

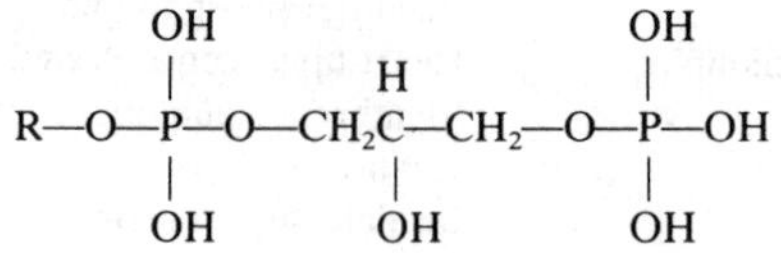

diphosphatidylglycerol (cardiolipin)

R = 1,2-diacylglycerol, the remaining portion of L-phosphatidic acid

Figure 3.21 Chemistry of the phospholipids and glycolipids.

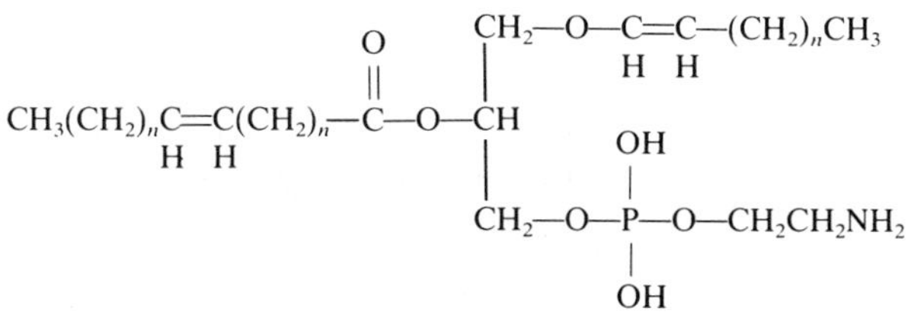

$$CH_3(CH_2)_nC=C(CH_2)_n-\overset{\overset{\displaystyle O}{\|}}{C}-O-CH$$

with substituents: $\underset{H\ H}{}$ and

$$CH_2-O-C=C-(CH_2)_nCH_3 \quad (\underset{H\ H}{})$$

$$CH_2-O-\overset{\overset{\displaystyle OH}{|}}{\underset{\underset{\displaystyle OH}{|}}{P}}-O-CH_2CH_2NH_2$$

a plasmalogen

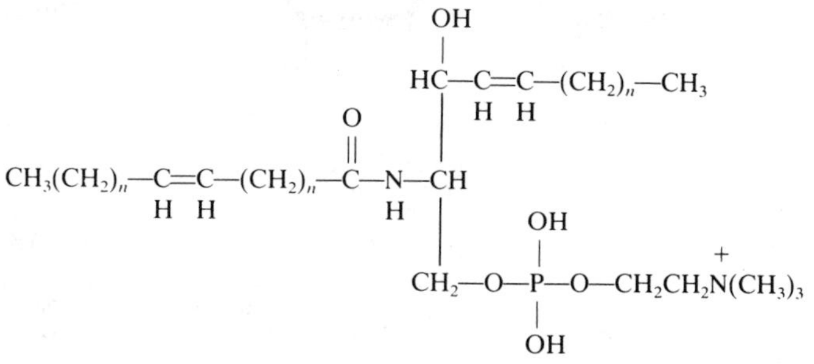

$$CH_3(CH_2)_n-C=C-(CH_2)_n-\overset{\overset{\displaystyle O}{\|}}{C}-\overset{}{N}-CH \quad (\underset{H\ H}{})(\underset{H}{})$$

$$HC-C=C-(CH_2)_n-CH_3 \quad (\overset{\displaystyle OH}{|})(\underset{H\ H}{})$$

$$CH_2-O-\overset{\overset{\displaystyle OH}{|}}{\underset{\underset{\displaystyle OH}{|}}{P}}-O-CH_2CH_2\overset{+}{N}(CH_3)_3$$

sphingomyelin

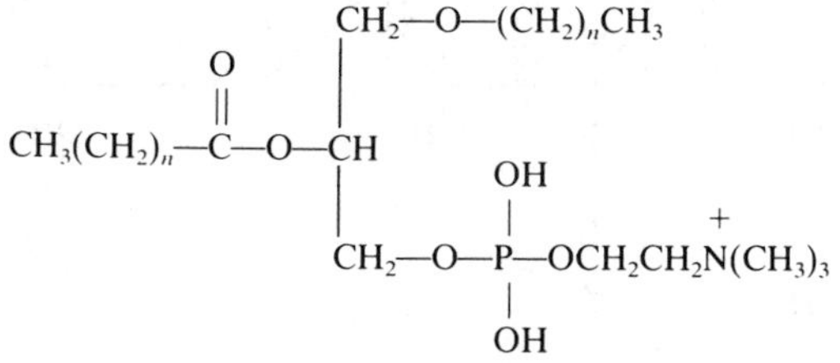

$$CH_3(CH_2)_n-\overset{\overset{\displaystyle O}{\|}}{C}-O-CH$$

$$CH_2-O-(CH_2)_nCH_3$$

$$CH_2-O-\overset{\overset{\displaystyle OH}{|}}{\underset{\underset{\displaystyle OH}{|}}{P}}-OCH_2CH_2\overset{+}{N}(CH_3)_3$$

alkylphospholipid

$$CH_3-(CH_2)_{14}-\overset{\overset{\displaystyle O}{\|}}{C}-\overset{}{N}-CH \quad (\underset{H}{})$$

$$HC-C=C-(CH_2)_{12}-CH_3 \quad (\overset{\displaystyle OH}{|})(\underset{H\ H}{})$$

$$CH_2-OH$$

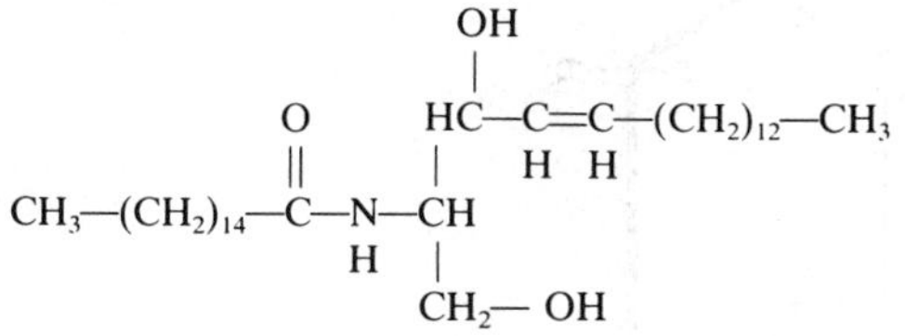

ceramide

Figure 3.21   (continued)

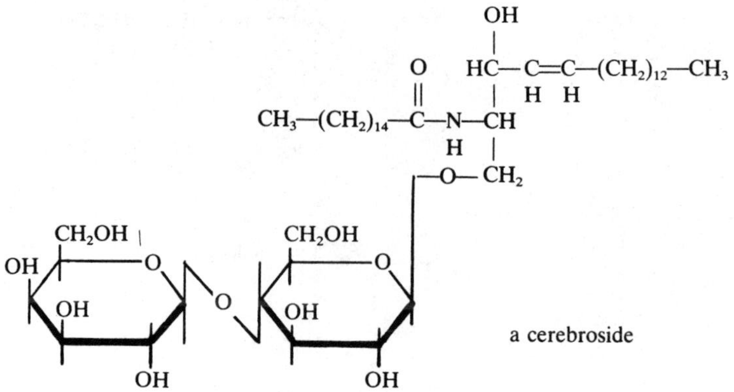

a cerebroside

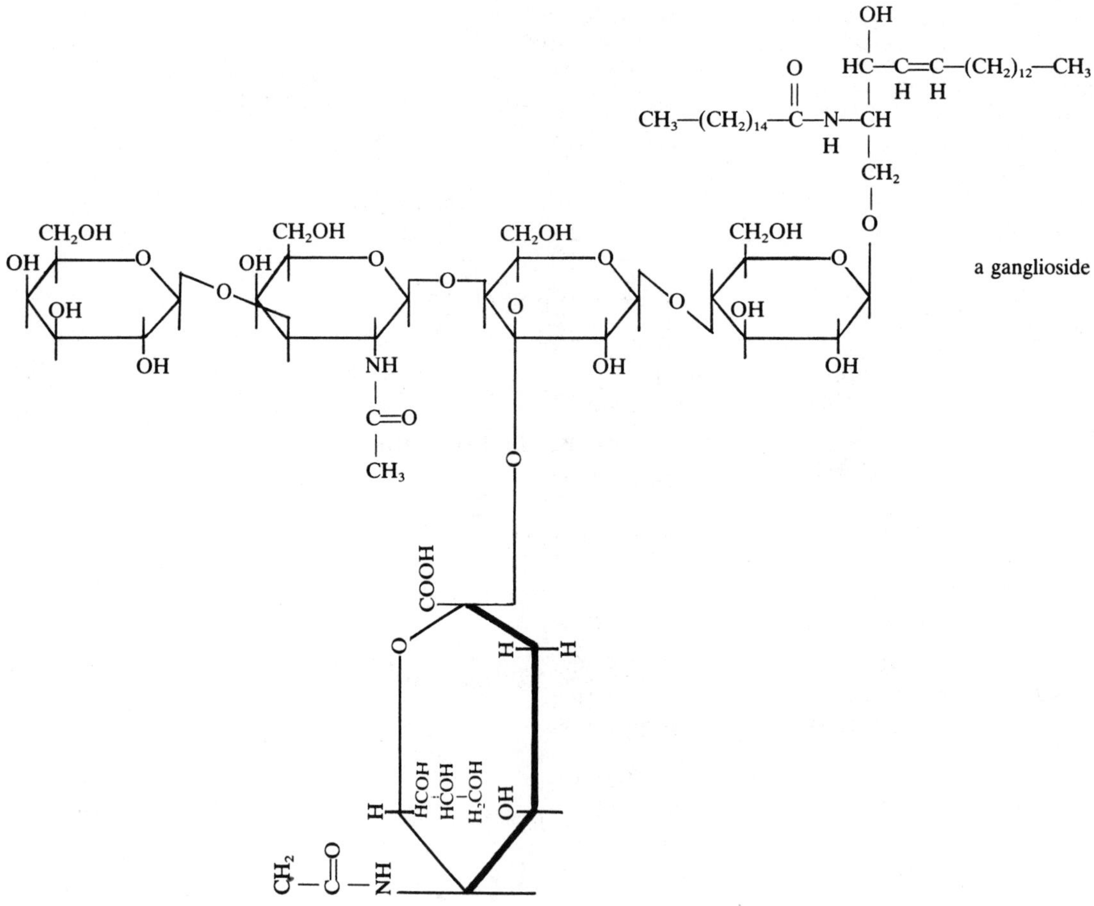

a ganglioside

Figure 3.21 (continued)

teristics and functions of the more important phospholipids, and Figure 3.21 provides their chemical structures.

Glycolipids

Conjugates of carbohydrates—glucose, galactose, *N*-acetylglucosamine, and *N*-acetylneuraminic acid with sphingosine (or dihydrosphingosine)—are all glycolipids. Ceramide is the common component of all glycolipids. To ceramide is affixed the carbohydrate moiety, forming cerebrosides and gangliosides (Figure 3.21). The glycolipids are common membrane components of the central nervous system and peripheral nerve tissues (Table 3.9).

VITAMINS

> *Vitamin:* any of a number of unrelated complex organic substances found variously in most foods and essential in small amounts for the functioning of the body (*Webster's New World Dictionary*).

Throughout history, in certain places at certain times, people have suffered not always from a lack of food but also from a dietary lack of certain nutrients. Populations of the ancient world were frequently susceptible to the dietary absences and deficiencies of the organic factors the body needed but was not receiving. We know these organic dietary factors today as the vitamins. The lack of these dietary organic factors, as the vitamin-deficiency diseases, were known to the ancient Chinese and Greeks; the Crusaders of the Middle Ages; the seafaring explorers of Portugal, Spain, Italy, and England; the Japanese; and even to Americans living in the South in this century. The lack of vitamins in the diet of peoples have at times no doubt altered the course of history. Many cultures developed dietary and remedial practices to prevent vitamin-deficiency diseases. Such practices have been passed through the generations and are referred to today as traditional medicine, folklore, and "old wives' tales." Within this century modern Western cultures have replaced such seemingly primitive practices with fortified foods available year round, and vitamin tablets. (Table 3.10).

No specific chemical knowledge of any vitamin was known before 1900. With the advent of purification of proteins, carbohydrates, and inorganics the stage was set for the discovery of the trace essential dietary organic factors which soon followed. The discovery of these organic dietary factors we now call vitamins is by any historical measure a contemporary event. Dietary growth factors were initially discovered and separated based on their solubility in oils (fat) or water. By 1920, E. V. McCullum had identified a fat-soluble vitamine (*sic*) A and a water-soluble B vitamine. Ascorbic acid was soon discovered and became vitamine C in a growing vitamine alphabet. In 1912, Casimir Funk coined the term "vitamine" to describe the newly discovered growth factors because they were thought to *be*

TABLE 3.10 COMPOSITION OF A MULTIVITAMIN, MULTIMINERAL SUPPLEMENT[a]

Ingredient	Chemical form	Quantity	Percent RDA
Vitamin A	As acetate and β-carotene	5000 IU	100
Vitamin E	As DL-α-tocopheryl acetate	30 IU	100
Vitamin C	As ascorbic acid	60 mg	100
Folic Acid	—	400 mcg	100
Vitamin B₁	As thiamin mononitrate	1.5 mg	100
Vitamin B₂	As riboflavin	1.7 mg	100
Niacinamide	—	20 mg	100
Vitamin B₆	As pyridoxine hydrochloride	2 mg	100
Vitamin B₁₂	As cyanocabolamin	6 mg	100
Vitamin D	—	400 IU	100
Vitamin K₁	As phytonadione	25 mcg	[b]
Biotin	—	30 mcg	10
Pantothenic acid	As calcium pantothenate	10 mg	100
Calcium	As dibasic calcium phosphate	162 mg	16
Phosphorus	As dibasic calcium phosphate	125 mg	13
Iodine	As potassium iodide	150 mcg	100
Iron	As ferrous fumerate	18 mg	100
Magnesium	As magnesium oxide	100 mg	25
Copper	As cupric oxide	2 mg	100
Zinc	As zinc oxide	15 mg	100
Manganese	As manganese sulfate	2.5 mg	[b]
Potassium	As potassium chloride	40 mg	[b]
Chloride	As potassium chloride	36.3 mg	[b]
Chromium	As chromium chloride	25 mcg	[b]
Molybdenum	As sodium molybdate	25 mcg	[b]
Selenium	As sodium selenate	25 mcg	[b]
Nickel	As nickelous sulfate	5 mcg	[c]
Tin	As stannous chloride	10 mcg	[c]
Silicon	As sodium metasilicate	10 mcg	[c]
Vanadium	As sodium metavanadate	10 mcg	[c]

[a]This is an example of modern multivitamin, multimineral formulation. Note the chemical forms and quantity of each ingredient. The formulation contains 30 nutrients, 15 present at 100% of the RDA for that nutrient, 4 at less than 25% of the RDA, and 11 nutrients having no established RDA, provided at the manufacturer's discretion, based on present nutrition evidence.

[b]Recognized as essential in human nutrition, but no RDA established.

[c]Not recognized as essential in human nutrition.

Source: Composition of *Centrum*, reproduced by permission of Lederle Laboratories Division of American Cynamid Company, Pearl River, NY 10965.

vital to life and quite mistakenly *amines*. The term "vitamine" stuck, and with the omission of the "e," deleting the reference to any chemical constituent, the reference to these organic dietary factors as vitamins continues today.

Today, we recognize vitamin C and eight members of the B-complex of vitamins as the dietary essential water-soluble vitamins. Thiamin, vitamin B₁, was first isolated in 1926, but its chemical structure was not fully elucidated until 1936. As the water-soluble vitamins were identified as individual dietary factors, each was designated with a subscript numeral—B_1, B_2, B_3, and so on—following a convention introduced by the British. Along the way of vitamin discoveries, compounds once believed to be water-souble vitamins and so designated were later found not to be vitamins at all. Examples include choline, *p*-aminobenzoate, inositol, lipoic acid, vitamins P (for permeability) and M (for monkey), and coenzyme Q (ubiquinone). Even pangamic acid and laetril have been designated as water-soluble vitamins B_{15} and B_{17}, for which no vitamin function is known. The Food and Drug Administration prohibits the sale of these compounds as vitamins.

From early research, beginning with the identification of a fat-soluble growth factor in milk (vitamin A), four fat-soluble factors have now been identified as the vitamins A, D, E, and K. These vitamins possess characteristics which in addition to their solubility are much different from those of the water-soluble vitamins. The water-soluble B vitamins all function as coenzymes with enzymes, are required in the diet, do not exhibit appreciable tissue storage, and are relatively nontoxic. In contrast, fat-soluble vitamins do not knowingly function like the classical coenzymes, and all but vitamin A or β-carotene are not obligatory in the human diet. Provitamin D, 7-dehydrocholesterol, is synthesized in the skin and is converted to vitamin D in the presence of adequate sunshine. Vitamin E can experimentally be replaced in animal diets with other antioxidants, such as BHA or BHT (Chapter 2), and vitamin K, synthesized by the intestinal flora of mammals, is absorbed from the human intestinal tract. When ingested in large amounts, fat-soluble vitamins A and D can be quite toxic, as they will continuously accumulate in lipid tissues, due to their solubility.

Vitamins as Coenzymes

All B vitamins and many nonvitamin organic factors (e.g., lipoic acid and ubiquinone) function as coenzymes with enzymes. Unlike enzymes, which do not participate directly in biological reactions but affect the rates of reactions, coenzymes participate in the reactions directly and are required for catalysis to occur. Most enzymes are of moderate to large molecular weight, but in comparison, coenzymes are of very small molecular weight. Most coenzymes are found loosely bound to enzymes and can be separated with ease from enzymes by either dialysis or molecular sieve chromatography. All enzymes act catalytically on substrates to produce products. In Equation 3.3, an enzyme (E) combines with its substrate (S) at the active site to form a transient enzyme–substrate (E-S) association complex. Catalysis occurs within this (E-S) complex, resulting in dissociation of a product(s), renewing the enzyme for further catalysis. In enzyme reactions that require coenzymes (Equation 3.4), the enzyme (E) must first combine with the coenzyme (Co-E), as in association 1, to complete the structural integrity of the active site of the enzyme for the binding of the substrate (association 2).

Equation 3.3

$$E + S \xrightarrow{\text{association}} [E - S] \xrightarrow{\text{disassociation}} E + P$$

Equation 3.4
Enzyme–coenzyme (vitamin) catalysis.

$$E + Co\text{-}E \xrightarrow{\text{association 1}} [E\text{-}Co\text{-}E] + S \xrightarrow{\text{association 2}} [E\text{-}Co\text{-}E\text{-}S] \xrightarrow{\text{disassociation 1}}$$

$$P + [E\text{-}Co\text{-}E] \xrightarrow{\text{dissociation 2}} E + Co\text{-}E$$

The enzyme–coenzyme–substrate complex (E-Co-E-S) is functionally analogous to the (E-S) complex of equation 3.3. A product or products are produced from this complex (disassociation 1). The (E-Co-E) complex may recycle and combine with another substrate molecule (S) or disassociate as in disassociation 2. In enzymatic reactions requiring coenzymes, the reactions do not take place without participation of the coenzyme in a continuous recycling manner.

The functions of the water- and fat-soluble vitamins are individually described for their predominant biological roles. Some vitamins function without biochemical modification. Other vitamins, however, have to be converted by the body into their metabolically active form(s), while other vitamins serve as components of even larger coenzymes. The vitamins are presented in Table 3.11 in chrono-

TABLE 3.11 CHRONOLOGY OF VITAMIN DISCOVERIES BY PUBLICATION DATE

	Vitamin	Year of isolation	Year synthesized	Human deficiency disease	RDA[a]
B_1,	thiamin	1926	1935	Beriberi	1.1–1.5 mg
A,	retinal (precursor, β-carotene)	1931	1947	Xerophthalmia, night blindness, dermatitis	800–1000 units retinal, 4800–6000 mg β-carotene
D_2, D_3,	ergocalciferol cholecalciferol	1931	1936	Rickets	10 μg
C,	ascorbic acid	1932	1933	Scurvy	60 mg
B_2(G),	riboflavin	1934	1935	Ariboflavinosis	1.4–1.8 mg
H,	biotin	1935	1942	—	100–200 μg
K_1, K_2,	phylloquinone menaquinone	1935	1939	Antihemorrhagic factor	100 μg
E,	α-tocopherol	1936	1937	—	10 mg
Nicotinic acid (niacin)		1937	—	Pellagra	12–20 mg
B_6(P),	pyridoxal	1938	1939	Varied symptoms	2.0 mg
Pantothenic acid		1938	1940	—	4–7 mg
Folic acid (folicin)		1945	1945	Megaoblastic anemia	400 μg
B_{12},	cobalamin	1948	1973	Megloblastic anemia, pernicious anemia	3 μg

[a]Approximate for the adult; see RDA tables in the Appendix for RDA requirements based on age, sex, and so on.

logical order of their published discovery, accounting for the lack of a strict alphabetical listing.   Descriptions of each vitamin are presented in the text in the same chronological order.

Thiamin (B₁)

> *Name:* Thiamin hydrochloride
> *Molecular weight:* 337
> *Form:* White crystals
> *Composition:* $C_{12}H_{18}ON_4SCl_2$
> *Active form:* Thiamin pyrophosphate
> *Function:* Decarboxylation and transketolations

Dietary deficiency of thiamin may lead to a neurological condition known as beriberi.   The disease sometimes involves atrophy of cardiac muscles and paralysis of involuntary muscles.   The Dutch physician C. Eijkman is credited with the 1897 discovery that rice polishings prevented nutritional polyneuritis in chickens fed polished rice and that the disease in chickens was similar to beriberi in humans. The antineuritic factor in rice bran and yeasts was indirectly investigated until its isolation and identification as thiamin by B. C. P. Jansen and W. F. Donath in 1926.   Its organic synthesis was completed in 1936 by R. R. Williams and J. K. Cline. Thiamin is comprised of pyrimidine and thiazole rings connected by a methylene (—CH₂—) bridge.   The active form of thiamin as a coenzyme is thiamin pyrophosphate (TPP), which is formed by phosphorylation of thiamin with ATP *in vivo* (Equation 3.5).

Equation 3.5
Phosphorylation of thiamin.

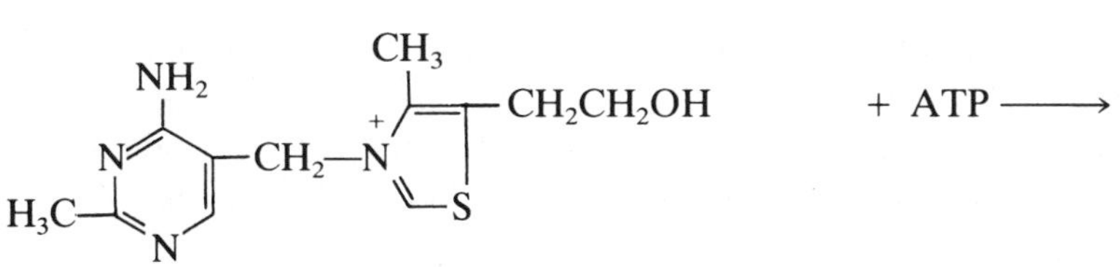

thiamin

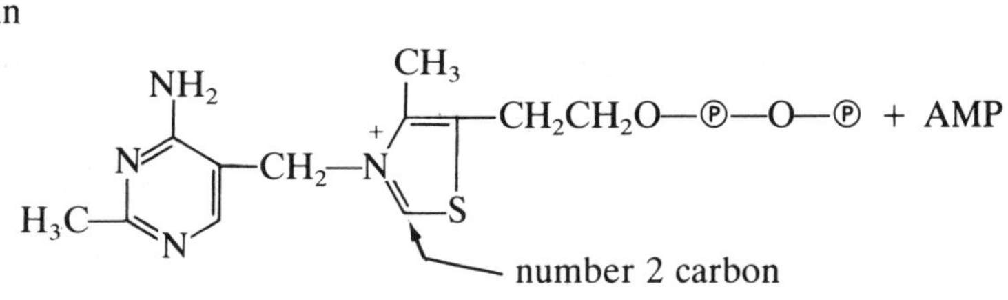

thiamin pyrophosphate (TPP)

The best known coenzyme functions for TPP are:

1. The oxidative decarboxylation of α-keto acids
2. The transfer of ketones (—C=O) from an α-keto acid in transketolase reactions.

The functional portion of TPP is carbon 2 of the thiazole ring. This carbon carries an aldehyde moiety. The decarboxylase and transketolase reactions usually require a divalent cation, either Mg^{1+} or Mn^{2+}.

Oxidative decarboxylations and transketolase reactions. The oxidative decarboxylation of pyruvic acid and α-ketoglutaric acid are examples of α-keto acid decarboxylations (Equation 3.6).

Equation 3.6
Oxidative decarboxylation pyruvate by TPP.

TPP—"active aldehyde"

In this reaction CO_2 is liberated and the methyl ketone

$$CH_3-\overset{\overset{\textstyle O}{\|}}{C}-$$

is transferred to TPP-C-2 as an "active aldehyde." The liberated CO_2 is to become respiratory CO_2. The active aldehyde in the oxidative decarboxylation of pyruvate is transferred to another coenzyme lipoamide (which is not a vitamin), forming an acetyl lipoamide. The acetyl is transferred again, this time to coenzyme A (Equation 3.7).

Equation 3.7
Formation of acetylcoenzyme A from TPP and acetyllipoamide.

TPP—"active aldehyde" +   oxidized lipoamide   acetyl lipoamide

$$+ \; HS\text{—coenzyme A} \longrightarrow \underset{\underset{\text{reduced lipoamide}}{}}{\overset{HS}{\underset{HS}{\rightthreetimes}}} \quad + \; CH_3\overset{\overset{O}{\|}}{-C}\text{—S coenzyme A} + NAD^+$$

reduced lipoamide   acetylcoenzyme A

Analysis of this reaction reveals that a three-carbon acid (pyruvate) is shortened by one carbon which is eliminated as CO_2, and two carbons are transferred to coenzyme A as "active aldehyde." This is one of the most important reactions in metabolism for almost all carbohydrates; glucose, sucrose, fructose, starch, and so on, are metabolized in part through this reaction with thiamin for the formation of energy (see Figures 7.1 and 7.2).

Transketolase reactions involve the hexose monophosphate shunt (HMP shunt), which uses TPP to transfer a ketol

$$\overset{\overset{O}{\|}}{-C}\text{—CH}_2\text{OH}$$

to an aldose (aldehyde carbohydrate), thereby adding two new carbons to the carbohydrate. In this manner ribose-5-phosphate, a five-carbon carbohydrate, is converted to sedoheptulose, a seven-carbon carbohydrate (Equation 3.8).

Equation 3.8
Transketolase reaction by TPP.

$$\underset{\underset{\text{ribulose-5-}\textcircled{P}}{OH \quad OH \; OH}}{\overset{O \quad H \quad H}{CH\text{—}C\text{—}C\text{—}C\text{—}CH_2\text{—}\textcircled{P}}} \quad \underset{\overrightarrow{NADP^+ \qquad NADPH_2}}{\overset{\text{TPP—"active aldehyde"}}{\curvearrowright}} \quad \underset{\underset{\text{sedoheptulose-7-}\textcircled{P}}{OH \quad H \quad OH \; OH \; OH}}{\overset{O \; OH \; H \quad H \quad H}{CH_2\text{—}C\text{—}C\text{—}C\text{—}C\text{—}CH_2\text{—}\textcircled{P}}}$$

Thiamin, like the other water-soluble vitamins, is relatively nontoxic. Daily doses of thiamin in humans have been administered up to 1 g per day for extended periods without adverse effects. This is undoubtedly due to a regulation of absorption of thiamin being limited to about 5 mg per dosage by its intestinal transport and the rapid excretion of excess thiamin in urine.

Retinol (A₁)

Name: Retinol
Molecular weight: 286
Form: Yellow prisms

Composition: $C_{20}H_{30}O$
Active form: Retinol, retinal
Function: Antioxidant, visual cofactor
Activity: 1 IU = 0.300 μg of vitamin A
                1 IU = 0.344 μg of vitamin A acetate
Precursor: β-Carotene

Vitamin A, as one may guess, was the "first" fat-soluble vitamine (*sic*) to be recognized. E. V. McCollum had by 1920 separated a fat-soluble A vitamine and a water-soluble B vitamine. McCollum was later to discover that his vitamine A also contained another lipid-soluble factor, vitamine D (see "Cholecalciferol").

Night blindness, a vitamin A deficiency, had been recognized and historically was treated by the ancient Chinese, the early Egyptians, and even Hippocrates himself. A more severe vitamin A deficiency can lead to xerophthalmia (dry eye) and if untreated, permanent blindness. Xerophthalmia among children of southeast Asia remains an almost permanent contemporary problem.

Vitamin A, in addition to preventing night blindness, and xerophthalmia, is required for normal growth, reproduction, and the integrity of epidermal and epithelial tissues. Vitamin A is a major antioxidant (see Chapter 12) of skin, lung, and intestinal mucosa. Vitamin A, β-carotene, and some analogs of vitamin A have been shown to be very effective in reducing naturally occurring cancers in humans and experimental cancers in laboratory animals.

Vitamin A, retinol, some vitamin A analogs, and previtamin A, β-carotene, are shown in Figure 3.22. Retinol and β-carotene are formed in plants from isoprene. Most retinol ingested is in the form of retinyl esters, usually retinyl palmitate (Figure 4.6), in which the ester stabilizes the molecule from peroxidation. Also found in plants is β-carotene. Both vitamin A and β-carotene are absorbed from the gastrointestine along with the other lipid components of the diet. After ingestion, vitamin A (retinol, retinal, or retinyl esters) is transported and stored with retinal binding proteins (RBP), raises the plasma levels of vitamin A, and if consumed in excess over time, can be toxic. Stored in the liver and eye bound to protein, toxic vitamin A symptoms are variable but may include dry skin, loss of hair, and enlarged liver and spleen, among others. β-Carotene, on the hand, when ingested in excess, is rather nontoxic and is stored in the epidermis, producing a orange-yellowish color in the appearance of the skin. β-Carotene does not contribute to plasma vitamin A unless plasma vitamin A falls below homeostatic levels. When this happens, a dioxygenase found in both the intestines and liver cleaves β-carotene, theoretically yielding two molecules of retinol, raising levels of plasma vitamin A. Sission of β-carotene is shown in Figure 3.23.

The best known function for vitamin A is its role as a coenzyme with the protein opsin, found in rods and cones, the photoreceptor cells of the eye. The visual protein pigments, rhodopsin (rods), responsible for low light vision, and iodopsin (cones), responsible for color and bright light vision, both contain 11-*cis*-

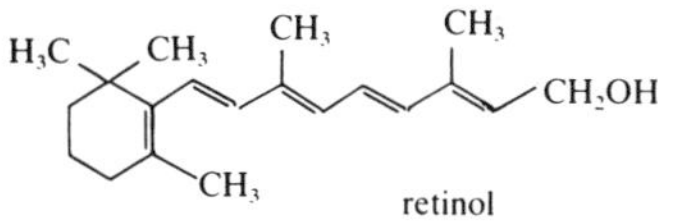

retinol

Vitamin A_1 toxic in excessive amounts, antioxidant, functions in visual cycle

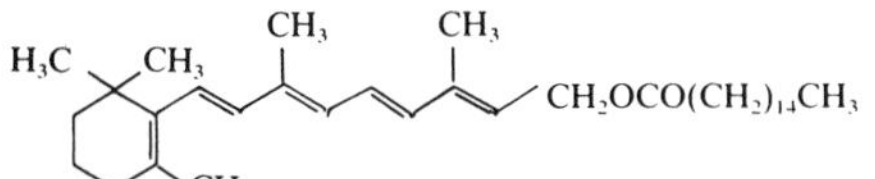

retinyl palmitate

Major storage form of vitamin A in body

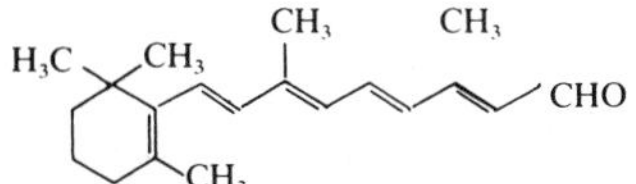

retinal

All-*trans* form of vitamin A in visual cycle, oxidized form of retinol

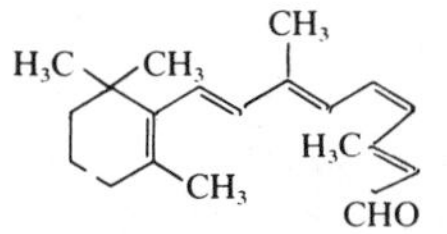

11-*cis*-retinal

Active form of vitamin A in visual cycle, combines with opsin to form visual pigments rhodopsin and iodopsin

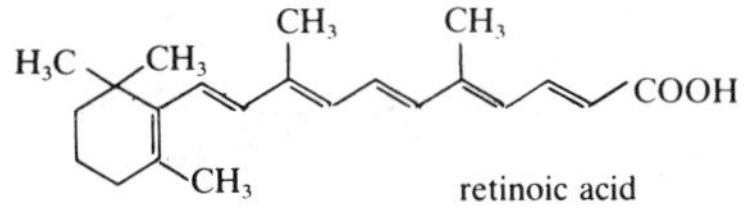

retinoic acid

Oxidation product of retinal, toxic, metabolite excreted in urine, used in dermatology

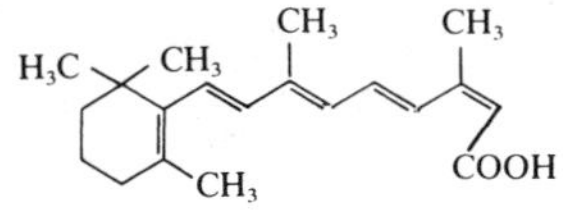

13-*cis*-retinoic acid

Isomer of retinoic acid used in the prevention and treatment of some cancers

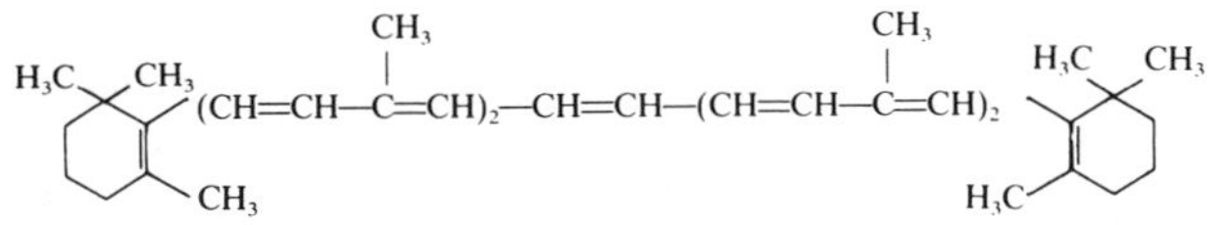

β-carotene

Major plant previtamin A, nontoxic, theoretically converted to two-molecules of vitamin A (retinal) antioxidant; biologically, β-carotene has one-sixth the value of retinol

Figure 3.22 Vitamin A, some analogs, and β-carotene.

retinal (see Figure 3.24), attached through amide linkages to a lysyl residue

$$\text{11-}\textit{cis}\text{-retinal}-\overset{\overset{\displaystyle O}{\|}}{C}-\underset{\displaystyle H}{N}-(CH_2)_4\text{-opsin.}$$

Rhodopsin and iodopsin are the "visual pigments" of the eye, which in the presence of light are "bleached." Bleaching results in the conversion of vitamin A to the all-*trans*-retinal by light energy, release of opsin, and the interruption of optic nerve

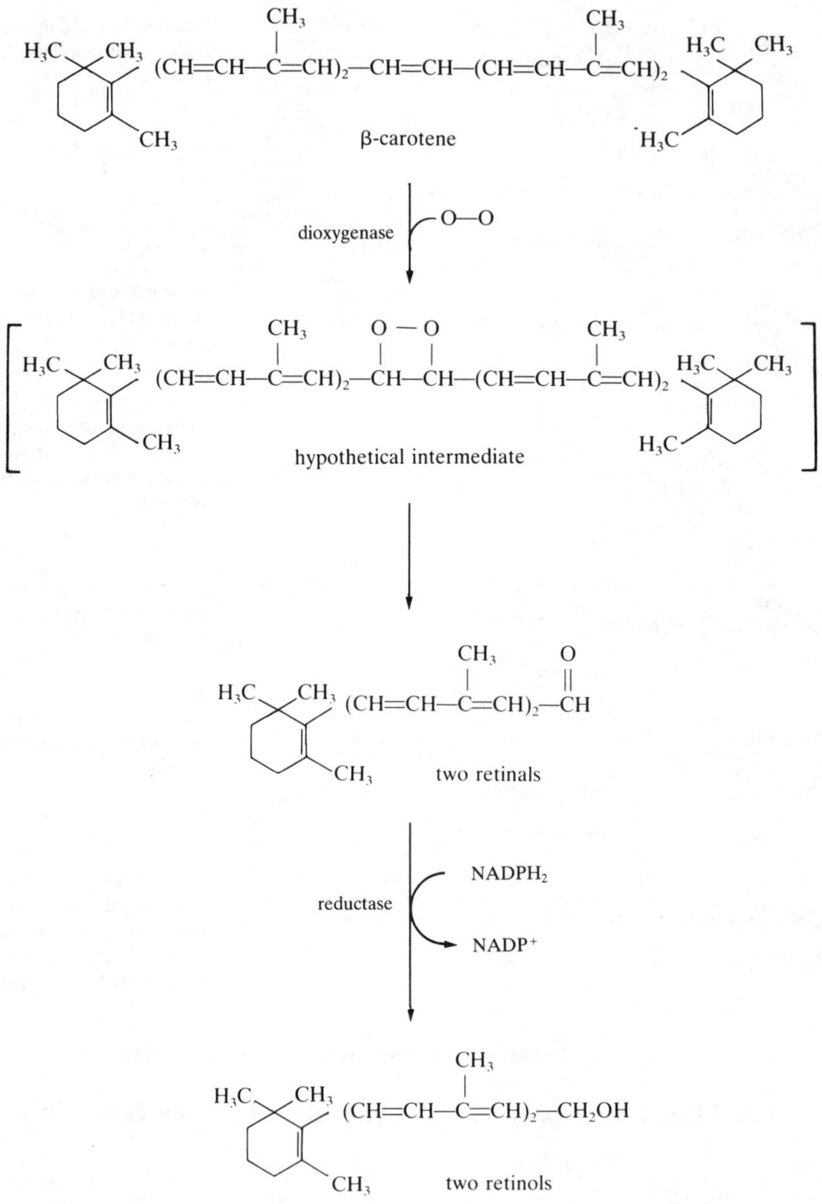

Figure 3.23 Sission of β-carotene by dioxygenase.

electric impulses by Ca^{2+} (dark current), which are amplified and interpreted as light (Figure 3.24). Lack of rhodopsin because of a retinol deficiency causing night blindness is a sensitive indicator of vitamin A status. β-Carotene, in addition to being a source of retinal, protects the skin from ultraviolet light, a known carcinogen

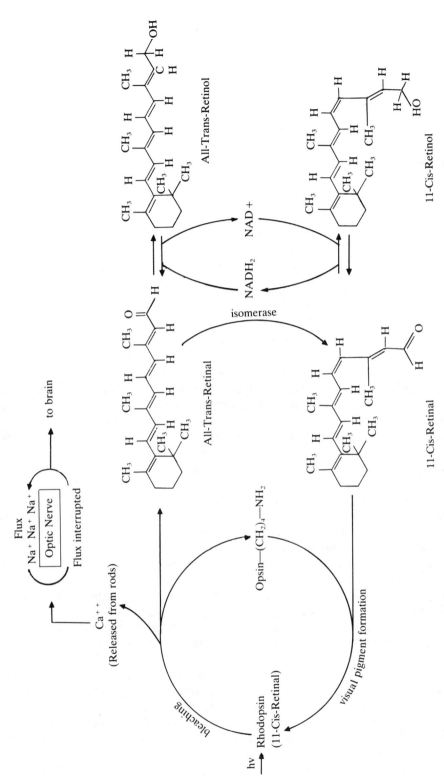

Figure 3.24 Vitamin A in the visual cycle. Release of all-*trans*-retinal from rhodopsin causes Ca²⁺ to be released from rods interrupting a continuous flux of Na⁺ within the optic nerve. The interruption of Na⁺ flux is interpreted by the brain as vision by the pattern of rods and/or cones so affected by light (*hv*). Rhodopsin is regenerated from retinal, retinol, or hydrolysis of retinyl esters.

responsible for the relatively common occurrence of skin cancer.   Because of β-carotene's unique structure of alterating double bonds (π-bonding system), it alone absorbs ultraviolet light (see Chapter 12) and disperses the ultraviolet-light energy falling on the skin as heat.   In this respect, β-carotene is nature's original sunscreen.

Cholecalciferol (D₃)

Name:	Cholecalciferol
Molecular weight:	385
Form:	Needles
Composition:	$C_{27}H_{44}O$
Active form:	1,25-dihydroxy D_3
Function:	Facilitates absorption of calcium and some mobilization of calcium (antirachitical)
Activity:	1 IU–0.025 µg D_3
Precursors:	7-dehydrocholesterol

Vitamin D deficiency is the cause of rickets, a crippling disease of children caused by the lack of calcium absorption and subsequently, failure of the collagen matrix of bone to calcify.   In adults, vitamin D deficiency is expressed as osteomalacia, an inability of reabsorbed bone to recalcify.   These diseases have been a scourge on humankind throughout history.   Especially plagued with the disease have been those people living in the northernmost latitudes of Europe, Asia, and North America.   The Industrial Revolution and its extensive use of coal added to the number of cases of rickets in both Europe and the United States.   Why? Because modern nutritional science has demonstrated that vitamin D is not a vitamin at all in the classic sense of dietary need and coenzyme function.   Vitamin D is a vitamin-hormone produced in the skin of people in amounts adequate to prevent rickets and osteomalacia when exposed directly to the ultraviolet light of the sun.   Those factors necessary to produce rickets and osteomalacia were all present for people living in northern latitudes in cities of the Industrial Revolution. Long winters, indoor confinement, overcast skies, heavy clothing, and polluted cities all contributed to reduced ultraviolet light exposure and vitamin D synthesis. Such environmental circumstances were compounded by the lack of significant vitamin D in the diet.   Vitamin D is a vitamin in the classic sense as a result of environmental life-style.

In the early part of this century, Edward Mellanby both produced and cured rickets with cod-liver oil in dogs.   E. V. McCollum in 1922 found the "anti-rachitic factor" in cod-liver oil not to be vitamin A (which he had also discovered; see "Retinol") and named the fat-soluble substance vitamin D—vitamins A, B, and C having been so designated at that time.   The ultraviolet-light conversion of fat-soluble factors into vitamin D came into practice and was made possible by H. Steenbock and A. Black in 1924.   Their discovery followed the 1919 observations of K. Huldskinsky, who was curing rachitic children with ultraviolet light. A U.S. patent (1,680,818) covering the irradiation of ergosterol for the synthesis of vitamin D was issued in 1928.

The precursors of vitamin D, ergosterol in plants and 7-dehydrocholesterol in the skin of animals and humans, are synthesized from acetyl-CoA and isoprene and have chemical structures nearly identical to cholesterol (Figure 3.25). As described above, in the presence of ultraviolet light of 250 to 310 nm, ergosterol is converted into vitamin D_2 and 7-dehydrocholesterol into vitamin D_3 (Figure 3.25). As shown in Figure 3.25, ultraviolet light results in the sission of the β-sterol ring containing the 5,7-diene. The chemical structures of vitamins D_2 and D_3 differ only with respect to unsaturation occurring between C_{22} and C_{23} in ergosterol. Vitamin D_2, known as ergocalciferol, has been the major form of vitamin D as a supplement to human foods and animal feeds. Vitamin D_3 is known as cholecalciferol and is the natural human form of the vitamin. It has also been used as a food and feed supplement.

Vitamins D_2 and D_3 are prohormones to the active vitamin derivative. In a series of brilliant experiments by J. Lund and H. F. Deluca, beginning in 1966,

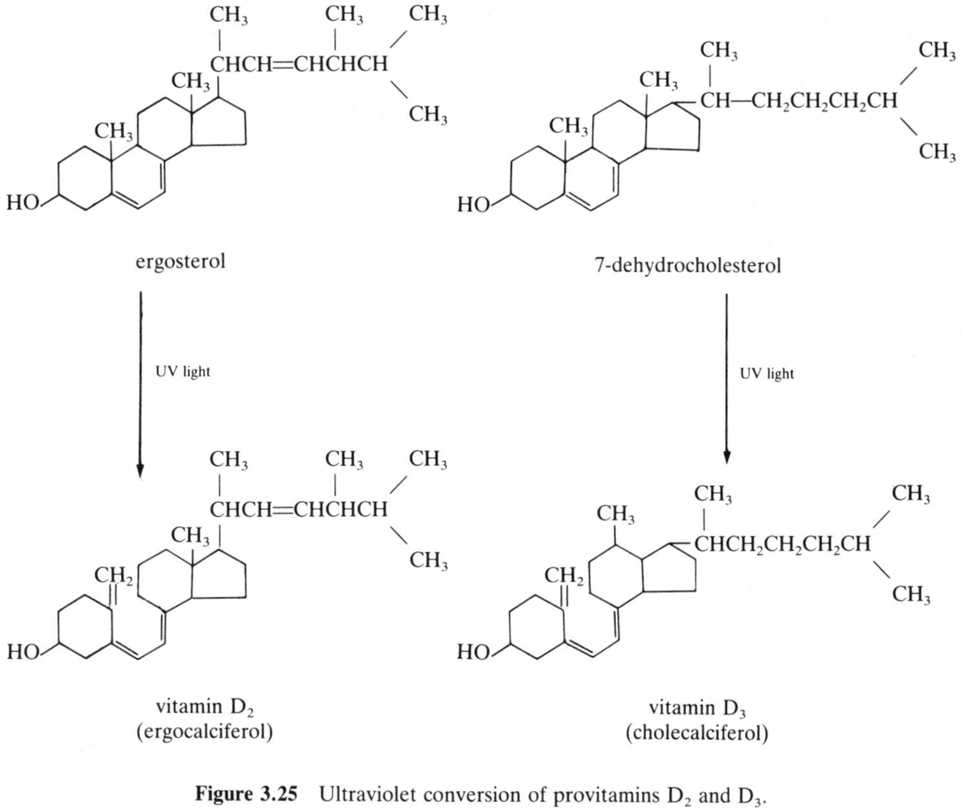

Figure 3.25 Ultraviolet conversion of provitamins D_2 and D_3.

the metabolism of vitamin D began to unfold. Following dietary absorption of vitamin D_2 or D_3 or synthesis of vitamin D_3 in the integument, vitamins D_2 and D_3 in mammals are hydroxylated in the liver by enzymes requiring molecular oxygen, Mg^{2+}, and $NADPH_2$, producing 25-OH-vitamin $D_2(D_3)$. This derivative of vitamin D is not yet the metabolically active form. The 25-OH-vitamin $D_2(D_3)$ transported by the α-globulin from the liver to the kidney undergoes a second renal hydroxylation by a mixed-function oxygenase to yield $1,25\text{-}(OH)_2$-vitamin $D_2(D_3)$, calcitrol. Although $1,25\text{-}(OH)_2$-vitamin $D_2(D_3)$ may undergo further metabolism, all evidence suggests that this is the biologically active form of vitamin D. It is

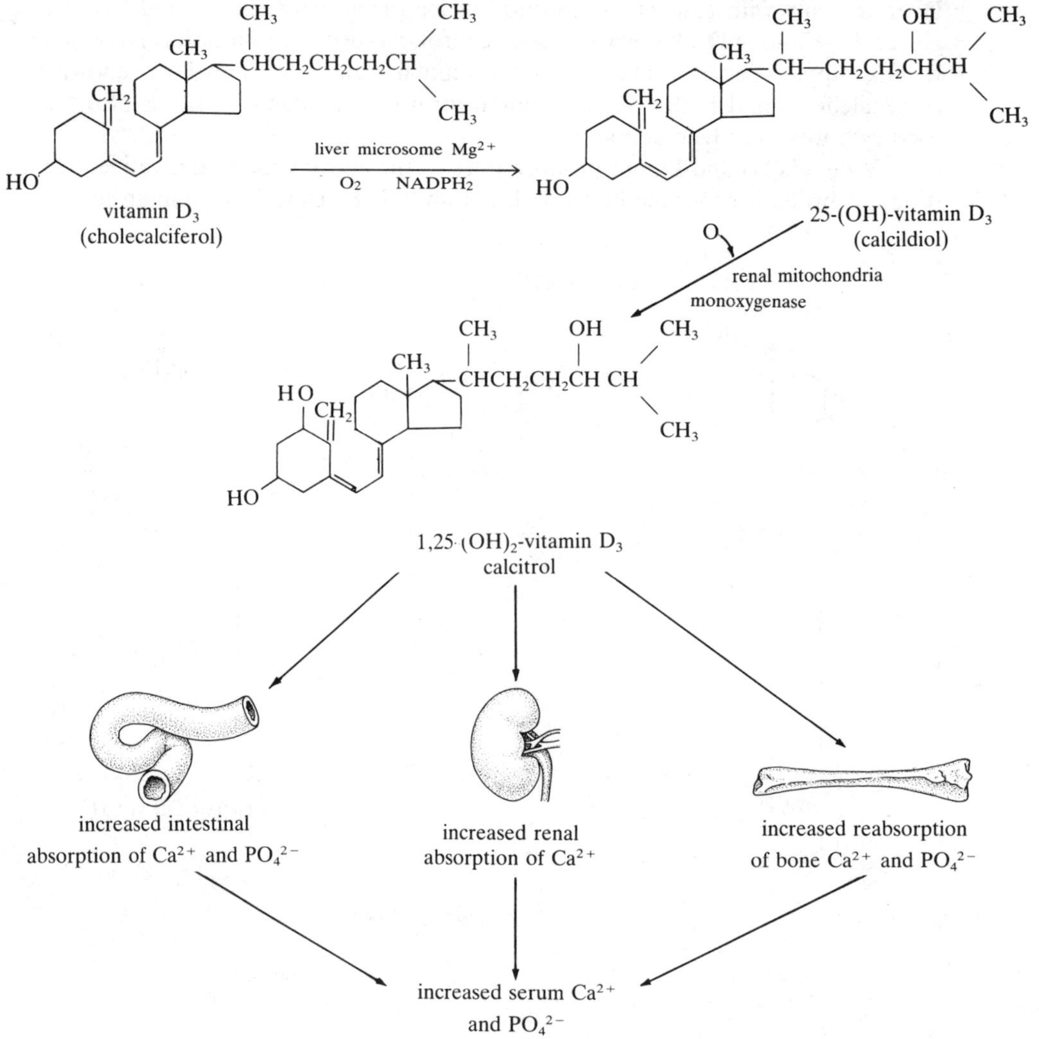

Figure 3.26 Metabolism of vitamin D_3.

responsible for intestinal calcium and phosphate uptake, renal reabsorption of calcium, and bone demineralization (Figure 3.26). Serum levels of both calcium and phosphorus effectively regulate 1,25-$(OH)_2$-vitamin D renal synthesis.

While vitamin D deficiencies are of concern, vitamin D toxicity is a serious consequence of excessive vitamin intake. Only vitamin D and vitamin A pose serious toxic consequences when ingested in excess over extended periods. Consequences of vitamin D toxicity include hypercalcemia and hypercalciuria, with death possible from calcification of the heart, major arteries, and kidney.

Ascorbic Acid (C)

Name:	Hydroascorbic acid
Molecular weight:	176
Form:	Usually plates
Composition:	$C_6H_8O_6$
Active form:	Reduced ascorbic acid
Function:	Hydrogen carrier, hydroxylations, antioxidant

A human ascorbic acid, vitamin C inadequacy produces scurvy, a nutritional deficiency disease described by ancient authors, including Hippocrates, the Greek physician of the fifth century. Scurvy ravaged the thirteenth-century French (crusaders) in Palestine, and it became perilous for sailors of the sixteenth and seventeenth centuries to be at sea for more than four or five months. A voyage of six months or more meant almost certain death. One hundred Portuguese sailors led by Vasco da Gama died of scurvy. The French explorer Jacques Cartier described the disease in 1535 while waiting out the long North American winter on the St. Lawrence River, near Quebec City.

> The unknown sickness began to spread itself amongst us accompanied by the most marvelous and extraordinary symptoms . . . inasmuch as some did lose all their strength and could not stand on their feet. Their legs became swollen, the sinews contracted and turned black as coal. . . . Others had their skin spotted with spots of blood of a purple color; then did it creep up to their hips, thighs, shoulders, arms and neck. Their mouths became stinking, their gums so rotten that all the flesh did fall off, even to the root of the teeth. . . . The disease spread out . . . so widely that, by February, out of our group of 110, there were not 10 left in good health. . . . We had already 8 men dead and there remained over 50 whom we had given up for lost.

Many other observations of scurvy were later to be made and recorded. Admiral Richard Hawkins of the British Royal Navy wrote in 1662 "that sour oranges and lemons" were effective against the disease, but scurvy continued to be the primary cause of death of sailors at sea. It was the great sea plague. Not until Royal Navy Surgeon James Lind did his human experiments with scorbutic sailors using oranges, lemons, cider, and seawater aboard the *Salisbury* at sea (May

20, 1747) were the value of citrus fruits appreciated. Published in 1753, Lind's *Treatise on the Scurvy* and other publications led the British admiralty in 1795 to order rations of lemons to sailors at sea. Lemons, often referred to as limes by the British, resulted in future sailors of the Royal Navy being called limeys.

The principal factor contributing to scurvy was the lack of dietary ascorbic acid. This anti-scorbutic factor was isolated in 1932 by C. G. King and W. A. Waugh and independently by J. L. Surbely and A. Szent-Györgyi, who was to receive the Nobel Prize in 1937. Ascorbic acid's molecular composition was determined and its synthesis were both accomplished in 1933.

Vitamin C, ascorbic acid, is similar in structure but functionally different from D-glucose or D-galactose (Figure 3.27). Synthesized by plants, vitamin C is dietarily required by only a few species of animals and primates, including humans. The guinea pig is most often employed in vitamin C research in the laboratory. Most animals possess the enzyme L-gulono-γ-lactone oxidase, responsible for the oxidation of L-gulono-γ-lactone into L-2-oxogalactono-γ-lactone and ascorbic acid. Humans and animals like the guinea pig lack this renal and/or hepatic enzyme and therefore cannot synthesize vitamin C from glucose via the hexose-monophosphate shunt (Figure 3.28).

Ascorbic acid is a strong reducing agent and upon oxidation, dehydroascorbic acid is formed (Figure 12.3). One of the major functions of ascorbic acid is therefore that of an antioxidant protecting cells and cellular components from free-radical attack (see Chapter 12). As a strong reducing agent, vitamin C may

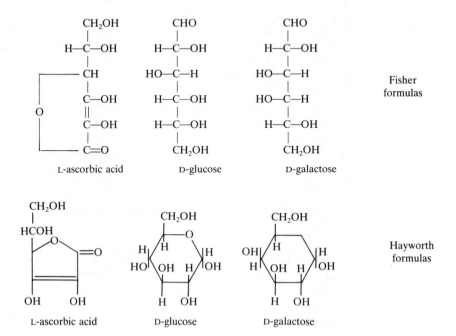

Figure 3.27 Hexoses: ascorbic acid, glucose, and galactose.

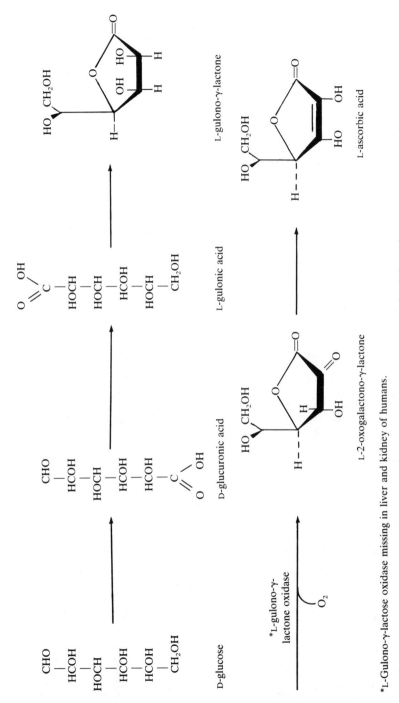

Figure 3.28 Synthesis of ascorbic acid by animals from glucose.

*L-Gulono-γ-lactose oxidase missing in liver and kidney of humans.

facilitate the absorption of ferric iron (Fe^{3+}) by its reduction to ferrous iron (Fe^{2+}). Metabolically, ascorbic acid may cause reduction of iron as well as other metals.

A major function of vitamin C is its coenzyme role with hydroxylases. The hydroxylation of the amino acids proline and lysine to hydroxyproline and hydroxylysine are important reactions in the formation of collagen (Figure 3.29).

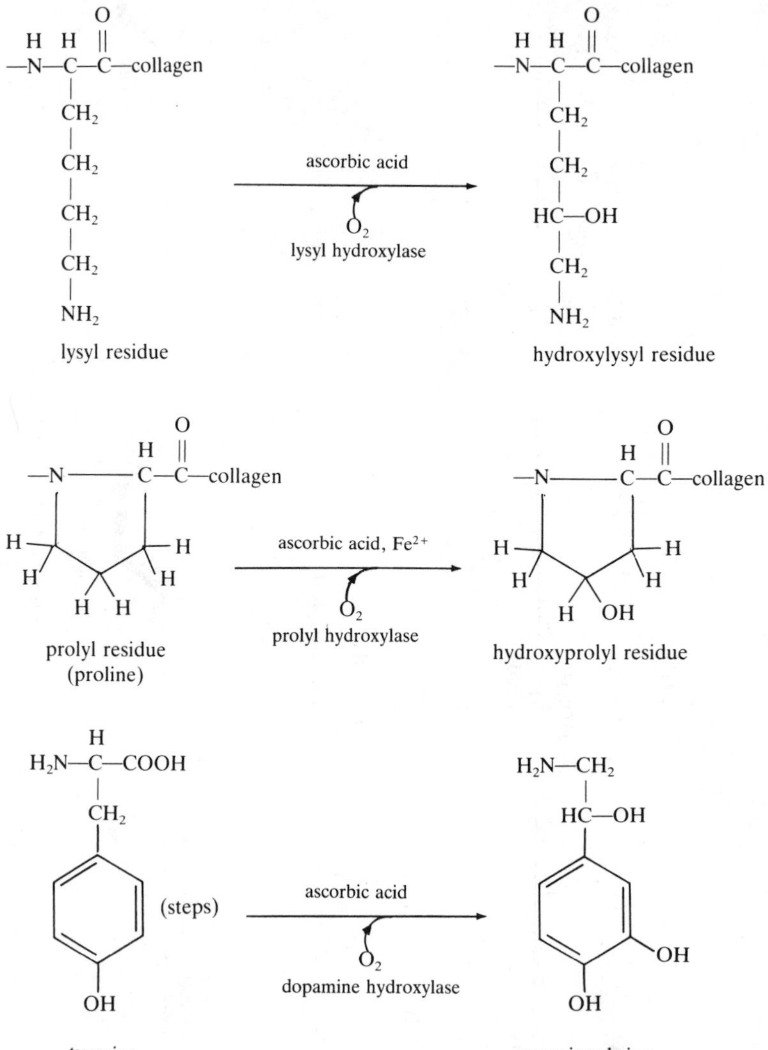

Figure 3.29 Some hydroxylation reactions with ascorbic acid (abbreviated). (See also bile acid synthesis and xenobiotic metabolism hydroxylation reactions in Fig. 13.4.)

Collagen is a matrix protein of skin and connective tissues whose cross-linked structural formation is dependent on vitamin C. Other hydroxylations that require vitamin C include the hydroxylation of cholesterol in bile acid formation (Figure 4.7) and the formation of hydroxylated steroids and hydroxylated xenobiotics (Figure 13.4), rendering them more water soluble. The metabolism of tyrosine and its hydroxylation, forming norepinephrin, is also dependent on ascorbic acid (Figure 3.29).

The prevention of diseases other than scurvy has been attributed to vitamin C. Higher-than-adequate intakes of vitamin C have been suggested to accelerate healing, increase immunoresistance, prevent or reduce the severity of the common cold, and reduce the risks of cardiovascular disease and cancer. The true effective value of higher-than-recommended dietary intake of vitamin C remains to be elucidated more fully.

Riboflavin (B₂, G)

Name:	D-Riboflavin
Molecular weight:	376
Form:	Orange-yellow needles
Composition:	$C_{17}H_{20}N_4O_6$
Active form:	Flavin mononucleotide, flavin adenine dinucleotide
Function:	Hydrogen carrier

Riboflavin is a bright orange-yellow compound. Its color gives the slight yellow color to egg "whites," where it is found as ovoflavin. One of only two highly colored vitamins, it is strongly fluorescent in solution, and its ability to absorb ultraviolet light causes it to be chemically unstable. A lack of dietary riboflavin leads to ariboflavinosis. Riboflavin consists of a conjugated isoalloxazine ring (flavin) and a five-carbon carbohydrate, ribitol (Figure 3.30).

Riboflavin was recognized early as a separate entity often found in the presence of thiamin. As a separate growth factor for animals, it was named vitamin B₂, following the convention established for naming the vitamins by the British,

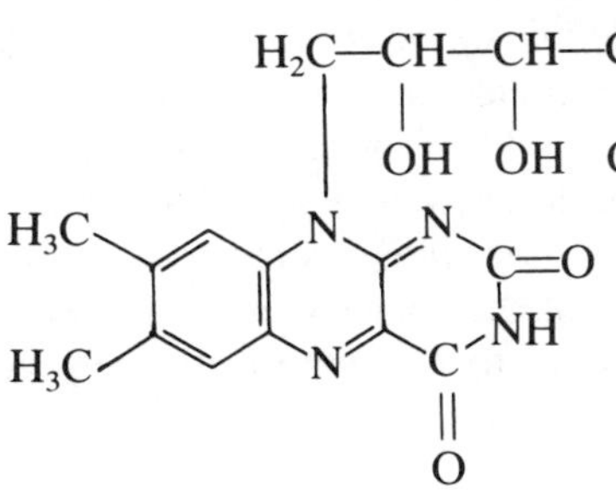

Figure 3.30 Structure of riboflavin.

and as vitamin G in the United States. Riboflavin was first isolated in 1934 from egg whites by P. Gyorgy and was synthesized by R. K. Khun and P. Karrer in 1935.

Riboflavin forms part of and is the functional moiety of two larger coenzymes. Both coenzymes are functional with a large number of enzyme systems, including amino acid oxidases, xanthine oxidase, and many dehydrogenase enzyme systems. The first of two riboflavin coenzymes is flavin mononucleotide (FMN), formed by the phosphorylation of riboflavin by ATP (Equation 3.9).

Equation 3.9
Phosphorylation of riboflavin.

The second coenzyme containing riboflavin is formed by the addition of adenosine diphosphate (ADP) to ribitol. Flavin adenine dinucleotide (FAD) is thus formed. FMN and FAD are structurally different coenzymes that participate in different coenzymes systems. Functionally, however, FMN and FAD both serve as hydrogen carriers in oxidation (i.e., dehydrogenation) reactions. FMN and FAD designate the oxidized forms of the respective riboflavin coenzymes, while $FMNH_2$ and $FADH_2$ designate the reduced forms of the coenzymes. The two hydrogens in the reduced forms of both coenzymes are to be found at the nitrogens of the isoalloxazine ring of riboflavin (Equation 3.10).

Equation 3.10
Oxidation–reduction of riboflavin coenzymes.

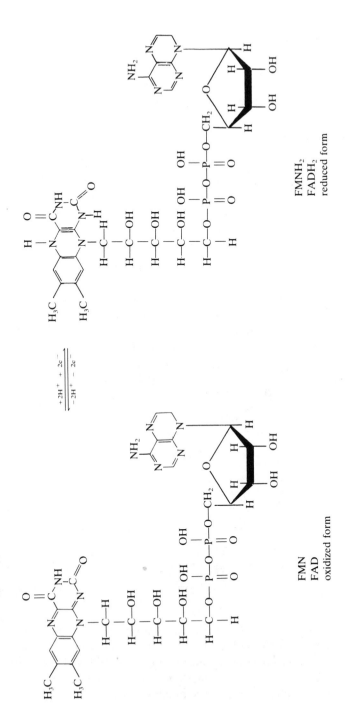

FMN
FAD
oxidized form

FMNH₂
FADH₂
reduced form

Nutritionally, these coenzymes participate with enzymes primarily in the oxidations of carbohydrates, fatty acids, and amino acids, as well as other metabolites as carriers of hydrogen. Reduced riboflavin coenzymes are oxidized in mitochondria by coenzyme Q, from which ATP is ultimately synthesized. Excreted in and regulated by urinary output, riboflavin has no known toxicity in humans.

Biotin (H)

Name:	Biotin
Molecular weight:	244
Form:	Fine long needles
Composition:	$C_{10}H_{16}N_2O_3S$
Active form:	Carboxybiocytin
Function:	Carboxylations

Biotin, one of only two vitamins to contain sulfur (Figure 3.31) was first isolated from egg yolks by F. Kogl and B. Tonnis in 1936. The chemical structure of biotin was determined by Kogl in 1937 and by du Vigneaud in 1941. The egg white glycoprotein avidin binds biotin and can lead to a biotin deficiency. This biotin binding protein was first observed by Bateman in 1916 and was observed again in rats in 1927. The chemical synthesis of biotin was first accomplished by S. A. Harris and co-workers in 1945.

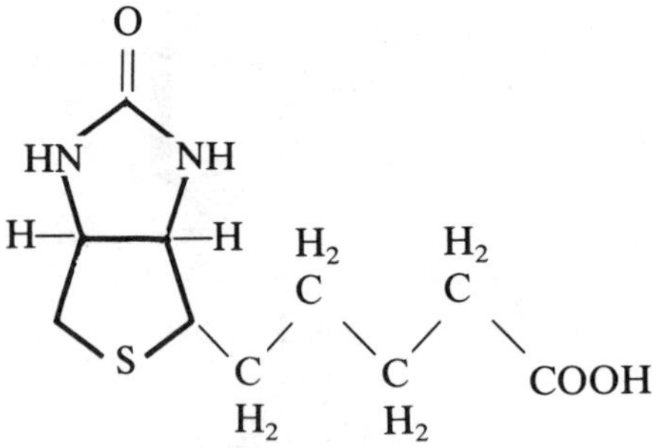

D-biotin

Figure 3.31 Structure of D-biotin.

Biotin has been isolated or chemically synthesized in eight isomeric forms. Only D-biotin is biologically active as a coenzyme. In tissues, D-biotin is covalently attached to enzymes by an amide bond linking the vitamin to a lysine residue of the enzyme. This conjugation is probably facilitated by ATP (Equation 3.11), and the vitamin–enzyme conjugate is known as biocytin.

Equation 3.11
Conjugation of D-biotin to apoenzyme.

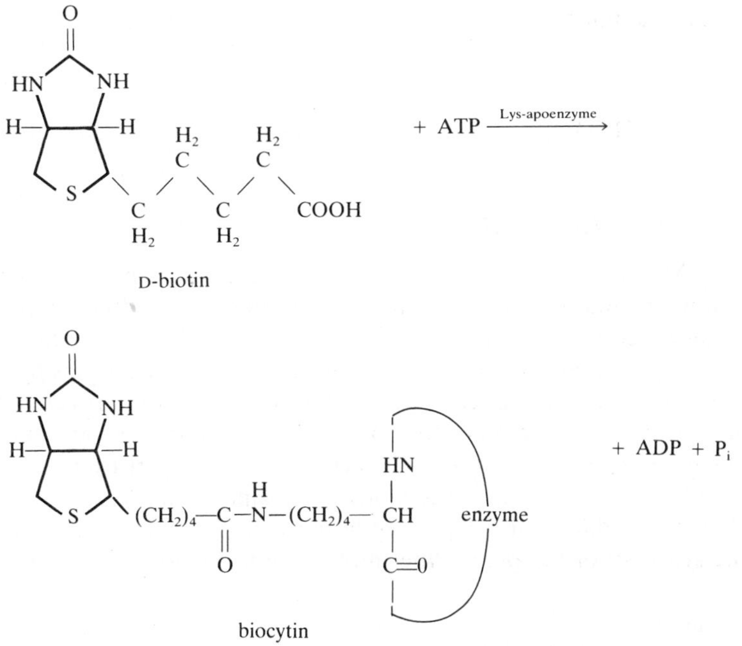

D-biotin

+ ATP $\xrightarrow{\text{Lys-apoenzyme}}$

biocytin

+ ADP + P$_i$

Biotin as biocytin functions in carboxylation reactions, one-carbon metabolism, whereby bicarbonate in the presence of ATP and Mg^{2+} is covalently attached to biotin, forming carboxybiocytin (1'-N-carboxy-D-biotin-enzyme; Equation 3.12).

Equation 3.12
Carboxylation of biotin to form carboxybiocytin.

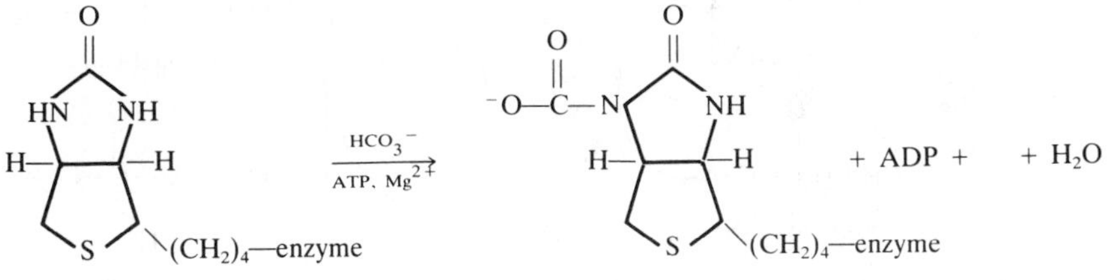

carboxybiocytin

$\xrightarrow[\text{ATP, Mg}^{2+}]{\text{HCO}_3^-}$

+ ADP +   + H$_2$O

Carboxybiocytin in a carboxylation reaction transfers the activated carboxyl moiety to one of several substrates, thereby increasing the size of the substrate by one carbon and regenerating biocytin. This reaction is summarized in Equation 3.13.

Equation 3.13
Coenzyme function of biocytin in carboxylation reactions.

$$HCO_3^- + ATP \diagdown \quad \text{biocytin} \longleftarrow \qquad \diagup \text{substrate} - \overset{\overset{\displaystyle O}{\|}}{C} - O^-$$

$$P_i + ADP + H_2O \diagup \quad \text{carboxybiocytin} \diagdown \quad \text{substrate}$$

Major carboxylation reactions involving biocytin permit the conversion of odd-numbered hydrocarbons into even-numbered hydrocarbons which are then metabolized in the major metabolic pathways. Both odd-numbered amino acids and fatty acids are converted to even-numbered hydrocarbons by carboxybiocytin. Major carboxylase reactions include the conversion of pyruvate into oxaloacetate, acetylcoenzyme A into malonylcoenzyme A, and propionylcoenzyme A into methylmalonylcoenzyme A. These reactions are shown in Equation 3.14 and can be found again in sections on carbohydrate, amino acid, and fatty acid metabolism. Biocytin is additionally important in the synthesis of carbamoylphosphate, used in the synthesis of the pyrimidines and in the formation of urea (Figure 7.7).

Equation 3.14
Major carboxylations utilizing biocytin.

Biotin is rapidly excreted in the urine intact, with a small number of additional metabolites having been discovered. A small number of these additional metabolites involve side-chain modifications of biotin. Biotin is relatively nontoxic, with doses of 2 mg of biotin per kilogram of body weight not demonstrating any adverse effects.

Phylloquinone (K₁) and Analogs

Name:	Phylloquinone
Molecular weight:	451
Form:	Viscous yellow oil
Composition:	$C_{31}H_{46}O_2$
Active form:	Unknown
Function:	Cofactor in synthesis of prothrombin
Activity:	Nondietarily required vitamin synthesized by microflora

Phylloquinone, vitamin K, was the first of a series of fat-soluble compounds derived from 2-methyl-1,4-naphthoquinone to be isolated and identified by E. A. Doisey in 1939 (Figure 3.32). The vitamin had earlier been observed as an unidentifiable lipid-soluble factor that produced hemorrhaging in chicks fed a fat-free diet. This lipid-soluble factor present in plants was recognized in 1935 by H. Dam and named vitamin K after the Dutch word *koagulation*. In 1939, Dam isolated vitamin K from alfalfa. Doisey, having isolated an analog of vitamin K from fish, designated phylloquinone vitamin K₁ and menaquinone isolated from fish meal,

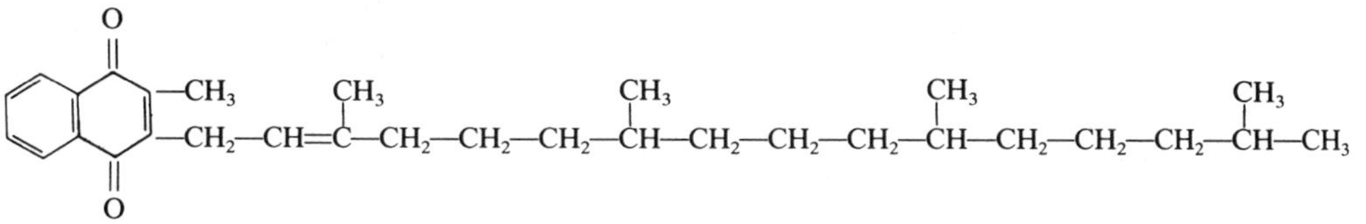

vitamin K₁

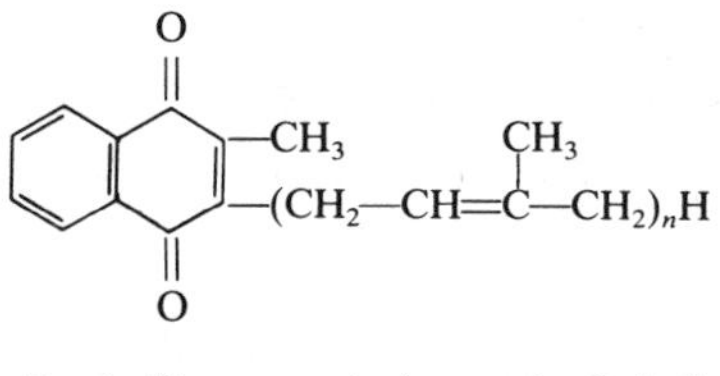

vitamin K₂ menaquin (*n* may be 6, 7, 8, 9, or 10, depending on the species)

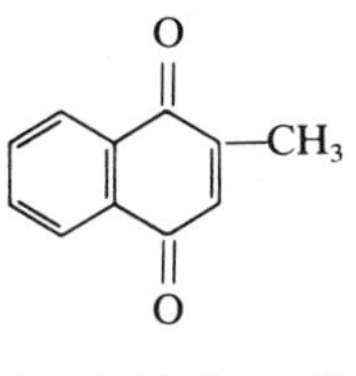

vitamin K₃ (menadione)

Figure 3.32 Phylloquinone (vitamin K₁) and analogs.

vitamin K_2. Menadione, observed to have vitamin K activity upon being converted to the active menaquinone by liver *in vivo*, has been designated vitamin K_3.

With the exception of chicks, monogastric animals and humans normally absorb sufficient quantities of vitamin K synthesized by the microflora of the gastrointestinal tract and plant foods, such that vitamin K deficiencies are uncommon. As with the other lipid-soluble vitamins, vitamin K absorption can be affected by the lack of bile secretion and gastrointestinal disorders that impair lipid absorption. Due to poor placental transfer of vitamin K and an initial sterile intestinal tract following birth, attention to vitamin K nutrition among newborns may be required. Supplements of vitamin K may be indicated in patients on long-term antibiotic therapy, as wide-spectrum antibiotics may reduce the gastrointestinal flora vitamin K synthesis sufficiently to require the use of vitamin K supplements.

The process of blood coagulation (clotting) involves a highly complex and not fully understood process involving cells: thrombocytes, platelets and erythrocytes, numerous protein factors, and Ca^{2+} ion (Figure 3.33). The net result of this complex process is the conversion of a highly soluble protein, fibrinogen, into a highly insoluble protein matrix, insoluble fibrin. Four protein factors are known to be reduced in plasma by a vitamin K deficiency. These proteins are coagulation factors II, VII, IX, and X (Figure 3.33). In 1974, prothrombin (factor II) was found to contain many residues of carboxylated γ-glutamate. In the following two years it was demonstrated using *in vitro* systems that vitamin K was a necessary coenzyme in a γ-carboxylase enzyme system. In this biotin-independent system, reduced vitamin K (hydroquinone) is the hydrogen donor for a microsomal electron-

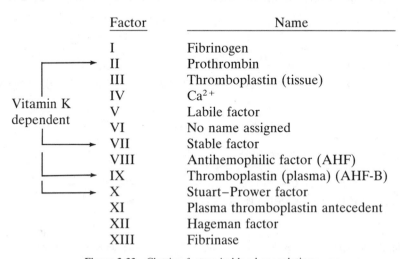

Factor	Name
I	Fibrinogen
II	Prothrombin
III	Thromboplastin (tissue)
IV	Ca^{2+}
V	Labile factor
VI	No name assigned
VII	Stable factor
VIII	Antihemophilic factor (AHF)
IX	Thromboplastin (plasma) (AHF-B)
X	Stuart–Prower factor
XI	Plasma thromboplastin antecedent
XII	Hageman factor
XIII	Fibrinase

Vitamin K dependent → II, VII, IX, X

Figure 3.33 Clotting factors in blood coagulation.

transport system and serves to transfer CO_2 to glutamate residues, forming γ-carboxyglutamate (Equation 3.15).

Equation 3.15
Scheme for the γ-carboxylation of glutamate residues by vitamin K.

$$\text{vitamin K} \cdot H_2 + CO_2(HCO_3) + O_2 + R\!-\!\underset{\underset{\overset{|}{CH_2}}{\overset{H}{N}}}{}\!-\!\underset{\underset{\underset{COOH}{|}}{\overset{|}{CH_2}}}{\overset{H}{C}}\!-\!\overset{\overset{O}{\|}}{C}\!-\!R \xrightarrow{\text{microsomes}}$$

glutamyl residue

$$\left[\begin{array}{c}\text{vitamin K} \cdot H \cdot CO_2 \\ \text{(hypothetical)}\end{array}\right] \longrightarrow H_2O + R\!-\!\underset{\overset{H}{N}}{}\!-\!\underset{\underset{\underset{CH}{|}}{\overset{|}{CH_2}}}{\overset{H}{C}}\!-\!\overset{\overset{O}{\|}}{C}\!-\!R + \text{vitamin K}$$

$$^-OOC \diagup \quad \diagdown COO^-$$

γ-carboxyglutamate

Equation 3.15 is a hypothetical, yet plausible scheme to account for vitamin K's role as both electron donor and coenzyme. The exact chemistry of how vitamin K functions as a coenzyme in carboxylation of glutamate residues remains to be elucidated. The importance of this reaction resides in the ability of γ-carboxyglutamate to bind calcium ions in the coagulation chemistry of prothrombin binding to platelets.

Two compounds (Figure 3.34) are extensively used as inhibitors of vitamin K activity which serve as effective anticoagulants. Dicumarol, found in spoiled clover and the cause of a hemorrhagic disease in cattle, suppresses prothrombin (factor II) synthesis. Its use as a human anticoagulant is quite extensive. Warfarin, an analog of dicumerol, also depresses prothrombin levels, in addition to causing capillary fragility and hemorrhage. Warfarin became a proprietary drug of the Wisconsin Alumni Research Foundation in 1966 and has been applied as a rodenticide.

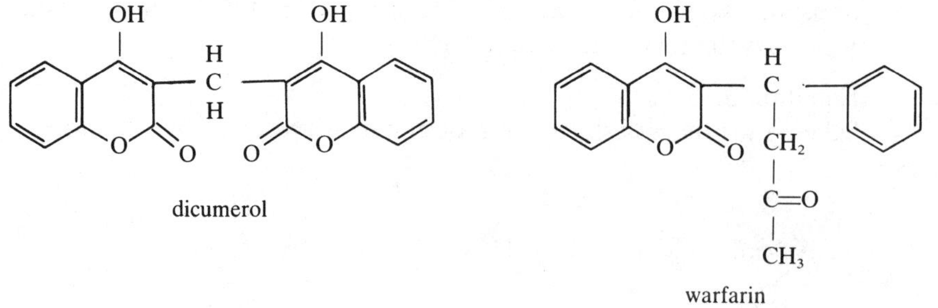

Figure 3.34 Anticoagulants: dicumarol and warfarin.

α-Tocopherol (E)

Name(s):	Tocopherols
Molecular weight:	(α-) 431
Form:	Pale yellow oil
Composition:	$C_{29}H_{50}O$
Active form:	Unoxidized
Function:	Membrane antioxidant
Activity:	1 IU–1 mg *dl*-α-tocopheryl acetate

Vitamin E was recognized and named by Herbert Evans in 1925 as the fertility factor that prevented reproductive failure in female rats fed a rancid diet and whole wheat.   Present in the oil of the wheat germ was vitamin E.   Isolated as a pale yellow oil, and identified structurally in 1938 by Fernholz, vitamin E was found to be a derivative of tocol and was named α-tochopherol, meaning childbirth (*tokos*, Greek) and to carry or bear (*pherein*).   In usual chemical nomenclature, -ol refers to the hydroxyl moiety of vitamin E.   *d*-α-Tocopherol is the most active of a series of tocopherols (tocotrienols and tocols) (Figure 3.35).   In plants and seeds (oils) α-tocopherol may constitute only 10 to 15% of the total tocopherols, but in animals and fish, α-tocopherol normally accounts for >90% of all tocopherols.   In addition to the conjugated rings, tocopherols contain isoprene units.   Commercial tocopherols are stabilized and supplied as either the acetate or succinate esters which are hydrolyzed by intestinal esterases prior to absorption.   Absorption of dietary tocopherols is only 20 to 40% complete and is facilitated by triglycerides and bile salts.   Absorbed into the lymph and subsequently, the blood, vitamin E circulates with the lipoproteins and membranes of erythrocytes.   In general, vitamin E penetrates and is found associated with the lipid fraction of cells and membranes.   Its concentration is particularly high in association with adipose tissue and adrenal glands.

The major function attributed to vitamin E is its role as an antioxidant (see Chapter 12).   In concert with the antioxidant enzymes, vitamin E protects those

Structure	Common name	Biological activity in international units per milligram
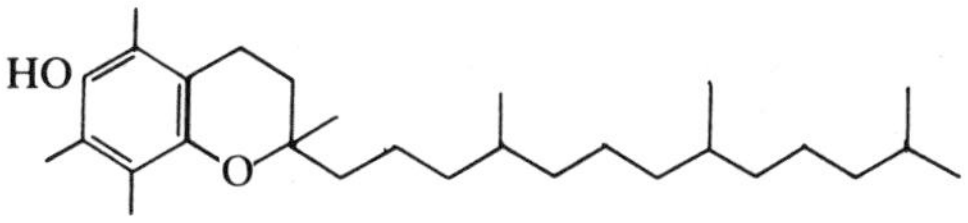	*d*-α-tocopherol (5,7,8 trimethyltocol)	1.49
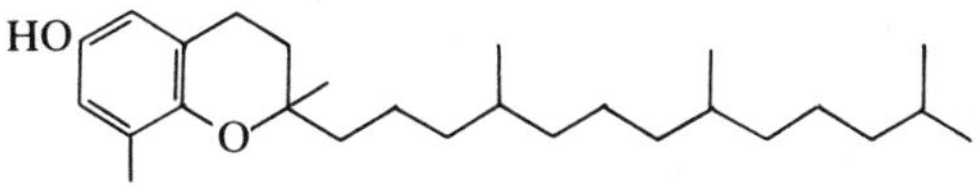	*d*-β-tocopherol	0.75
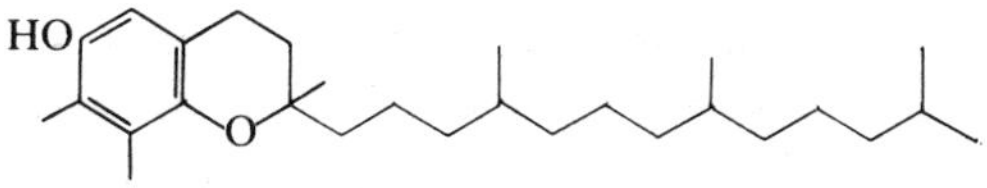	*d*-γ-tocopherol	0.15
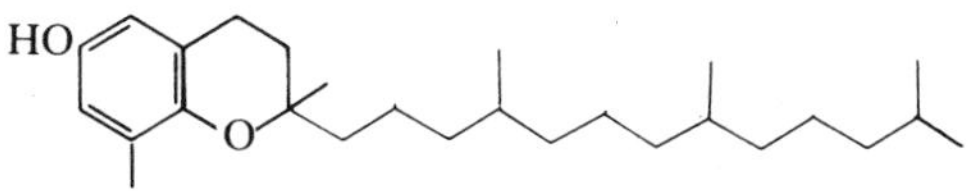	*d*-δ-tocopherol	0.05
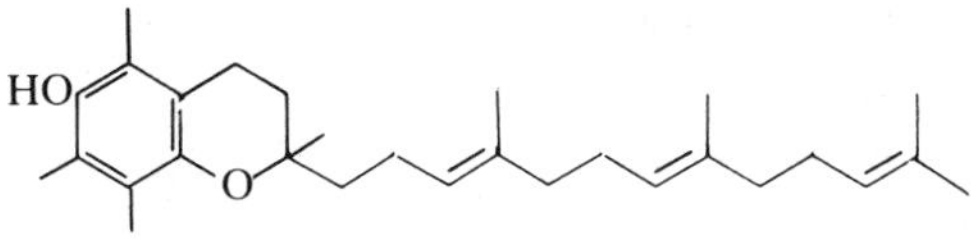	*d*-α-tocotrienol	0.45
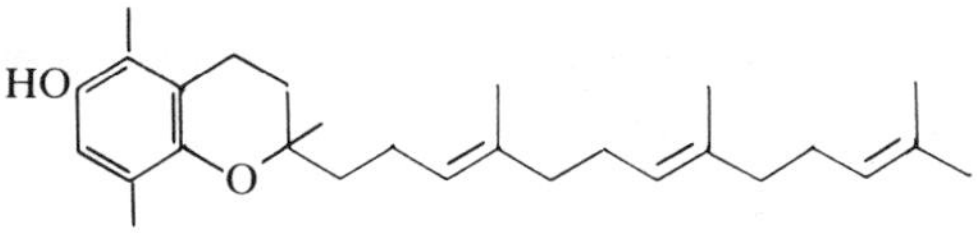	*d*-β-tocotrienol	Not determined
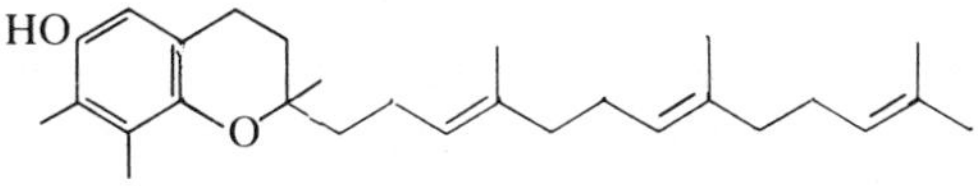	*d*-γ-tocotrienol	Not determined
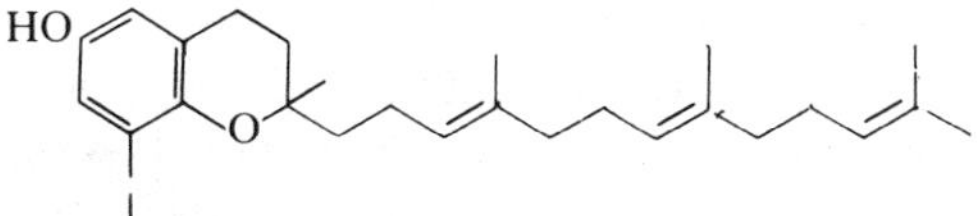	*d*-δ-tocotrienol	Not determined
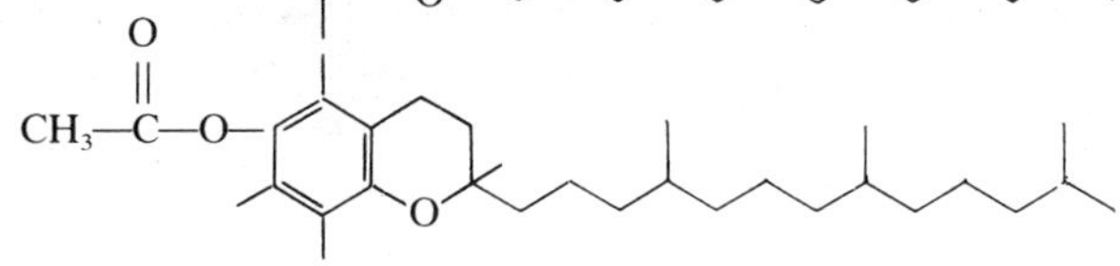	*d*-α-tocopherol acetate	1.36
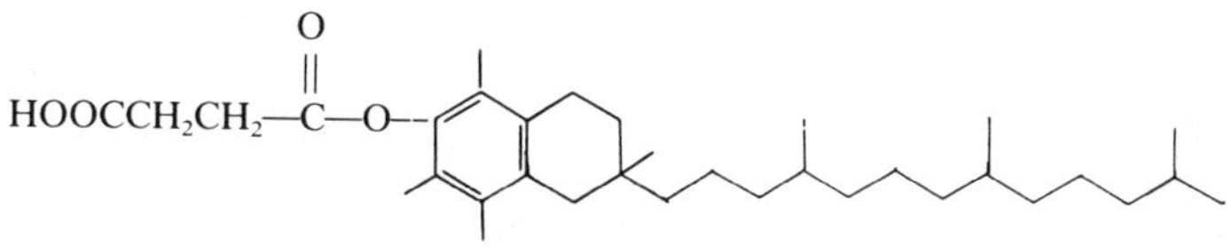	*d*-α-tocopherol succinate	1.21

Figure 3.35 Natural and synthetic occurring forms of vitamin E.

lipid components of cells from free-radical attack by itself becoming oxidized. Rats made dietarily deficient of both vitamin E and the trace element selenium are subject to liver necrosis and death from peroxidation. In other animal species, conditions attributed to vitamin E deficiency included muscular myopathies, accumulation of tissue lipofusin pigments, anemia, *in vitro* hemolysis, cataracts, and retinal degeneration. Although dietary vitamin E deficiency in humans is rare and occurs only under extremes of malnutrition and malabsorption of lipids, conditions such as increased susceptibility to peroxidation have been observed. Vitamin E is protective against the hepatotoxicity of acetaminophen, alcohol, and certain chlorinated hydrocarbons such as carbon tetrachloride. It may also reduce the toxicity of the metals iron (owing to its peroxidative property) and lead, which accumulates in erythrocytes.

Unlike all other vitamins, vitamin E has not been definitively shown to possess any coenzyme function. It is possible that in the future a specific coenzyme function for vitamin E will be found. Until that time, vitamin E remains a relatively nontoxic antioxidant of the lipid portion of cells.

Niacin (B_3, B_5)

Name:	Niacinamide
Molecular weight:	122
Form:	Needles
Composition:	$C_6H_6N_2O$
Active form:	Nicotinamideadenine dinucleotide/nicotinamide dinucleotidephosphate
Function:	Hydrogen carrier

The discovery of niacinamide as a vitamin was tied to the search for the cause of human pellagra (meaning "rough skin") in the southern United States by Joseph Goldberger of the U.S. Public Health Service just prior to World War I. Believing that pellagra was an infectious disease, Goldberger and four assistants failed at attempts to transfer pellagra to healthy individuals. In dogs, a disease comparable to human pellagra, black tongue, developed when animals were fed human diets

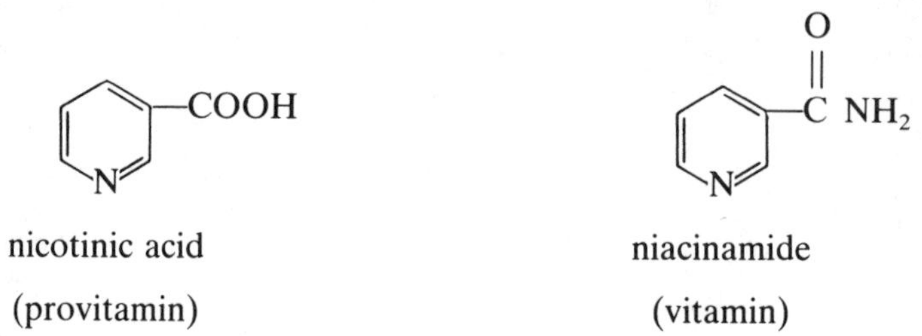

nicotinic acid

(provitamin)

niacinamide

(vitamin)

Figure 3.36 Structure of nicotinic acid and niacinamide.

that knowingly caused the disease. At the University of Wisconsin in the 1930s, C. A. Elvehjem and associates were feeding nicotinic acid and niacinamide (Figure 3.36) to dogs with black tongue. Nicotinic acid, then packaged in bottles with a skull and crossbones, and liver-isolated niacinamide both cured black tongue in dogs and were later found to prevent human pellagra.

Nicotinic acid is known to be converted to niacinamide by liver in a series of reactions involving ATP, ADP, and glutamine, which provides the amine in the conversion of nicotinic acid to niacinamide. Tryptophan, an essential amino acid, in a series of biochemical transformations, is also capable of being transformed by liver into niacinamide, as first demonstrated in rats. The conversion of nicotinic acid and tryptophan into niacinamide is shown in abbreviated chemistry in Equation 3.16.

Equation 3.16
Conversion of nicotinic acid and tryptophan into niacinamide (niacin) of NAD^+ (Abbreviated).

nicotinic acid

tryptophan   quinolinic acid

Niacin, or more specifically, niacinamide, like riboflavin, forms a portion of two larger redox coenzymes common to the metabolism of carbohydrates, lipids, and proteins: nicotinamide adenine dinucleotide (NAD^+) and nicotinamide adenine dinucleotide phosphate ($NADP^+$) (Figure 3.37). These two coenzyme molecules, both shown in their reduced form, differ only by the addition of the phosphate ester supplied by ATP to the 2'-hydroxyl of ribose. This phosphate added to

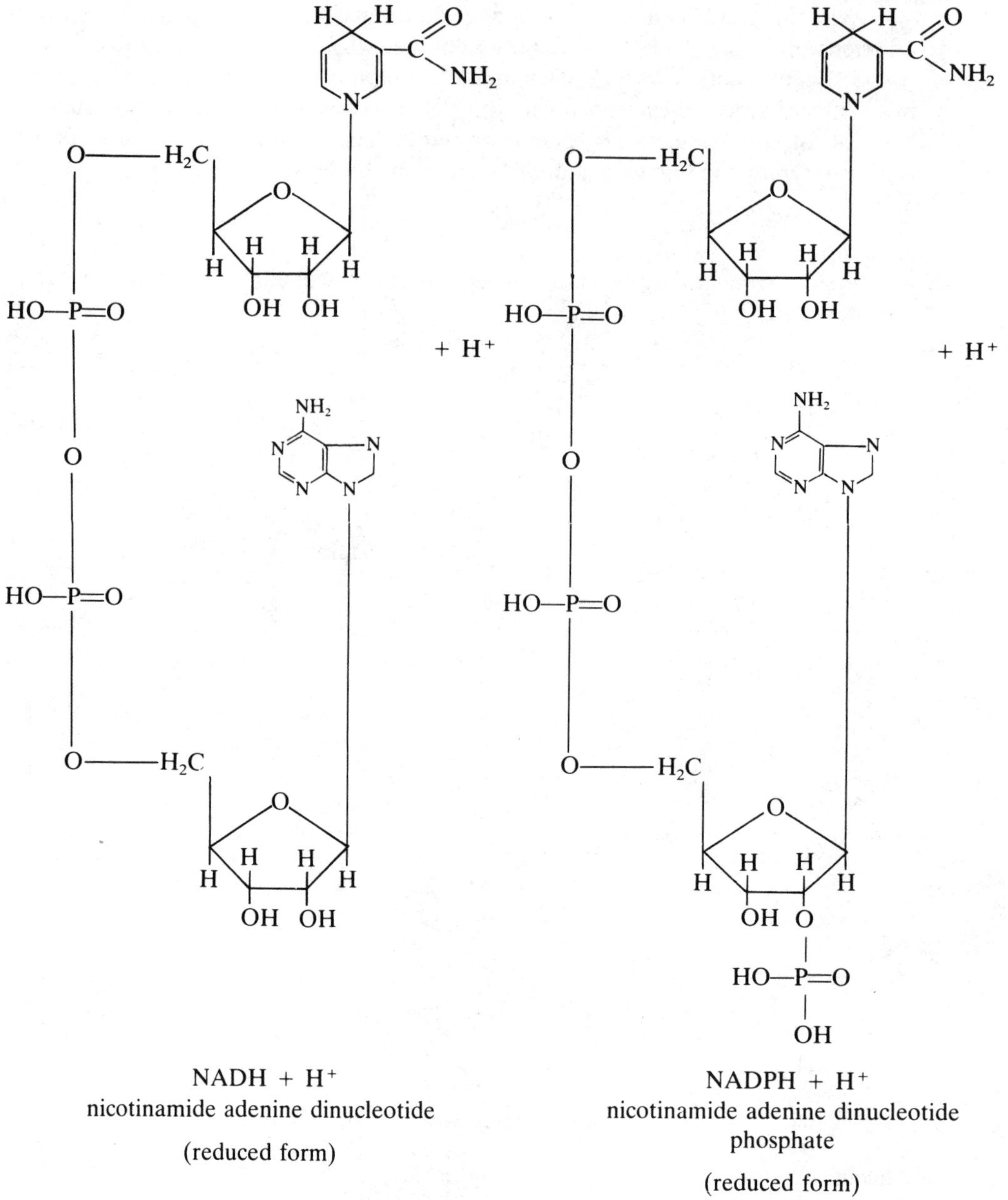

NADH + H^+
nicotinamide adenine dinucleotide

(reduced form)

NADPH + H^+
nicotinamide adenine dinucleotide phosphate

(reduced form)

Figure 3.37 Coenzymes of niacinamide.

$NADH_2$, forming $NADPH_2$, is significant, for it allows for the metabolic separation of anabolic and catabolic process through enzymatic recognition of functionally similar coenzymes. NAD^+ is utilized in most catabolic (oxidations) reactions, while $NADPH_2$ is the coenzyme for most anabolic (reductions) reactions (see Table 5.1). The redox reactions characteristic of these coenzymes occur on the niacinamide ring with stereospecificity mediated by dehydrogenases and reductases. As shown in Equation 3.17, oxidation of substrate SH_2 by NAD^+ or $NADP^+$ is a two electron–two hydrogen process. Only one hydrogen, but two electrons, are accepted by niacinamide during reduction. The second hydrogen becomes a proton given up in the reaction to the aqueous environment. The reverse reactions will take place during oxidation of $NADH_2$ or $NADPH_2$.

Equation 3.17
Oxidation–reduction reactions of nicotinamide coenzymes.

Like other water-soluble vitamins, niacin appears in the urine following methylation, forming N^1-CH_3-nicotinamide. Other niacin metabolites excreted include the oxidation products of methylnicotinamide, 2- and 6-pyridone-N^1-methylnicotinamide. Although nicotinamide is not toxic when ingested in the range 3 to 9 g per day, nicotinic acid may produce a "flush" and itching above doses of 50 mg, and liver damage may occur above doses of 3 gm of nicotinic acid per day.

Pyridoxal (B₆)

Name:	Pyridoxal, pyridoxamine, pyridoxine
Molecular weight:	167
Form:	Rhombic crystals

Composition: $C_8H_9NO_3$
Active form: Pyridoxal phosphate, pyridoxamine phosphate
Function: Transamination, deamination reactions

Vitamin B_6 was initially recognized as an antidermatitis factor in rats by J. Goldberger and R. Lillie in 1926 and was again recognized as the same antidermatitis factor by P. Gyorgy, who in 1934 proposed the vitamin's name. Independently isolated by three research teams in 1938, vitamin B_6 was then synthesized in the following year (1939). Since 1945 it has been known that vitamin B_6 could be isolated in three different forms: two in animal tissues, pyridoxal and pyridoxamine, and from plants, pyridoxine (also known as pyridoxol). These three forms of vitamin B_6 are shown in Figure 3.38.

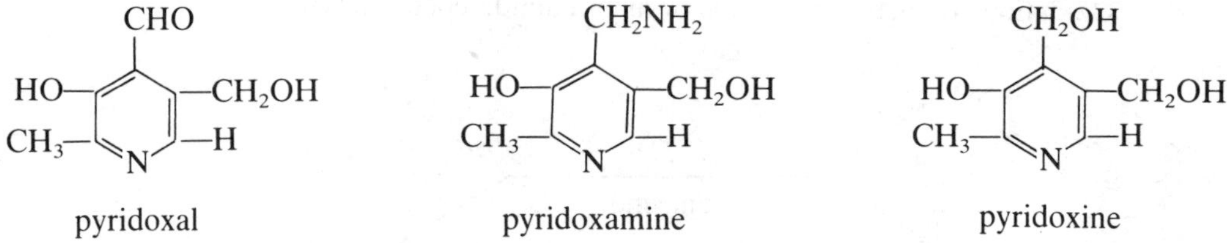

pyridoxal   pyridoxamine   pyridoxine

Figure 3.38   Three naturally occurring forms of vitamin B_6.

Vitamin B_6, like other B vitamins, participates in enzymatic reactions as a coenzyme. Its coenzyme function in the metabolism of predominately amino acids occurs only when vitamin B_6 has been converted to its active form, pyridoxal (or pyridoxamine) phosphate (PLP). Pyridoxal phosphate is formed by the phosphorylation of pyridoxal by ATP (Equation 3.18).

Equation 3.18
Phosphorylation of pyridoxal.

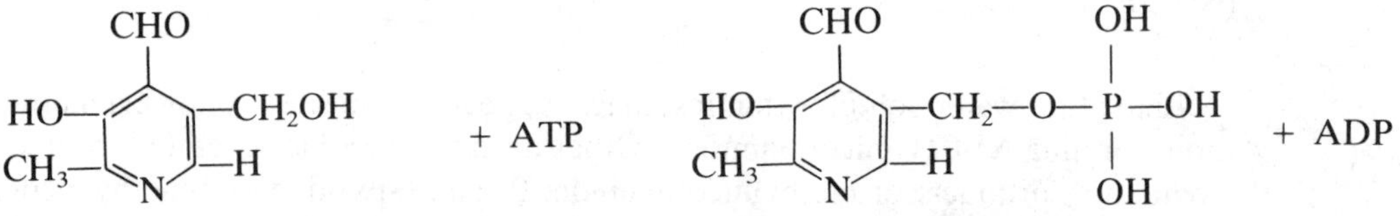

Pyridoxal phosphate (as well as pyridoxalamine) participates as a cofactor in four major classes of enzymatic reactions in the metabolism of the essential and nonessential amino acids. The enzymatic reactions in which PLP participates are transamination reactions, in which α-amino acids are converted to α-keto acids with the concurrent transfer of the amino moiety to a different α-keto acid, forming a second and usually different amino acid. Such transaminatition reactions, as shown in Equation 3.19, are responsible for the synthesis of the nonessential amino acids from the α-keto acids. These α-keto acid substrates exist as metabolic intermediates of carbohydrate and lipid catabolism.

Equation 3.19
Transamination reaction.

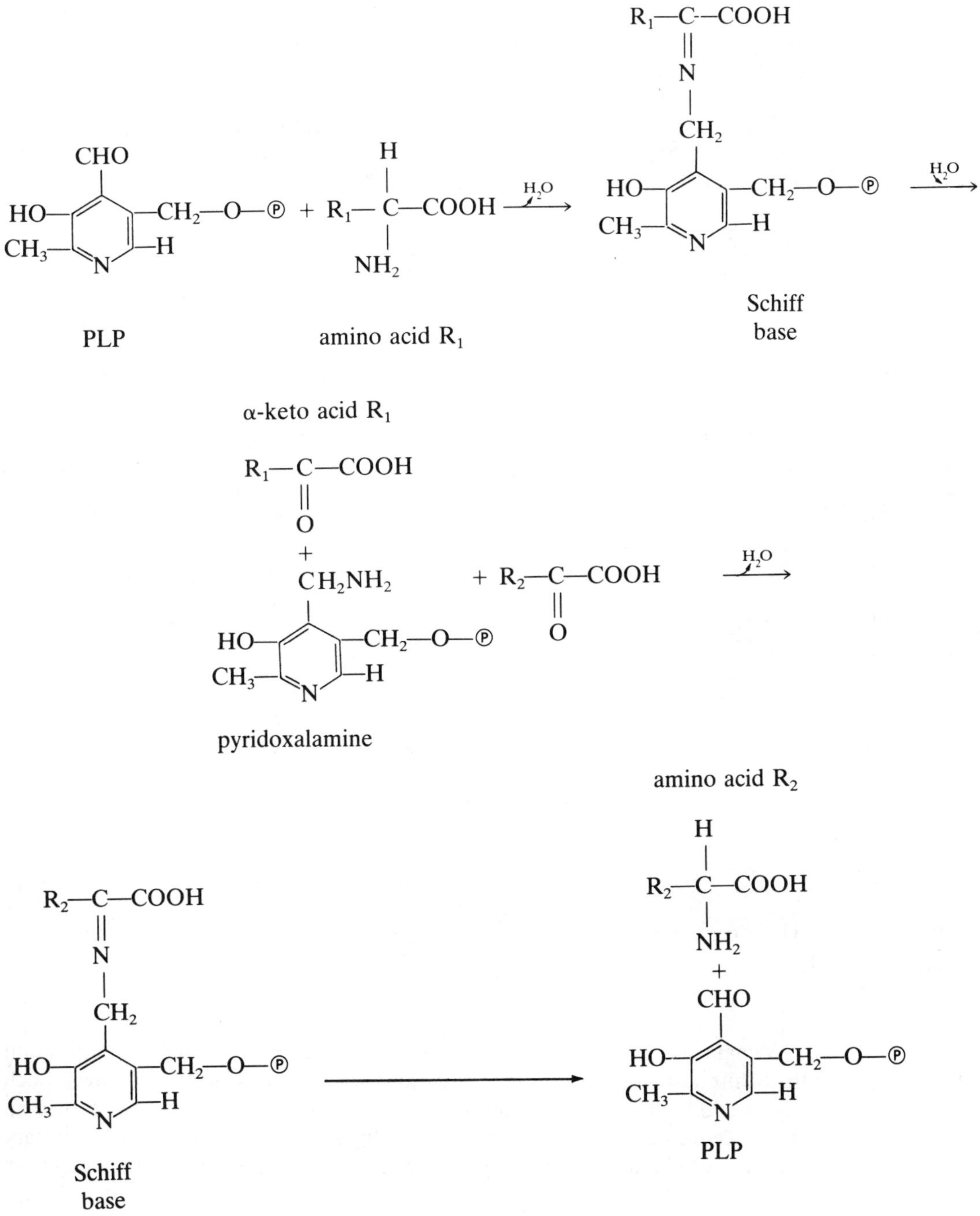

PLP   amino acid R₁   Schiff
                                                        base

α-keto acid R₁

pyridoxalamine

Schiff
base

amino acid R₂

PLP

Almost all enzymatic and nonenzymatic reactions of amino acids with vitamin B_6 stem from the condensation of an amino acid and the aldehyde of PLP (as pyridoxamine phosphate with the α-keto acid) forming a Schiff base —C=N—CH= $\rightleftharpoons$ —C—N=CH—, permitting the amino moiety to be transferred between amino and α-keto acids. In such reactions with pyridoxamine phosphate, oxaloacetate is converted to glutamic acid and pyruvate is converted to alanine.

The formation of the Schiff base also allows for the decarboxylation of amino acids by PLP. Mediated by a decarboxylase, amino acids are converted to amines upon the loss of carbon dioxide (Equation 3.20).

Equation 3.20
Decarboxylation reaction.

Vitamin B_6 as a cofactor with other enzymes, again through the formation of the Schiff base, participates in additional reactions involving amino acids. Such reactions add hydrocarbons or cleave the side chain (R) of amino acids, providing for the racemization, deamination, or desulfhydration of amino acids. Urinary metabolites of vitamin B_6 include pyridoxic acid, the major metabolite; along with lesser amounts of pyridoxic acid phosphate, pyridoxol, pyridoxine, and pyridoxal, among others. Pyridoxal is relatively nontoxic and has been administered up to 25 mg/kg body weight per day without measurable toxicity.

Pantothenic Acid (B₃, B₅)

Name:	Pantothenic acid
Molecular weight:	219
Form:	Hydroscopic pale yellow oil
Composition:	$C_9H_{17}NO_5$
Active form:	Coenzyme A
Function:	Forms portion of coenzyme A; two-carbon metabolism

Pantothenic acid (Equation 3.21), discovered by R. J. Williams in 1933, is one of the B-complex of vitamins thought to be formed by the condensation of β-alanine and pantoic (dihydroxybutyric) acid. It had at one time been identified as either vitamin B_3 or B_5. Unlike the other B vitamins, pantothenic acid does not function independently as a coenzyme; rather it forms a portion of a much larger coenzyme, coenzyme A (Figure 3.39).

Equation 3.21
Synthesis of pantothenic acid.

$$\underset{\substack{\text{pantoic acid}\\ \text{(dihydroxybutyric acid)}}}{\overset{\displaystyle\text{OH CH}_3\text{ OH}}{\text{H}-\overset{|}{\underset{|}{C}}-\overset{|}{\underset{|}{C}}-\overset{|}{\underset{|}{C}}-\text{COOH}}}\quad + \quad \underset{\text{β-alanine}}{NH_2CH_2CH_2COOH} \xrightarrow{\;H_2O\;}$$

$$\underset{\text{pantothenic acid}}{\overset{\displaystyle\text{OH CH}_3\text{ OH O}}{\text{H}-\overset{|}{\underset{|}{C}}-\overset{|}{\underset{|}{C}}-\overset{|}{\underset{|}{C}}-\overset{||}{C}-\underset{H}{N}-CH_2CH_2-COOH}}$$

The remaining components comprising coenzyme A are β-mercaptoethyl-amine and adenosine diphosphate (ADP). Coenzyme A, often abbreviated CoA or CoASH, is perhaps the most important coenzyme in intermediate metabolism, as it resides in a pivotal position in the metabolism of carbohydrates, amino acids,

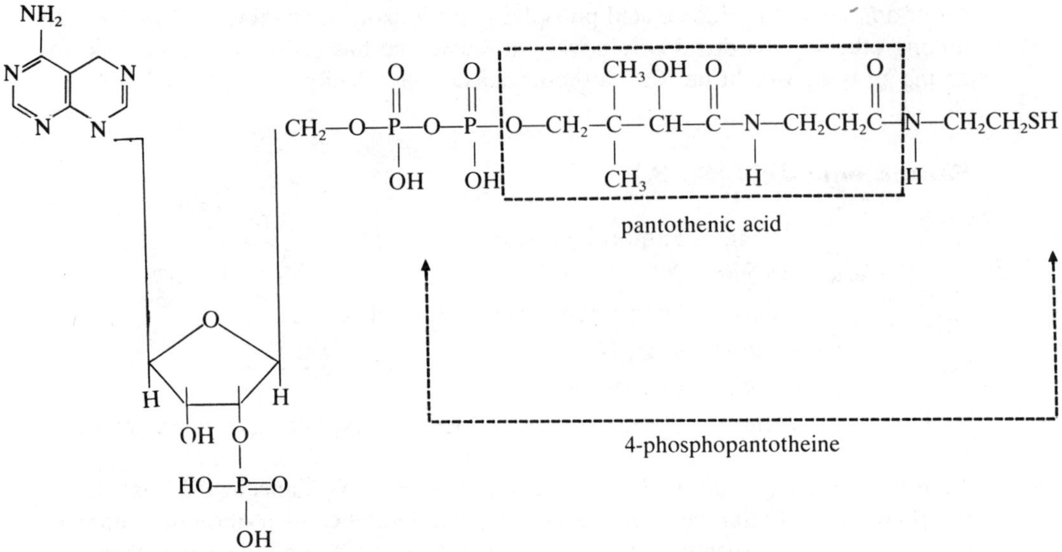

Figure 3.39 Coenzyme A containing pantothenic acid.

fatty acids, and other biomolecules. Coenzyme A readily forms with its sulfhydryl, thiol esters, such as with pyruvate, forming acetylcoenzyme A:

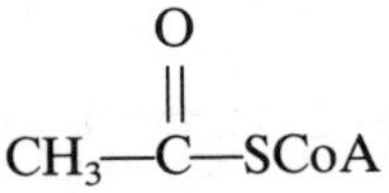

$$CH_3-\overset{\overset{\displaystyle O}{\|}}{C}-SCoA$$

Coenzyme A is the major regulatory coenzyme for two-carbon metabolism and accepts or donates substrates, fatty acids principally, with 4 to 13 carbons.

Pantothenic acid, as 4-phosphopantotheine (Equation 3.22), is also responsible for the synthesis of fatty acids (see also Figure 7.10). Attached to a protein via a serine residue, forming a phosphodiester, 4-phosphopantotheine is a cofactor capable of forming thioesters with fatty acids, providing the site of attachment for fatty acid elongations. The complex of protein and 4-phosphopantotheine is known as the acyl carrier protein, or ACP (Equation 3.22).

Equation 3.22
Formation of acyl carrier protein (ACP).

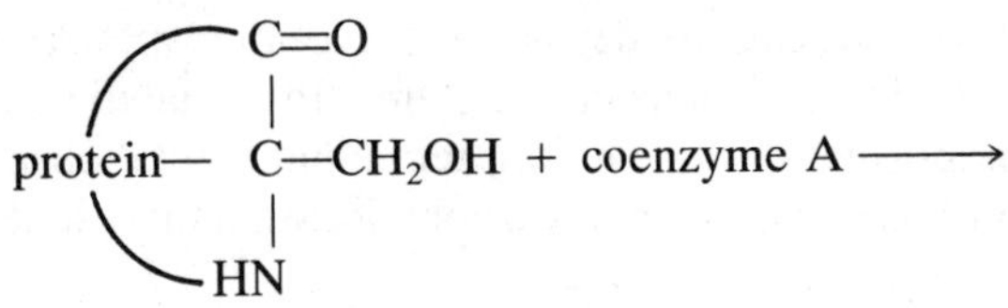

$$\text{protein}-\ \overset{\overset{\displaystyle C=O}{|}}{\underset{\underset{\displaystyle HN}{|}}{C}}-CH_2OH\ +\ \text{coenzyme A}\longrightarrow$$

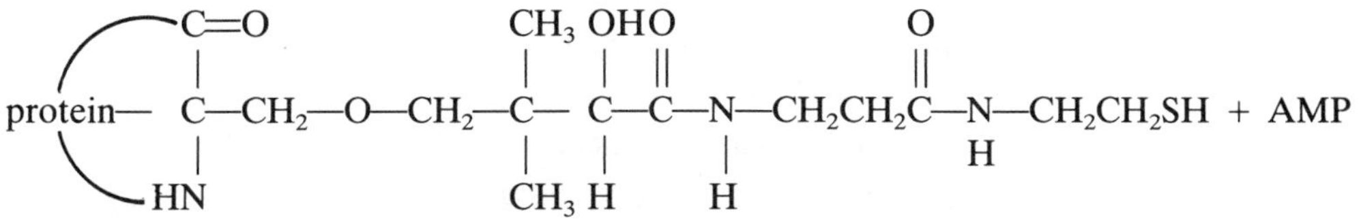

$$\text{protein} - \begin{array}{c} \overset{\displaystyle\frown}{} \\ C \\ | \\ HN \end{array} \overset{\displaystyle C=O}{\underset{|}{}} - CH_2 - O - CH_2 - \overset{CH_3}{\underset{CH_3}{\overset{|}{\underset{|}{C}}}} - \overset{OH}{\underset{H}{\overset{|}{\underset{|}{C}}}} - \overset{O}{\overset{\|}{C}} - \overset{N}{\underset{H}{}} - CH_2CH_2C - \overset{O}{\overset{\|}{}} - N - CH_2CH_2SH + AMP$$

protein-4-phosphopantotheine

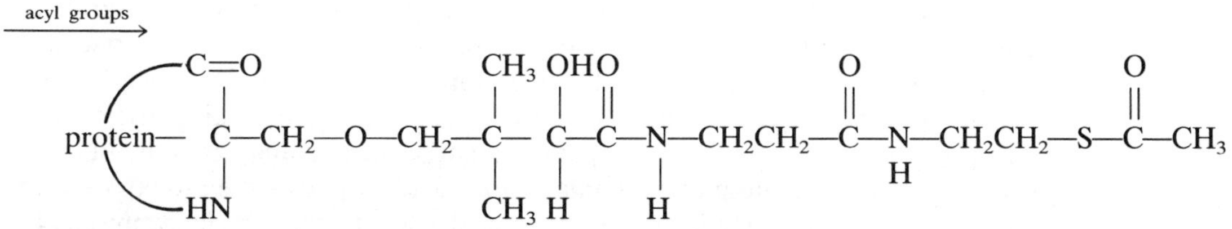

$\xrightarrow{\text{acyl groups}}$

$$\text{protein} - \begin{array}{c} \overset{\displaystyle\frown}{} \\ C \\ | \\ HN \end{array} \overset{\displaystyle C=O}{\underset{|}{}} - CH_2 - O - CH_2 - \overset{CH_3}{\underset{CH_3}{\overset{|}{\underset{|}{C}}}} - \overset{OH}{\underset{H}{\overset{|}{\underset{|}{C}}}} - \overset{O}{\overset{\|}{C}} - \overset{N}{\underset{H}{}} - CH_2CH_2 - \overset{O}{\overset{\|}{C}} - N - CH_2CH_2 - S - \overset{O}{\overset{\|}{C}} - CH_3$$

acyl carrier protein (ACP)

Other acyl group carriers as thiol esters

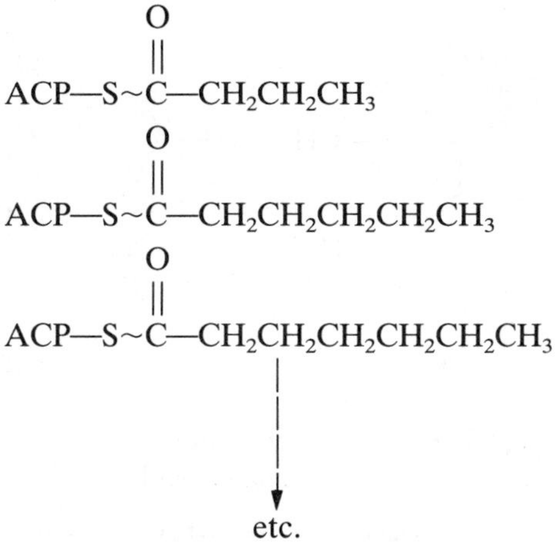

$$ACP - S \sim \overset{O}{\overset{\|}{C}} - CH_2CH_2CH_3$$

$$ACP - S \sim \overset{O}{\overset{\|}{C}} - CH_2CH_2CH_2CH_2CH_3$$

$$ACP - S \sim \overset{O}{\overset{\|}{C}} - CH_2CH_2CH_2CH_2CH_2CH_3$$

etc.

fatty acid—ACP complexes

Hydrolysis of the acyl moiety from the ACP yields a free fatty acid.

In cells, most pantothenic acid is quantitatively found present as coenzyme A followed by lesser amounts of ACP. Free pantothenic acid is found in the least amount in cells. A pantothenic acid deficiency in humans is indeed rare, if ever seen, and would occur only during extreme malnutrition.

Folic Acid (M, Bc)

Name: Folic acid
Molecular weight: 441

> *Form:* Yellow-orange crystals
> *Composition:* $C_{19}H_{19}N_7O_6$
> *Active form:* Tetrahydrofolic acid
> *Function:* One-carbon metabolism

Folic acid, also known as folicin, formally called vitamin M or Bc, is chemically named pteroylmonoglutamic acid (the "p" is silent). It is composed of pteridine, *p*-aminobenzoic acid, and glutamic acid (Figure 3.40). Found in plants, folic acid was both identified as an animal and bacterial nutrient factor and was synthesized in 1946. Natural folates can be isolated with oligo- and poly-γ-glutamyl chains. Polyglutamates of folic acid are capable of supporting animal growth, but not bacterial growth. Folate monoglutamate (folic acid) supports the growth of both animals and bacteria. Deficiency of folic acid leads to the classic symptoms of megaloblastic anemia in humans. Known also as vitamin M (formally) and vitamin Bc (c for "chicken"), folic acid also prevents hematological defects in other animal species.

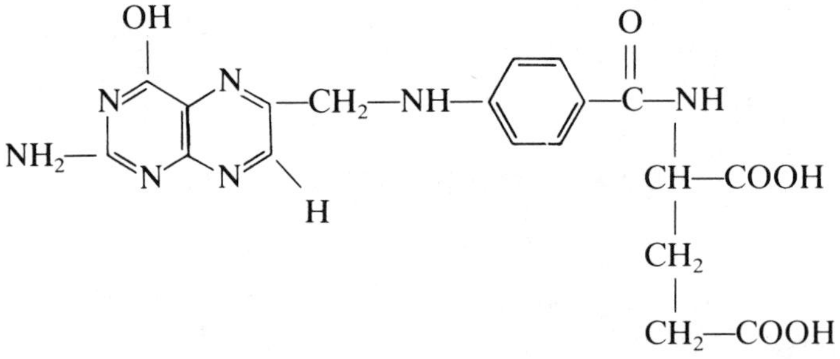

pteryl ring   *p*-amino-   glutamic acid
                     benzoic acid

Figure 3.40   Structure of folic acid.

Folic acid is absorbed from food in the gastrointestinal tract as polyglutamates, which are converted by the jejunal epithelial cells to the monoglutamylfolate. As either monoglutamylfolate or 5-methylmonoglutamylfolate, the folates are transported to the liver, where they are converted and stored as pentaglutamylfolate or hexaglutamylfolate. Serum folates circulate predominantly as 5-methylmonoglutamate.

Metabolic active folates exist in the reduced tetrahydro form of the coenzyme. Reduction of folic acid by two molecules of $NADPH_2$ yields tetrahydrofolic acid (THFA), the active form of the coenzyme. THFA is responsible for both acceptance and donation of single-carbon units from and for a variety of organic substrates. This function is often referred to as one-carbon metabolism. The

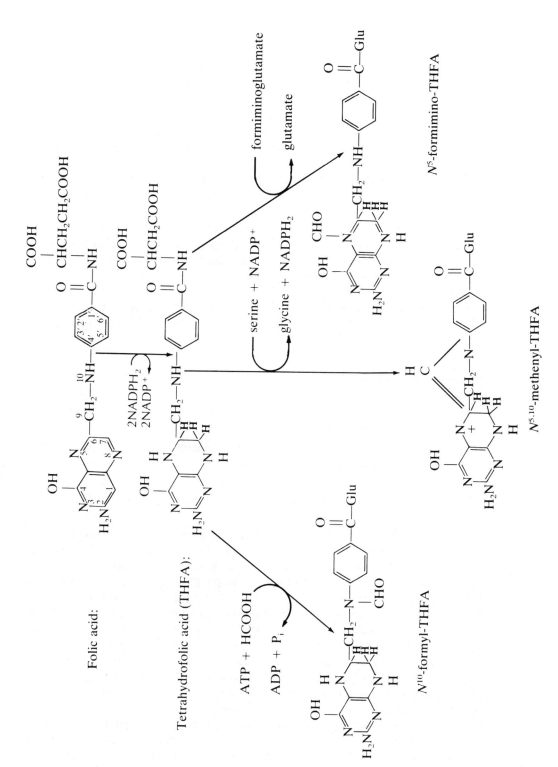

Figure 3.41 Reduction and coenzyme forms of folic acid.

single carbon units carried and transferred by THFA include a

methenyl $\left(=\underset{H}{C-}\right)$,   formyl (—CHO),   formylimino (>N—CHO)

and carbons of other oxidation states.   The formation of these THFA intermediates are shown in Figure 3.41.   These and other THFA derivatives that participate in one-carbon metabolism are most important in the synthesis of the purines and pyrimidines, precursors of the nucleic acids (see Chapter 12).   Drugs that interfere with THFA and its function in the *de novo* synthesis of nucleic acids are powerful inhibitors of cell division.   The THFA antagonist methotrexate (4-amino-N_{10}-methylfolate) is widely used in the treatment of cancer (see Figure 13.2).

THFA and its derivatives are also responsible for the metabolism of amino acids.   A primary source of single carbon units is serine, producing $N^{5,10}$-methylene-THFA.   This THFA derivative can be oxidized by NADP$^+$ to $N^{5,10}$-methenyl-THFA for the synthesis of purines.   Upon reduction, $N^{5,10}$-methylene-THFA is used to synthesize methionine and pyrimidines.   In conjunction with vitamin B_{12}, N^5-methyl-THFA is responsible for the conversion of homocysteine to methionine (see Equation 3.23).

Cyanocobalamin (B₁₂)

Name:	Cobalamin
Molecular weight:	1355
Form:	Hydroscopic dark-red crystals
Composition:	$C_{63}H_{88}CoN_{14}O_{14}P$
Active form:	Co(I)
Function:	Redox reactions, one-carbon metabolism with THFA

Vitamin B_{12}, cobalamin (Figure 3.42), was the last of the vitamins to be isolated in crystalline form.   It was first isolated on December 11, 1947, by Karl Folkers and Edward Rickers of Merck & Co. from a fermentation process using *Lactobacillus lactis*.   From a blood-red solution formed dark-red crystals of the long-sought antipernicious anemia factor named vitamin B_{12} by Folkers.   Vitamin B_{12} was also discovered to be the animal protein factor and its use in poultry and livestock feeds became extensive.   The dark-red color of vitamin B_{12} assisted others with its isolation.   Vitamin B_{12} is very different from all other water-soluble vitamins in that it possesses a mineral, cobalt, coordinate covalently bonded within a pyrrole ring system, strikingly similar to the iron porphyrins (hemoglobin) and magnesium porphyrins (chlorophyll).   Cobalt is sequestered within the corrin ring, filling four of cobalt's six coordinations.   A fifth coordination position is filled by a 5,6-dimethylbenzimidazole ribonucleotide, which is constant for a vitamin B_{12} molecule.   The sixth coordination position can be filled by cyanide (CN) used during the vitamin's isolation and purification, or by the hydroxyl (—OH), methyl

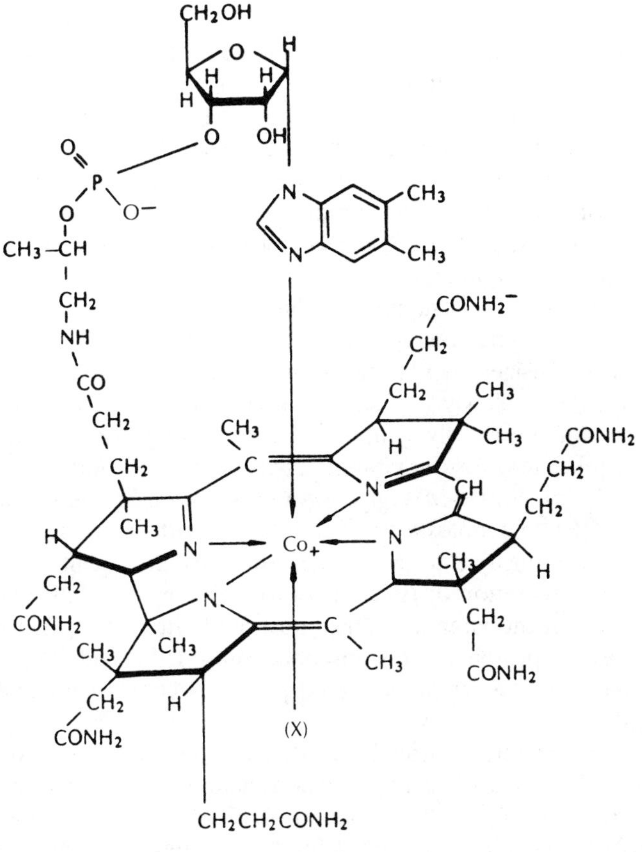

vitamin B$_{12}$

(X) = —NO$_2$ nitrocobalamin

    = —H$_2$O aquacobalamin

    = —CN in cyanocobalamin

    = —OH in hydroxycobalamin

    = —CH$_3$ in methylcobalamin   (coenzyme B$_{12}$)

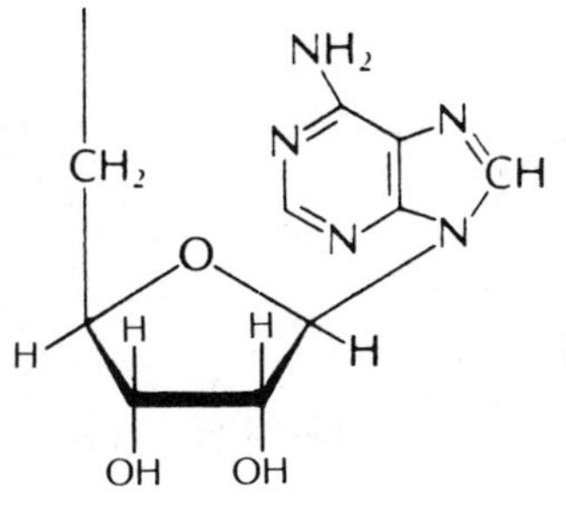

in 5'-deoxyadenosylcobalamin   (coenzyme B$_{12}$)

Figure 3.42 Structure of vitamin B$_{12}$ and coordinate substitutes.

89

(—CH_3), nitro (—NO_2), or water (H_2O) ligands. In size and structure, vitamin B_{12} is the most complex of all the vitamins. For this reason, many other analogs of vitamin B_{12} have been identified. When the sixth ligand is a coordinate of 5'-deoxyadenosine or a methyl group, vitamin B_{12} is known as coenzyme B_{12}. Years passed before its structure was determined and the vitamin was synthesized. The synthesis of vitamin B_{12} was completed in 1973 by R. B. Woodward and a team of many scientists. In 1975 the Nobel Prize in Chemistry was awarded for the synthesis of the vitamin.

Dietary vitamin B_{12} is supplied to humans and other carnivores principally by animal products, liver, kidney, heart, eggs, and some seafoods. In herbivores, vitamin B_{12} is synthesized by the microflora of the rumen and cecum when cobalt is present in the diet. Newly synthesized vitamin B_{12} is then absorbed and utilized. Vitamin B_{12} is not sufficiently synthesized by human gastrointestinal flora, hence the dietary requirement for the vitamin. Absorption of vitamin B_{12} is physiologically mediated by a 40,000-MW glycoprotein secreted by the stomach, known as intrinsic factor (IF). Complexation of vitamin B_{12} with two molecules of IF renders the glycoprotein insensitive to proteolytic enzymes and facilitates its absorption. Lack of intestinal secretion of IF can lead to a vitamin B_{12} deficiency even with a dietary adequacy of the vitamin. Once absorbed, vitamin B_{12} is found in plasma bound to transport proteins, the transcobalamins: I, II, and III. Impairment of gastrointestinal function for an extended period is concern for malabsorption of vitamin B_{12}.

Vitamin B_{12} is physiologically needed for the maturation of erythrocytes. Metabolically, vitamin B_{12} has a coenzyme function with several enzymes. Coenzyme B_{12} participates in (1) the reduction of ribose to 2'-deoxyribose in 2-deoxyribonucleoside triphosphates required for the synthesis of DNA, (2) a shift in a hydrogen atom from carbon 1 to an adjacent carbon, and (3) in methylation reactions which involve methylcobalamin. Methylcobalamin is formed by the methylation of the cobalt of cobalamin by N^5-methyl THFA (see "Folic Acid"). This reaction results in the enzymatic methylation of homocysteine in the synthesis of methionine (Equation 3.23).

Equation 3.23
Vitamin B_{12}—THFA—mediated synthesis of methionine.

$$N^5—CH_3—THFA \qquad B_{12}—Co \qquad CH_3—S—CH_2CH_2\overset{\overset{\displaystyle NH_2}{|}}{C}—COOH$$

methionine   H

$$THFA \qquad B_{12}—Co—CH_3$$

$$HS—CH_2CH_2—\overset{\overset{\displaystyle NH_2}{|}}{\underset{\underset{\displaystyle H}{|}}{C}}—COOH$$

homocysteine

MINERALS

The mineral content of plants, animals, and humans is inorganic and is that material which remains after either thermal (fire or high temperature) or chemical (nitric, perchloric acid) oxidation. The mineral content that remains following oxidation is often called "ash." In animals and humans, minerals constitute about 4% of the total body weight (70-kg man). Calcium, phosphorus, magnesium, the highly concentrated minerals of bone, represent about 80% of the total mineral content of the human body. Sodium, chlorine, potassium, and sulfur complete the largest group of minerals, called the macrominerals. The macrominerals comprise approximately 99.7% of all the essential minerals of the body (Figure 3.43).

TABLE 3.12 MINERALS

Macrominerals	Micro (trace) minerals	Newer trace minerals	
Calcium	Iron	Fluorine[a]	Toxic metals
Phosphorus	Fluorine[a]	Silicon	Cadmium
Magnesium	Zinc	Nickel	Lead
Sodium	Selenium	Tin	Mercury
Potassium	Manganese	Arsenic	Silver
Chlorine	Iodine	Vanadium	Gold
Sulfur	Copper	Boron	
	Molybdenum		
	Chromium		
	Cobalt		

[a]Fluoride is essential for hardening the enamel of the teeth and perhaps bone; its metabolic function has not been determined.

The remaining minerals, constituting about 0.3% of the total minerals of animals and humans, are the microminerals, more commonly referred to as the "trace minerals." Trace minerals* were so named during the time when analytical procedures and instrumentation were insufficiently sensitive to measure and quantitate accurately minerals found in tissues in very small amounts. Thus their detection was often quantitatively reported as "trace" amounts. There are 10 elements having general scientific acceptance as being essential trace elements for higher animals and humans. These are, in order of descending body concentration: iron, fluorine, zinc, copper, selenium, manganese, molybdenum, iodine, chromium, and cobalt. Boron is essential for growth of higher plants, but no known function has with certainty been attributed to it in animals. Silicon forms the elaborate and beautiful shells of the diatoms and along with boron is one of the newer trace elements. The newer essential trace elements are those elements that

*Some authors consider the least concentrated trace minerals to be the ultramicro trace minerals, cadmium, germanium, gold, lead, mercury, platinum, and silver. Aluminum, bromine, rubidium, and other nonessential minerals are often found in some tissues in higher concentrations than some of the essential trace elements. Cadmium, lead, mercury, and to a lesser degree gold and silver are toxic metals (Table 3.12).

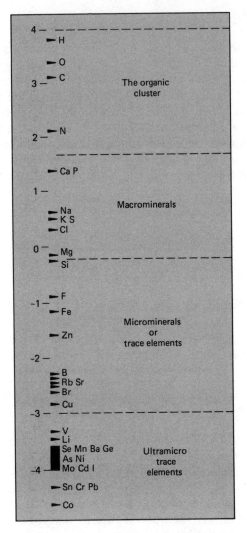

Figure 3.43 Elemental composition of the adult human (log gram-moles for 75-kg man). [Adapted from G. Schrauzer, *Biochemistry of the Essential Ultratrace Elements*, E. Frieden, ed. (Plenum Publishing Co., 1984), Chapter 2, p. 18.]

have been demonstrated to have some biological function associated with them in plants or experimentally in animals but for which there is no specifically known biological function in humans. The newer trace elements are fluorine, silicon, nickel, tin, arsenic, boron, and vanadium.

There are 90 naturally occurring elements in the periodic table and 78 elements have been reported to occur in animals or human tissues. In light of present knowledge, many of these elements are nonessential. Presently, the list of nonessential elements includes aluminum, antimony, germanium, rubidium, and the remaining elements of the periodic table for which no biological function has been demonstrated.

General Nutritional Functions of Minerals

The macrominerals function to provide to higher primates (1) strength to the organic endoskeleton through the deposition of calcium, phosphorus, and magnesium in bone, (2) principal electrolytes (sodium, potassium, and chlorine as the chloride anion) for ionic and osmotic balance and electrical gradients, and (3) sulfur to provide structure to proteins. Macrominerals have in addition to these primary functions other vital metabolic regulator roles in cells.

Micro (trace) elements found in tissues and cells in parts per million (ppm) or parts per billion (ppb) function primarily with enzymes as components of the active site of enzymes or as regulators of enzymatic activity. As components of enzymes and proteins, trace elements are frequent participants in redox reactions with the metal often functioning as the electron carrier. Several of the earliest evolved proteins of primordial cells may have been metalloproteins and enzymes containing iron, copper, sulfur, or manganese. These minerals, along with selenium and molybdenum, function in a variety of redox and respiratory chain enzymes and proteins. Many of these redox proteins, both in plants and animals and humans, probably came into being when plants, simple at first, began to liberate oxygen from photosynthesis. The other trace elements, such as manganese and zinc, along with the macroelements, calcium and magnesium found nonredox functions in proteins and enzymes. They evolved with proteins and enzymes by contributing to their structural organization as binding sites for coenzymes and/or substrates as well as metabolic regulators of proteins, enzymes, and nucleic acids.

Many of the macroelements and trace elements are antagonistic to one another during absorption from the gastrointestinal tract, in which two or more minerals compete for absorption sites or interact chemically. Many examples of mineral antagonists are well known, both from natural observations and laboratory experimentation with animals. It is known, for example, that high dietary intake of copper reduces absorption of iron and in principle could lead to an iron deficiency if ingestion of a high dietary copper diet was sustained. Diets also contain organic factors that may either reduce or enhance mineral absorption from the digestive tract. Mineral absorption may be reduced by dietary fiber and phytic acid. Phytic acid, hexaphosphoinositol, found in whole grains where it serves the need of growing plants for phosphate, binds and can prevent the absorption of the minerals calcium, iron and zinc. There are also those organic factors in the diet that facilitate mineral absorption. Amino acids, organic acids such as citric and lactic acids, and some carbohydrates increase absorption of some minerals. Table 3.13 is a partial listing of mineral antagonists and organic facultative compounds for mineral absorption. Drugs and medicines may also adversely affect mineral absorption (see Chapter 13).

TABLE 3.13 MINERAL ANTAGONISTS AND ORGANIC FACILITATOR COMPOUNDS

Major mineral antagonists

```
Ca —[ P          P —[ Ca        Mg —[ Ca      Na —[ K       S —[ Se
       Al                Mg              P            S            Zn
       Zn                Mn                        Ag
       Mg                                          Cu          Mo —[ W
                                     Fe             Fe                 S
Fe —[ Mn         Mn —[ Cu        Zn —[ Ca    Cu —[ Mo                 Cu
       Cu                P               Cu           P                  Mn
       Co                Fe              Pb           Cd
       Mn                Co              Cd           Zn           [ S
       Zn                Mg                           Pb             As
                                  Cr —[ Zn            Se      Se —[ Hg
                                        V                            Cd
Cd —[ Zn                          I —[ Co                            Ag
       Cu         F —[ Al                      F —[ Al              Pb
       Fe               Ca        Sn —[ Fe           Ca              Au
       Hg               Mg              Cu           Mg
       Pb
       Se        Co —[ Fe
```

Organic inhibitors and facilitators of mineral absorption

Organic inhibitors of some minerals for absorption
  Phytic acid, fiber, some drugs
Organic facilitators of mineral absorption
  Vitamin C, citric acid, lactic acid, pyruvic acid, succinic acid,
  lactose, fructose, glucose, histidine, lysine, cysteine, valine

Essentiality and Bioavailability of Minerals

Almost all of the macrominerals, the trace minerals, the nonessential minerals, and the toxic metals are supplied to the body through the diet having once originated in soils. The soil's minerals are absorbed from the vegetables, fruits, grains, and animal products eaten. Lesser amounts of minerals are normally ingested in water; still lesser amounts are absorbed by the lungs from air. The elements derived from the soil, passed to us through plants and animals, are essential for humans if a dietary inadequacy results in a physiological or structural abnormality, and its addition to the diet prevents or reinstates normal health. Specific biochemical changes and defined functions for minerals which can be accurately measured lend credence to their essentiality. Lack of dietary adequacy of the essential macrominerals and trace elements results in the classic diseases, conditions, and afflictions: anemias (Cu and Fe), rickets (Ca), and goiter (I).

Essentiality is a qualitative feature of all minerals whose dietary deficiency or inadequacy over an extended period results in a disease condition, a feature shared with vitamins. Mineral deficiency, dietary adequacy, and mineral toxicity are quantitative values that can be assigned to each essential mineral over a dietary range beginning with no dietary intake. Each mineral will have its own quantitative

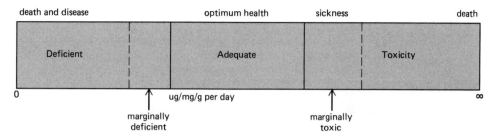

Figure 3.44 Deficiency, adequacy, and toxicity of essential minerals.

range of dietary adequacy and will vary in toxicity when excessive dietary intake exceeds excretory capacity. Almost all minerals can produce some toxicity when consumed in excess. These effects of dietary deficiency, adequacy, and toxicity that almost all essential minerals share are demonstrated in Figure 3.44.

Coordination and Chelation of Minerals

The key to understanding the general role of many of the macrominerals and the microminerals as metabolic regulators and as catalysts in proteins and enzymes is their ability to form coordination compounds, metal complexes, or what is often referred to as just "complexes." Coordination complexes usually contain a centrally located metal cation, surrounded by negative ions, molecules, or water. Coordination complexes are formed by coordinate covalent bonding (Chapter 1), and coordination positions may be from one to six, with two, four, six, and sometimes eight common. Molecules that have two or more coordinate positions or ligands are multidentate or chelating compounds. As the number of ligands increases about the central metallic cation, the stability of the metal complex is usually increased. Thus the stability of metal complexes is usually determined by the number of coordinating ligands about the metal cation, the size and charge of the metal ion, the ligating molecule, and the final structure of the chelate complex.

Surrounding the central metallic cation forming the coordination complex may be found ions, Cl^- (chloride) or PO_4^{2-} (phosphate) and SO_4^{2-} (sulfate), for example, which may be either inorganic or organic in form. Organic compounds forming complexes include $\ddot{N}H_3$ (ammonia), $\ddot{N}H_2CH_2CH_2\ddot{N}H_2$ (ethylenediamine) and

$$(\bar{:}O\!-\!\overset{\overset{\displaystyle O}{\|}}{C}\!-\!CH_2\!-\!\ddot{N}CH_2CH_2\ddot{N}\!-\!CH_2\overset{\overset{\displaystyle O}{\|}}{C}\!-\!O\!:\!\bar{\,})$$

(ethylenediaminetetraacetate, EDTA). Other organic compounds forming a variety of metallocomplexes include various amino acids, disulfides, and tetrapyrroles. Molecules containing amines, carboxyl anions, hydroxyl anions, thiols, sulfate and phosphate anions, and heterocyclic nitrogen compounds may also coordinate metals. Some of these metal complexes are shown in Figure 3.45. It is the coordi-

$$\begin{array}{c} H \\ CH_2 \!\!-\!\!-\!\! NH \\ | \qquad\quad \downarrow \\ C\!\!-\!\!O^- \!\!\rightarrow\!\! Cu^{2+} \\ \| \\ O \end{array}$$

copper glycinate

Nutritional/Physiological Significance
Amino acid metal complexes, especially cysteine and histidine for transport and mineral storage

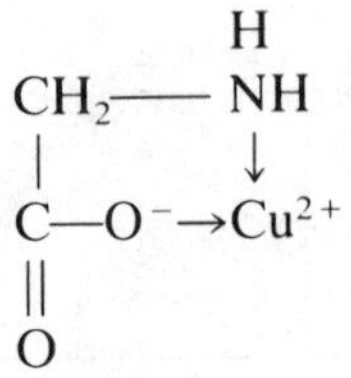

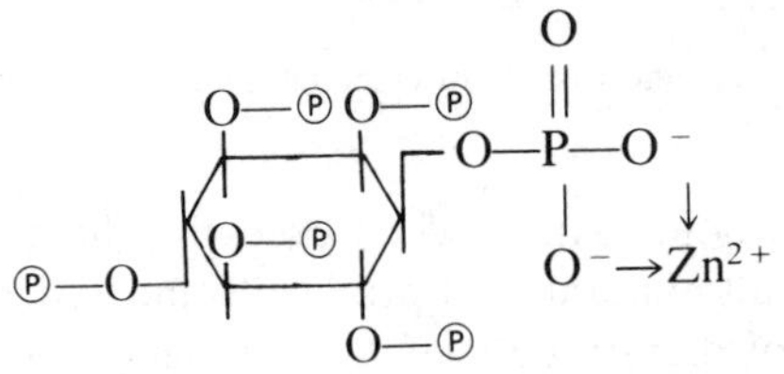

phytic acid
(hexaphosphomyoinositol)

Phytic acids binds Zn^{2+}, Fe^{2+}, Ca^{2+}, and may reduce absorption of these minerals

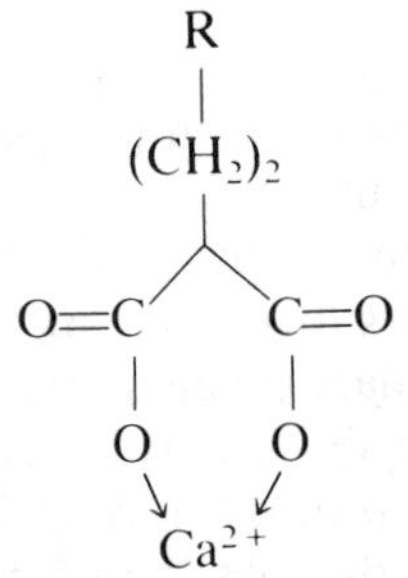

$$\begin{array}{c} R \\ | \\ (CH_2)_2 \\ | \\ O\!\!=\!\!C \qquad C\!\!=\!\!O \\ | \qquad\quad | \\ O \qquad\quad O \\ \searrow \quad \swarrow \\ Ca^{2+} \end{array}$$

calcium γ-carboxyglutamate

Calcium γ-carboxyglutamate binds Ca^{2+} precipitating prothrombins binding to blood platelets [see "Phylloquinone (K_1) and Analogs"]

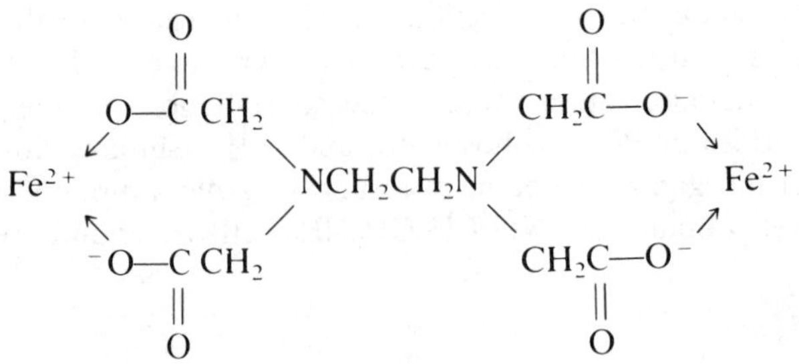

iron–EDTA
(ethylenediaminetetraacetic acid)

EDTA chelates Ca^{2+}, Zn^{2+}, Ca^{2+}, Fe^{2+}, Mn^{2+}, Mg^{2+}, sometimes used as food preservative

Figure 3.45 Nutritional ligands and chelates.

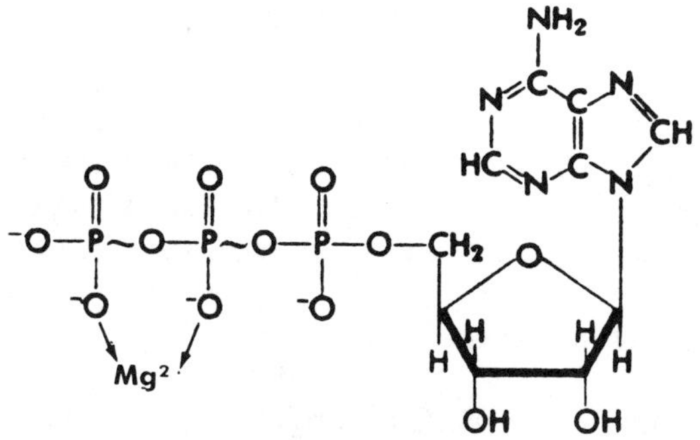

magnesium-ATP
(adenosine triphosphate)

Magnesium-ATP complex for the hydrolysis of ATP (ATP → ADP + P_i)

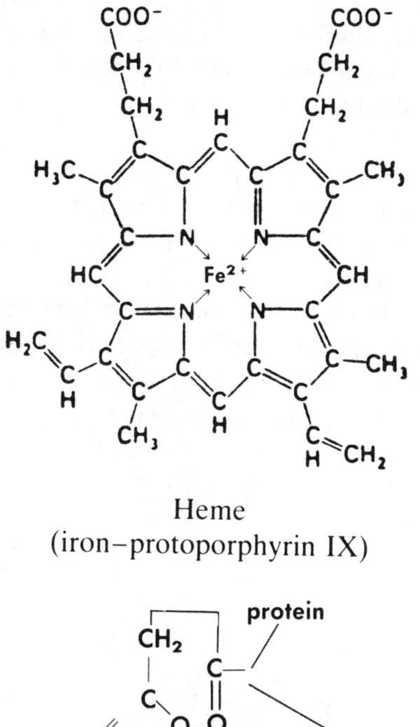

Heme
(iron–protoporphyrin IX)

Heme-tetrapyrrole complex containing Fe^{2+} in hemoglobin, myoglobin, and cytochromes. May complex Zn^{2+} in iron-deficiency anemia. Similar coordination complexes contain Mg^{2+} (chlorophyll) and Co^{2+} (vitamin B_{12})

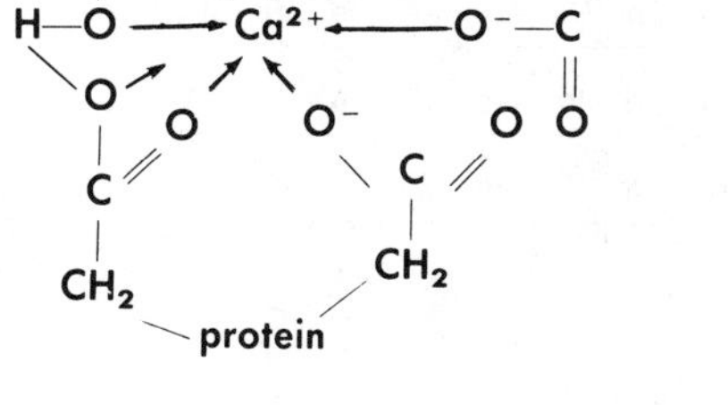

parvalbumin

Parvalbumin—shown is one of three calcium binding sites of this protein. Calcium binds to four acidic amino acid residues, one ketone, and a molecule of water occupies the eighth coordinate position

Figure 3.45 (continued)

nation chemistry of metal ions to ligands, forming either loosely or tightly bound metalloorganic complexes, that accounts for the absorption of minerals and the binding of cation minerals by fiber, by metallothionine, by DNA, by tetrapyrroles, and by the many proteins and enzymes requiring minerals for regulation and catalysis.

Absorption and Metabolism of Minerals

All minerals in the diet are not equally absorbed, nor are all different compounds and complexes of the same mineral absorbed with the same degree of efficiency. Such differences in absorption, along with factors such as age, sex, genetic variables, general health, nutritional status, and diet, affect mineral absorption and bio-availability.   Minerals become bioavailable from the diet following absorption, the process that predominates in mineral regulation.   Following mineral absorption across the intestinal mucosa, they enter their metabolic pool and are transported, often by a specific transport protein, to their storage, physiological, or biochemical site of action.

In the following section on minerals, beginning with calcium, the minerals are presented in decreasing order of abundance in the human body.   To each mineral is affixed the date of nutritional recognition, relative atomic size (H = 1.0) to hydrogen, its place within the periodic table, usual oxidation state(s), approximate RDA for an adult, and total body burden or content for an idealized 70-kg person.   Within the discussion of each mineral, tables have been included listing the known extent to which the mineral interacts with proteins, enzymes, and other molecules.   For each mineral (where known) an overview of its absorption, modes of excretion, and metabolism is presented in a final figure.

Calcium

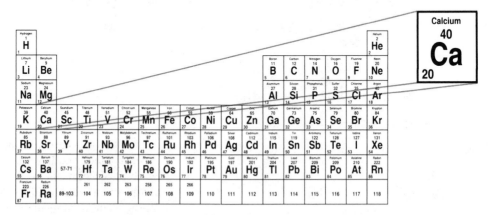

Date of nutritional recognition: 1842
Relative atomic size: 6.6
Oxidation state: +2

Recommended dietary allowance: 800 mg for adult male
Body burden: 1500 g

Calcium is the most abundant mineral of animals with a calcified skeleton and of humans, representing 52% of the body's mineral content. Almost all of this calcium is found in insoluble form in bone and teeth (99%) as an hydroxy-apatite, $Ca_{10}(PO_4)_6(OH)_2$, providing the structural support to the endoskeleton and dentition. The remaining 1% of calcium is found bound to proteins and ionized intra- and extracellulary, where it controls a wide variety of physiological and enzymatic controls. This small fraction of calcium is responsible for electrical cell potentials, muscle contraction, cell division, the clotting of blood (see "Phyllo-quinone and Analogs"), and adenyl cyclase formation. In many ways, ionized calcium is almost hormonelike in its varied functions.

Calcium is a rather abundant alkaline earth metal, often having been con-centrated in deposits of limestone as calcium carbonate. The metal was discovered in 1808 by Sir Humphry Davy, who gave it its name, calcium, after the Latin *calx*, meaning "lime." The nutritional importance of calcium was noted by M. Chossat in 1842, when he recognized the need for calcium for the development of the bones of pigeons.

The dietary absorption of calcium from the gastrointestinal tract is explicably tied to the physiological role of vitamin D (see "Cholecalciferol"). Indeed, there are at least two calcium deficiency diseases, rickets and osteoporosis. Rickets caused by a lack of bone calcification is in reality a vitamin D deficiency disease, which can occur in the face of adequate calcium nutriture. Osteoporosis, "porous bones," is an insidious loss of bone mineralization over a period of years which occurs most often in white, Anglo-Saxon, postmenopausal women of small bone stature. This disease leads to a loss in height, dowager's hump, and frequent fractures of vertebrae, wrists, and hips among the elderly. The course of osteo-porosis is not understood but increased calcium intake and exercise beginning about age 20 is being advocated as a preventative measure to slow or prevent this disease. In spite of recommendations for increasing one's dietary intake of calcium for osteoporosis, there are clearly no calcium deficiency diseases per se. Many elderly people do not exhibit fully developed osteoporosis, so it would appear that vitamin D, estrogens, parathyroid hormone, inactivity, and other unidentified factors are contributing to osteoporosis.

Calcium is absorbed from the gastrointestinal tract under control of vitamin D and calcium binding proteins (Figure 3.46). Although it is difficult to measure calcium absorption precisely, estimates of 20 to 30% calcium absorption of the 300 to 1000 mg ingested daily appears reasonable. The main storage site for calcium is bone, which constantly undergoes turnover by osteoclastic and osteoblastic cell-ular activity, with about 20% of bone being remolded each year. Bone calcium is the reservoir for serum calcium, which is carefully regulated and maintained by hormonal controls at around 10 mg/dl. PTH (parathyroid hormone) secretion controls the synthesis of renal 1,25-dihydroxyvitamin D, affecting intestinal ab-

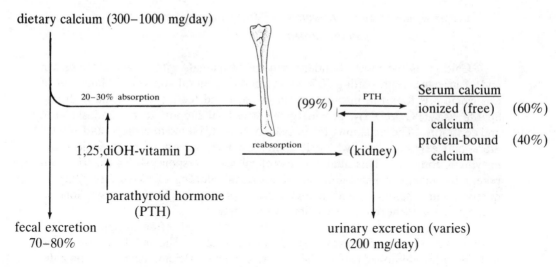

Figure 3.46 Calcium metabolism.

sorption of calcium and osteoclastic activity, effectively raising levels of serum calcium. When serum calcium levels are high, PTH secretion is decreased, reducing synthesis of 1,25-dihydroxyvitamin D and osteoclastic activity. Calcitonin, secreted by both the thyroid and parathyroid glands when PTH secretion is diminished, effectively lowers serum calcium levels. Serum and intracellular calcium bind to several calcium binding proteins, such as troponin-C, parvalbumin, and calmodulin (Table 3.14). Troponin-C within muscle binds calcium ion, permitting the contraction of muscle by the binding of the muscle proteins actin to myosin. Parvalbumin is an abundant calcium binding protein found in the muscle tissue of fish, reptiles, and amphibians. Its function remains unknown, but parvalbumin binds three calcium ions. Calmodulin, present in mammalian cells, binds four calcium ions, suggesting that the protein may have multiple functions when binding

TABLE 3.14 CALCIUM PROTEINS AND REGULATED ENZYMES

Enzyme/protein	Ca/molecule
Troponin-C	1
Parvalbumin	3
Calmodulin	4
Ca^{2+}-regulated enzymes and proteins via Ca^{2+} binding proteins	
Phosphorylases	
Adenylate cyclase	
Phosphatases	
Prothrombin	
Vitamin D dependent	
Ca^{2+} binding protein	

one, two, three, or four calcium ions.   In cells, calmodulin participates in the regulation of phosphorylation reactions, microtubule formation, and in the regulation of unbound intracellular calcium.   The intra- and extracellular concentrations of calcium ions bound to these proteins are important regulators of glycogenolysis, ATPase activity, ATP synthesis, membrane electrical potential, and calcium ion transport.   Excretion of dietary calcium is predominately in the feces (unabsorbed) and urine, and lesser amounts are lost through perspiration.

Reference

CHOSSAT, M. Note sur de système Ossent. *C.R. Acad. Sci. 14*, 451–454 (1842).

Phosphorus

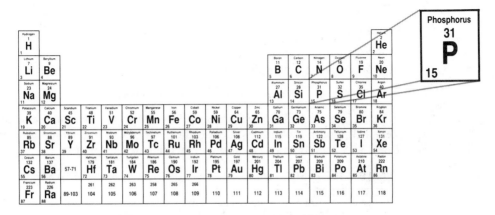

Date of nutritional recognition:	1842
Relative atomic size:	3.7
Oxidation state:	+5, ±3
Recommended dietary allowance:	800 mg
Body burden:	860 g

The element phosphorus was discovered by the German alchemist Hennig Brandt in 1669.   The first nutritional reference to phosphorus, like calcium, was made by M. Chossat (1842), who observed bone development in pigeons.   Phosphorus is the second most abundant element of the human body, which contains about 860 g or 30% of the total mineral content.

Most phosphorus (80%), like calcium, is stored in the bone and teeth in an inorganic mineral state, $Ca_{10}(PO_4)_6(OH)_2$, the hydroxyapatite (Figure 3.47).   The remaining 20% of body phosphorus is distributed throughout body cells in inorganic and various organic forms of great importance to the metabolic functioning of cells (Table 3.15).   In addition to the structural role of phosphorus in nucleic acids, coenzymes, and phospholipids, the function of phosphorus as phosphate in energy

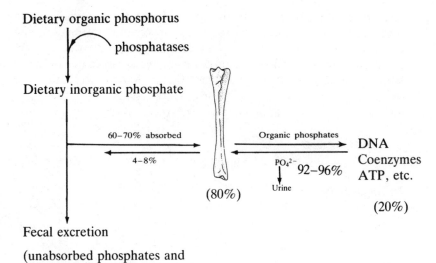

Dietary organic phosphorus

phosphatases

Dietary inorganic phosphate

60–70% absorbed

4–8%

(80%)

Organic phosphates

PO_4^{2-} 92–96%

Urine

DNA
Coenzymes
ATP, etc.

(20%)

Fecal excretion

(unabsorbed phosphates and
4–8% of systemic phosphates)

Figure 3.47   Phosphorus metabolism.

transfer (see Figure 7.4, Table 7.2) is singularly unique. Inorganic phosphorus within cells is the primary buffer system ($HPO_4^{2-}/H_2PO_4^-$) regulating intracellular pH. Table 3.15 lists some of the known functions of phosphorus.

TABLE 3.15   FUNCTIONAL ROLES OF PHOSPHORUS IN LIVING SYSTEMS

(Inorganic)	Structural component of mineralized tissues: bones, teeth Intracellular buffer: $H_2PO_4^- \rightleftarrows H^+ + HPO_4^{-2}$

(Organic)	Structural component of:
	    Nucleic acids
	        DNA, RNA
	Structural component of:
	    Coenzymes
	        $NADP^+$, NAD^+
	        FMN, FAD
	        Thiamin pyrophosphate
	        Pyridoxal phosphate
	        Coenzyme A
	Structural component of:
	    Lipids
	        Lecithin and other
	        Phosphatidic acid derivatives
	Energy transfer:
	        ATP and other trinucleotides
	        ADP and other dinucleotides
	        AMP and other mononucleotides
	        Creatine phosphate
	        Glucose-1-phosphate and other
	        Organophosphates

Phosphorus, being widely distributed in all foods, is ingested in both organic and inorganic forms. Phosphoric acid can be a major dietary source of phosphorus when carbonated beverages are consumed. Most phosphorus is absorbed with 60 to 70% efficiency, while some phosphorus, such as the organic phosphate of phytic acid, may go unabsorbed. Unabsorbed phosphorus is excreted in the feces, and most absorbed phosphorus is excreted in the urine as inorganic phosphate, PO_4^{2-}. Phosphate absorption can be adversely affected by ingestion of high amounts of antacids containing magnesium or aluminum hydroxides (see Chapter 13). Dietary deficiency of phosphorus in humans would be a rare event, and most common forms of phosphorus found in food are relatively nontoxic.

Reference

CHOSSAT, M. Note sur de système Ossent. *C.R. Acad. Sci. 14*, 451–454 (1842).

Potassium

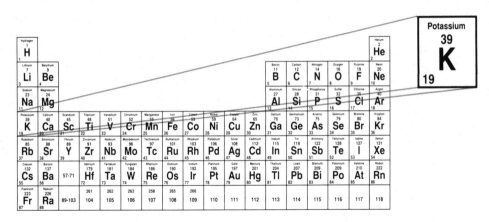

Date of nutritional recognition:	1926
Relative atomic size:	7.6
Oxidation state:	+1
Recommended dietary allowance:	1525–4515 mg
Body burden:	180 g

Potassium, third most abundant mineral within the human body, shares a number of similarities and some differences with its lighter sister mineral, sodium. Potassium was discovered in 1807 along with sodium, by Sir Humphry Davy, in an electrolysis of fused sodium chloride. The nutritional requirement for potassium was first described for the rat by H. G. Miller in 1926.

TABLE 3.16 ENZYMES REGULATED BY POTASSIUM

K$^+$-ATPase
Acetylkinase
Pyruvate phosphokinase

Potassium is the major intracellular cation, with 90% of all the body's potassium being in the ionized form.   The primary functions of potassium are control of muscle (along with sodium and calcium) contraction, enzyme regulation (Table 3.16), nerve excitation, and electrochemical transmission of nerve impulses.   Heart muscle is particularly susceptible to hypokalemia (low potassium), and it is for this reason that potassium supplements are often prescribed when diuretics are used or renal or peritoneal dialysis is required.   Extended diarrhea may lead to significant losses of potassium.   Potassium also contributes to osmolarity and the acid–base balance of cells.

Widely distributed in foods, there is no specific RDA for potassium, as the diet normally provides the 1.8 to 5.6 g of K/day suggested intake for the mineral. Potassium, like sodium, is almost completely absorbed by the intestinal tract, with the majority being excreted in the urine (Figure 3.48).   Potassium reabsorption is regulated by aldosterone, and normal renal reabsorption of K$^+$ is about 20% of total potassium filtration.

All dietary potassium contains a very small proportion (1 in every 10^4 potassium atoms) of a naturally occurring radioisotope, ^{40}K.   Having a half-life of 10^9

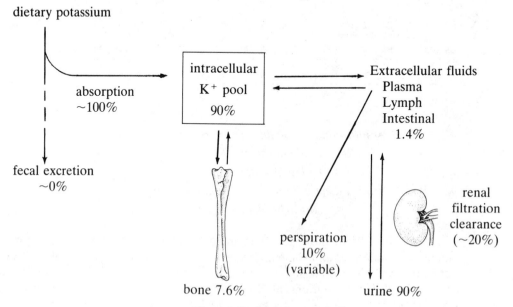

Figure 3.48 Potassium metabolism.

years, natural radioactive decay from this isotope can be used to measure total body potassium and can be employed to compute total body lean mass. Such measurement is performed by a whole-body gamma counter.

Reference

MILLER, H. G. Potassium in Animal Nutrition. IV. Potassium Requirements for Normal Growth and Maintenance. *J. Biol. Chem.* **70**, 587–591 (1926).

Sulfur

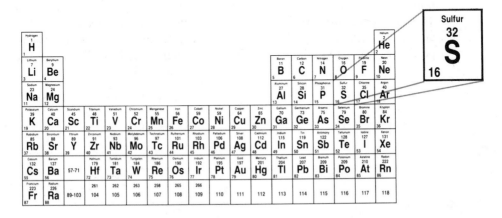

> *Date of nutritional recognition:* 1932
> *Relative atomic size:* 3.4
> *Oxidation states:* $-2, 0, +2, +4$
> *Recommended dietary allowance:* 15 mg/kg methionine and vitamins
> *Body burden:* 175 g

Sulfur is uniquely classified within the group of macrominerals, for all but sulfur and chlorine are metals. Chlorine is a halogen and sulfur is a nonmetal. All of the macrominerals exist *in vivo* in some inorganic form, whereas sulfur exists predominately in organic molecules, there being only very small amounts of free metabolic sulfite or sulfate. All of the macrominerals are absorbed from the gastrointestinal tract in their inorganic form, except for sulfur, which is absorbed predominately as the sulfur-containing amino acids methionine, cysteine, or cystine. There is no known dietary requirement for inorganic sulfur, and sulfates are poorly absorbed when ingested. Sulfites, sometimes used as antioxidants in foods, are absorbed by people sometimes with allergic (sulfite-sensitive) reactions.

Three forms of organic sulfur compounds exist which predominate in animals and humans. These forms of sulfur include (1) the thiomethyl of methionine residues in protein; (2) the sulfhydryl disulfides of protein; cysteine–cystine residues in proteins, and (3) a few other sulfur compounds containing ester or amide

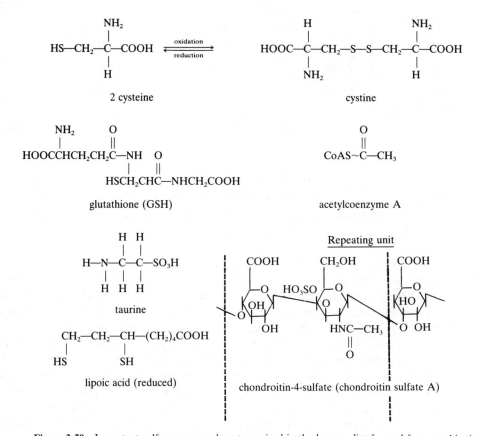

methionine   thiamin   biotin

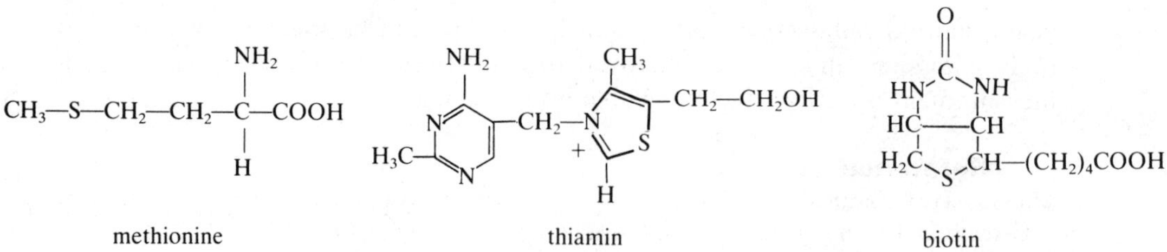

Figure 3.49   Sulfur compounds required in the human diet.

bound sulfates of glycosaminoglycans, a few steroids, and xenobiotic metabolites.
The dietary requirement for sulfur as methionine was described by R. W. Jackson
and R. J. Black in 1932.   While methionine is the only essential sulfur amino acid,
partial replacement of the methionine requirement can be met by cystine (cysteine).

Figure 3.50   Important sulfur compounds not required in the human diet formed from methionine.

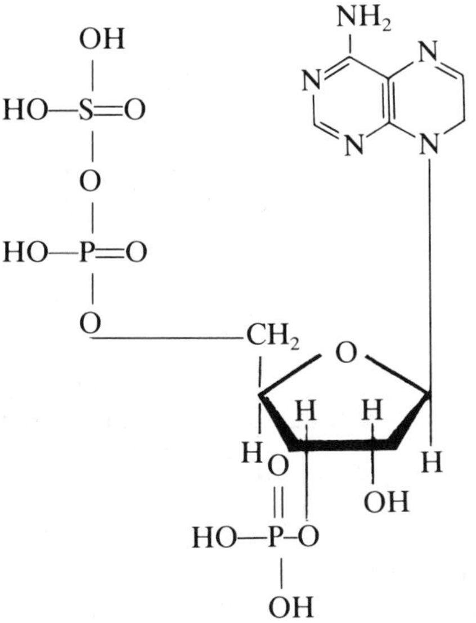

3'-phosphoadenosine-5'-phosphosulfate
(the donor of sulfate in biosynthesis)

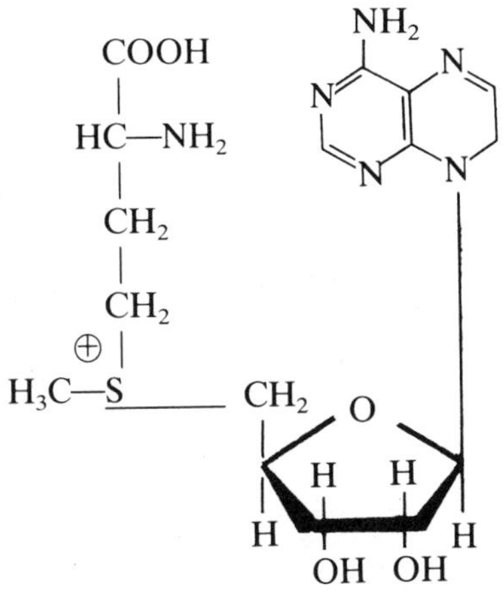

S-adenosylmethionine
(the donor of methyl groups in
biosynthesis)

Figure 3.51   Metabolic donors of sulfate and methyl groups.

In addition to methionine, the other sulfur-containing dietary nutrients required by humans are the vitamins thiamin and biotin (Figure 3.49).

From methionine are synthesized all the other important sulfur compounds, including cysteine (cystine), glutathione (see "Selenium") acetylcoenzyme A (see "Pantothenic Acid"), lipoic acid (see "Thiamin"), and taurine (see "Bile Acids and Bile Salts," Chapter 4) used in the synthesis of taurocholate (Figure 3.50). In the synthesis of these compounds methyl groups are donated by *S*-adenosylme-thionine, and the synthesis of sulfated glycosaminoglycans of connective tissues and sulfated xenobiotics is transferred by 3'-phosphoadenosine-5'-phosphosulfate (Figure 3.51).

During sulfur metabolism, sulfur is oxidized from its organic forms (sulfides, S^{2-}) to sulfites (SO_3^{2-}) and sulfates (SO_4^{2-}). A molybdenum-containing enzyme sulfite oxidase oxidizes the potentially toxic sulfite to sulfate, which is the major excretory form of sulfur found in urine (Figure 3.52).

Reference
JACKSON, R. W., and BLACK, R. J.   The Metabolism of Cystine and Methionine, *J. Biol. Chem.* **98**, 465 (1932).

dietary methionine,
thiamin, and biotin

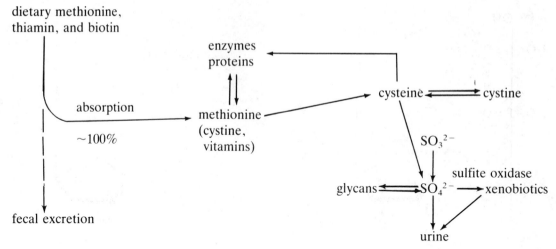

Figure 3.52   Sulfur metabolism.

Chlorine

Date of nutritional recognition: 1979
Relative atomic size: 3.3
Oxidation state: −1
Recommended dietary allowance: 1700–5100 mg
Body burden: 74 g

The element is chlorine but the nutritional need is for chloride (Cl^-), a major anion of numerous salts (e.g., NaCl, KCl, CaCl$_2$).   Chlorine was discovered in 1774 by C. W. Schelle and chloride was the anion found by Sir Humphry Davy in 1810 in those famous electrolysis experiments.

Since the diet is abundant in chloride, little interest in this element appears to have been expressed by research scientists over time.   During the late 1970s,

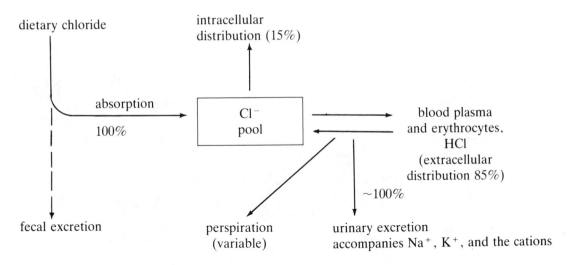

Figure 3.53 Chloride metabolism.

however, chloride-deficient infant formulas were inadvertently manufactured and distributed. Infants consuming only these formula diets developed varied degrees of a chloride deficiency. The deficiency resulted in alkalosis and growth retardation in some infants which was traced to the chloride deficiency of the formulas. This unfortunate event emphasized the nutritional need for chloride.

Chloride is the major extracellular anion which provides electrical neutrality for a multitude of mineral and protein cations. Chloride, together with the carbonic acid/bicarbonate anion, is most important in the maintenance of osmotic equilibria and for buffering the changes in pH (acid–base balance) of the blood. In erythrocytes, carbon dioxide from tissues and plasma is converted to carbonic acid by an enzyme, carbonic anhydrase. Disassociation of carbonic acid and diffusion of the bicarbonate anion (HCO_3^-) from the red blood cell into plasma is replaced by diffusion of Cl^- from plasma into the erythrocyte, contributing to electrical neutrality, referred to as the chloride shift. Large amounts of chloride are used by the chief cells in the synthesis and secretion of hydrochloric acid (HCl) (gastric juice) for the gastric digestion of protein by pepsin. The HCl lowers the pH of the stomach (pH 1 to 2), where pepsin is enzymatically active.

Dietary chloride is nearly totally absorbed and secretory Cl^- is reabsorbed from the digestive juices of the intestine. The major excretory route of Cl^- is accompaniment of Na^+, K^+, and other cations in urinary excretion (Figure 3.53). Chloride may also be lost in perspiration during diarrhea and in vomit (loss of HCl), losses that can vary greatly among individuals according to the severity of the condition.

Reference

Roy S., and Arant, B. S. Alkalosis from Chloride-Deficient Neo-Mull-Soy. *N. Engl. J. Med. 301*, 615 (1979).

Sodium

| | | | | | | | | | | | | | | | | | Sodium 23 **Na** 11 |

Date of nutritional recognition: 1847
Relative atomic size: 6.2
Oxidation state: +1
Recommended dietary allowance: 900–2700 mg
Body burden: 64 g

Sodium was first isolated, along with potassium, by the electrolysis of fused sodium chloride by Sir Humphry Davy in 1807. J. B. Boussingault described the need for sodium by cattle in 1847, but it was not until 1940 that E. Orent-Keiles and E. V. McCollum established a nutritional essentiality for sodium by feeding rats diets extremely deficient in sodium.

The adult human contains approximately 64 g of sodium. Not quite half of this sodium (ca. 40%) is associated with bone, with the remainder mostly in the extracellular fluids. Sodium is the most abundant extracellular cation responsible for the osmolarity and ionic balance of the extracellular fluids, the electrochemical gradient of nerve axions for electrical impulses to be transmitted, and the acid–base balance of cells and their organelles. Sodium is maintained as the primary extracellular cation by ATPase "sodium pumps." General homeostasis of sodium is carefully regulated by the adrenal corticosteroid, aldosterone, which controls renal reabsorption of sodium. Any alteration of the sodium homeostasis adversely affects the state of body hydration. Loss of excess sodium (hypoatremia) by the use of diruretics, diarrhea, vomiting, or perspiration may lead to dehydration, decreased blood pressure, and high hematocrits and possibly death. Sodium retention is thought to be a causative factor in hypertension among some people who are sensitive to salt and the edema often accompanying pregnancy. For such

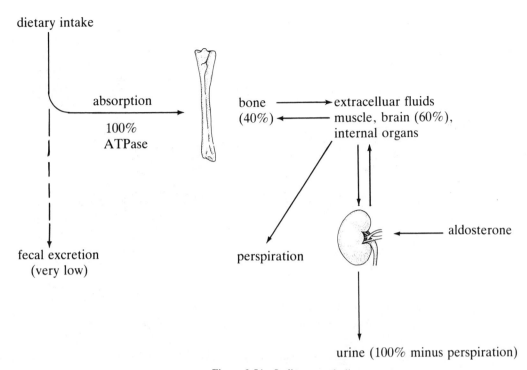

dietary intake

absorption

100%
ATPase

bone ──────→ extracelluar fluids
(40%) ◄────── muscle, brain (60%),
              internal organs

fecal excretion
(very low)

perspiration

aldosterone

urine (100% minus perspiration)

Figure 3.54 Sodium metabolism.

reasons, restricted-sodium diets are often prescribed to hypertensive and pregnant persons with edema.

Sodium intake, mainly as table salts of sodium chloride added to prepared foods is 10 to 15 g per day.   Since sodium chloride is 40% sodium, the daily ingestion of sodium is 4 to 6 g per day, considerably in excess of the RDA of 1.1 to 3.3 g of sodium per day.   Under normal physiologic conditions a sodium balance is sustained with a daily intake of approximately 200 mg of sodium.

Sodium is actively absorbed using ATP from the intestinal lumen with nearly 100% efficiency.   In addition to storage in bone (ca. 40%), 30% of the extracellular sodium is in skin; 18% is in muscle, where it counteracts calcium in muscular contraction; 8% is in blood plasma; and 3% is in the brain.   The major excretory route is via the urine and secondarily through perspiration during exercise (Figure 3.54).

References

BOUSSINGAULT, J. B.   *Ann. Chim. Phys. 71*, 113 (1847).

ORENT-KEILES, E, and MCCOLLUM, E. V.   Mineral Metabolism of Rats on Extremely Deficient Diets.   *J. Biol. Chem. 133*, 75–81 (1940).

Magnesium

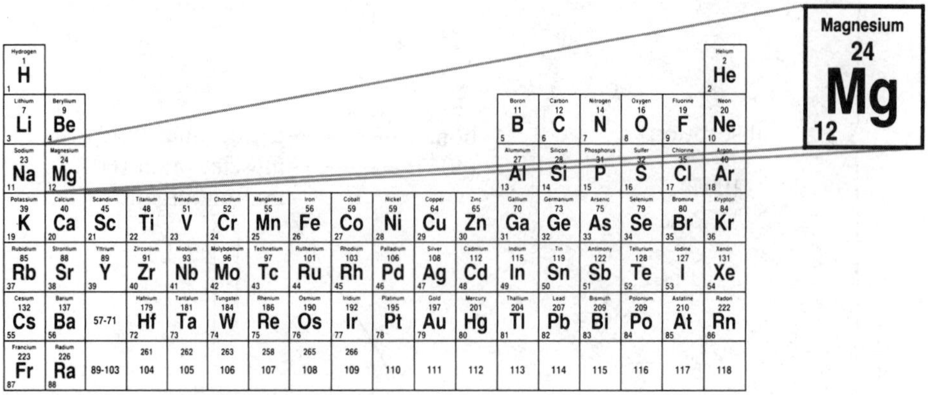

Magnesium
24
Mg
12

Date of nutritional recognition: 1932

Relative atomic size: 5.3

Oxidation state: +2

Recommended dietary allowance: 300 mg

Body burden: 25 g

Magnesium is the sixth and least abundant of the macrominerals of the human body. It comprises approximately 1% of the mineral content of the body, most (60%) being stored in bone along with calcium and phosphorus. Magnesium metal was discovered in 1808 by Sir Humphry Davy, and magnesium salts have been used as a medicine since the Renaissance. It was not until this century that H. D. Kruse and colleagues would, in 1932, demonstrate a nutritional need for magnesium in the rat. Experimentally, M. E. Shils was to describe magnesium deficiency in humans in 1964.

Much of the magnesium not associated with bone mineralization is complexed with phosphate or acts as a regulator of enzymatic activity (Table 3.17). It is the second most abundant mineral in cells after potassium. Magnesium participates

TABLE 3.17 ENZYMES/HORMONES REGULATED BY MAGNESIUM

ATPase
Adenylate cyclase
Enolase
Pyruvate kinase
Fructokinase
Creatine kinase
Some peptidases
May regulate insulin function
Thyroxine secretion regulated

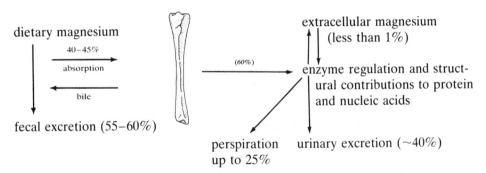

Figure 3.55 Magnesium metabolism.

as an enzymatic regulator of ATPase by complexing with the two terminal phosphates of ATP, forming Mg-ATP and all enzymatic reactions that involve phosphate transfer (see Figure 3.45). Magnesium is responsible for the structural integrity of the subunits forming ribosomes and the maintenance of the double-helical structure of DNA. In plants, magnesium complexes with a tetrapyrrole to form chlorophyll, which is necessary for photosynthesis (see Chapter 6).

Magnesium deficiency in healthy people is rare, as foods usually contain and provide for a dietary adequacy of the element. Magnesium is absorbed (40 to 45%) in the intestinal tract, is usually excreted in the urine, but may also be lost through perspiration (Figure 3.55). Magnesium salts appear not to be toxic.

References

KRUSE, H. D., ORENT, E., and McCOLLUM, E. V. Studies on Magnesium-Deficient Animals. I. Symptomology Resulting from Magnesium Deprivation. *J. Biol. Chem. 96*, 519–539 (1932).

SHILS, M. E. Experimental Human Magnesium Depletion. I. Clinical Observations and Gland Chemistry Attention. *Am. J. Clin. Chem. 15*, 133–143 (1964).

Iron

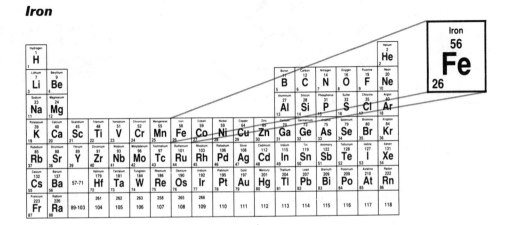

Date of nutritional recognition: Ancient Chinese; 1872
Relative atomic size: 4.1
Oxidation states: $+2, +3$
Recommended dietary allowance: 10–18 mg
Body burden: 4.5 g (4500 mg)

Iron is the most abundant of the trace elements with an estimated human body burden of 4 to 5 g and an RDA of 10 to 18 mg. A dietary need for iron may have been recognized by early civilizations, perhaps during an ancient Chinese dynasty, but such events went unrecorded until 1872, when J. B. Boussingault reported on the importance of iron. Iron is biologically important because of its inherent chemical properties, consisting of two oxidation states, Fe^{2+} (ferrous) and Fe^{3+} (ferric), and its ability to complex with organic molecules with a coordination number of 6. Iron's major functions in the body are: (1) the transport and storage of oxygen, (2) the transfer of electrons via the $Fe^{2+} \rightleftharpoons Fe^{3+}$ redox pair, and (3) the control of toxic oxygen species such as hydrogen peroxide, H_2O_2. The most important iron-containing protein is hemoglobin, both physiologically as the carrier of oxygen in the erythrocyte, and quantitatively, as it represents about 70% of the body's iron. The iron in hemoglobin is coordinated to four nitrogen atoms of a tetrapyrrole and to a ring nitrogen of a histidine residue within the protein chain. The sixth coordination position is for the free exchange of oxygen, as shown in Figure 3.56.

Myoglobin, a heme-Fe containing protein similar to hemoglobin, is found in

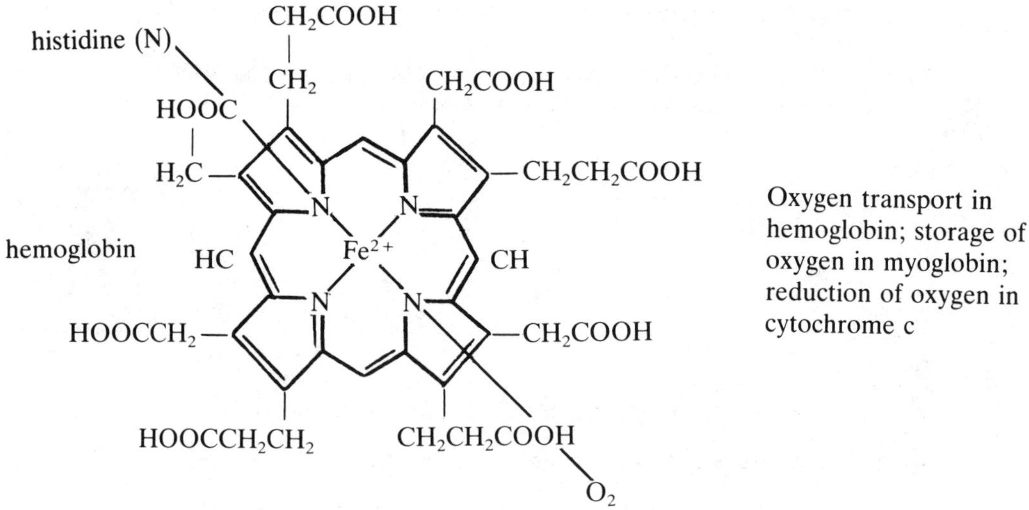

Oxygen transport in hemoglobin; storage of oxygen in myoglobin; reduction of oxygen in cytochrome c

Figure 3.56 Structure of heme-iron in hemoglobin/myoglobin/cytochromes.

TABLE 3.18 IRON ENZYMES AND PROTEINS

Enzyme/protein	Fe/molecule
Hemoglobin	4 hemes
Myoglobin	1 heme
Ferritin	20% $Fe(OH)_3$
Hemosiderin	35% $Fe(OH)_3$
Transferrin	2 Fe^{3+}
Cytochrome c	1 heme
Catalase	1 heme
Ferridoxins	1 Fe—S—Fe or 2 Fe—S—Fe
Rubedoxins	1 Fe or 2 Fe
Aldehyde oxidase	1 Fe—S—Fe, Mo, Flavin
Sulfite oxidase	1 heme, Mo

skeletal and cardiac muscle, where it serves as a storage site for oxygen having been transferred from hemoglobin. The iron found in myoglobin is about 3% of total body iron stores. Of the remaining iron in the body, less than 1% is found in the heme-Fe cytochromes a, a_3, b, b_5, c, c_1, located in the mitochondrian as electron ($Fe^{2+} \leftrightarrows Fe^{3+}$) carriers, microsomal cytochrome P-450, catalase, enzymes, and other iron proteins (Table 3.18). Remaining body iron, about 25%, is found stored principally in two liver proteins, ferritin and hemosiderin. Hemosiderin, representing the major store of iron, is believed to be an insoluble aggregate of ferritin.

Absorption of dietary iron is poor (20%; Figure 3.57). Its absorption is improved by reduction of Fe^{3+} to Fe^{2+} by the reducing agent ascorbic acid or by complexation of iron to organic compounds. Iron homeostasis is tightly controlled at the point of intestinal absorption and by the recycling of degraded iron proteins such as hemoglobin. Absorption of iron from the gastrointestinal tract results in transfer of iron to a serum protein aptly named iron transferrin. The iron is transported in the ferric (Fe^{3+}) state to tissues or is stored as hemosiderin. The oxidation of Fe^{2+} following absorption to Fe^{3+} in transferrin, is accomplished by reduction by the copper-containing protein ceruloplasmin.

Among bacteria, plants, and animals exist nonheme iron proteins in which iron is coordinated not to nitrogen but to sulfur. These are the iron-sulfur proteins, in which iron is often coordinated to the sulfur of the amino acid cysteine,

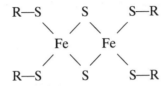

These proteins, the ferredoxins, are important electron carriers in plant chloroplasts

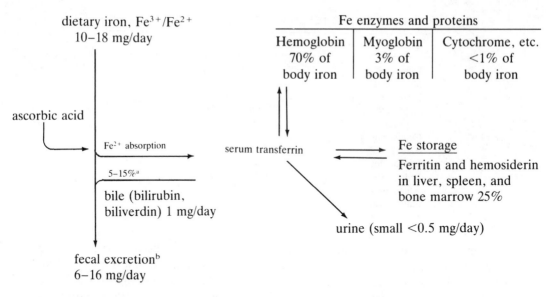

dietary iron, Fe^{3+}/Fe^{2+}
10–18 mg/day

Fe enzymes and proteins

| Hemoglobin 70% of body iron | Myoglobin 3% of body iron | Cytochrome, etc. <1% of body iron |

ascorbic acid

Fe^{2+} absorption

5–15%[a]

serum transferrin

Fe storage
Ferritin and hemosiderin
in liver, spleen, and
bone marrow 25%

bile (bilirubin,
biliverdin) 1 mg/day

urine (small <0.5 mg/day)

fecal excretion[b]
6–16 mg/day

[a] May double during iron-deficiency anemia.

[b] Other variable iron losses from desquamated cells, sweat, and menstrual blood losses, which can be significant for premenopausal women.

Figure 3.57 Iron metabolism.

during photosynthesis (Chapter 6) and participate in N_2 reduction by bacteria. Azoferridoxin contains only iron, whereas the bacterial protein, molybdoferridoxin, contains both iron and molybdenum.

With the many important biological oxidations mediated by iron and the relatively large dietary intake required because of poor absorption, it is perhaps not surprising that iron deficiency is quantitatively the leading trace mineral deficiency. Age, sex, health status, and dietary iron intake are factors contributing to adequate iron status. Under ordinary conditions iron is excreted in very small quantities through the urine and with even smaller amounts lost through perspiration. Larger amounts of iron are lost by desquamation of intestinal epithelial tissue in feces. Considerable loss of iron occurs during menstruation and when internal or external hemorrhaging is prolonged and protracted. Iron is one of the least toxic metals, with acute and chronic iron toxicity being uncommon events.

Reference

Boussingault, J. B. Du fer contenue dans le sang et dans les aliments. C. R. *Acad. Sci. Paris 74*, 1353–1359 (1872).

Fluorine

Periodic table highlighting Fluorine:

1	2	3	4	5	6	7	8	9	10	11	12	13	14	15	16	17	18
Hydrogen 1 **H**																	Helium 2 **He**
Lithium 7 **Li** 3	Beryllium 9 **Be** 4											Boron 11 **B** 5	Carbon 12 **C** 6	Nitrogen 14 **N** 7	Oxygen 16 **O** 8	Fluorine 19 **F** 9	Neon 20 **Ne** 10
Sodium 23 **Na** 11	Magnesium 24 **Mg** 12											Aluminum 27 **Al** 13	Silicon 28 **Si** 14	Phosphorus 31 **P** 15	Sulfur 32 **S** 16	Chlorine 35 **Cl** 17	Argon 40 **Ar** 18
Potassium 39 **K** 19	Calcium 40 **Ca** 20	Scandium 45 **Sc** 21	Titanium 48 **Ti** 22	Vanadium 51 **V** 23	Chromium 52 **Cr** 24	Manganese 55 **Mn** 25	Iron 56 **Fe** 26	Cobalt 59 **Co** 27	Nickel 59 **Ni** 28	Copper 64 **Cu** 29	Zinc 65 **Zn** 30	Gallium 70 **Ga** 31	Germanium 73 **Ge** 32	Arsenic 75 **As** 33	Selenium 79 **Se** 34	Bromine 80 **Br** 35	Krypton 84 **Kr** 36
Rubidium 85 **Rb** 37	Strontium 88 **Sr** 38	Yttrium 89 **Y** 39	Zirconium 91 **Zr** 40	Niobium 93 **Nb** 41	Molybdenum 96 **Mo** 42	Technetium 97 **Tc** 43	Ruthenium 101 **Ru** 44	Rhodium 103 **Rh** 45	Palladium 106 **Pd** 46	Silver 108 **Ag** 47	Cadmium 112 **Cd** 48	Indium 115 **In** 49	Tin 119 **Sn** 50	Antimony 122 **Sb** 51	Tellurium 128 **Te** 52	Iodine 127 **I** 53	Xenon 131 **Xe** 54
Cesium 132 **Cs** 55	Barium 137 **Ba** 56	57-71	Hafnium 179 **Hf** 72	Tantalum 181 **Ta** 73	Tungsten 184 **W** 74	Rhenium 186 **Re** 75	Osmium 190 **Os** 76	Iridium 192 **Ir** 77	Platinum 195 **Pt** 78	Gold 197 **Au** 79	Mercury 201 **Hg** 80	Thallium 204 **Tl** 81	Lead 207 **Pb** 82	Bismuth 209 **Bi** 83	Polonium 209 **Po** 84	Astatine 210 **At** 85	Radon 222 **Rn** 86
Francium 223 **Fr** 87	Radium 226 **Ra** 88	89-103	261 104	262 105	263 106	258 107	265 108	266 109	110	111	112	113	114	115	116	117	118

Callout: Fluorine 19 **F** 9

Dates of nutritional recognition:	1968, 1972
Relative atomic size:	2.4
Oxidation state:	-1
Recommended dietary allowance:	1.5–2.5 mg
Body burden:	2.6 g (2600 mg)

Fluorine (the element) is widely dispersed in biological tissues as the fluoride ion (F^-). Fluoride is found in mostly soft tissues dispersed mostly intracellularly, but it is also in the extracellular fluid space (Figure 3.58). Collectively, the total tissue fluoride represents about 1% of the adult fluorine content of 2.6 g. Most of the fluorine is present in bone and teeth (99%), where it combines with the calcium hydroxyapatite, forming a mixed calcium fluoroapatite. Deposition of fluoride in bone and teeth is dependent on the dietary or supplemental fluoride intake and the age of development of bone or dental enamel. Fluoride incorporated into bone and the dental enamel during development presumably decreases mineral solubility. Fluoridation of public water supplies began in the United States in 1945 (Newburgh–Kingston, New York; Grand Rapids–Muskegon, Michigan) following observations of people living in areas where natural fluorides in water already existed. Observations made in the 1930s suggested that natural fluorides (1 ppm) reduced dental caries, but when natural fluorides exceeded about 3 ppm, mottling of primary and secondary teeth could be expected of children prenatally exposed and postnatally consuming highly fluoridated waters. Use of fluorides to reduce dental cavities has been extended to topical fluoride applications, tablets of sodium fluoride, and inclusion of stannous fluoride and monofluorophosphates in dental pastes.

Dietary fluoride assists in increasing bone mass (density) and may help to prevent osteoporosis in some individuals. Fluoride supplements, along with vitamin D and calcium supplementation to adult women to decrease susceptibility to osteoporosis may be warranted.

Fluoride, if ingested in excessive amounts, is toxic, manifested by dental fluorosis (mottling). If ingested in very high amounts, skeletal fluorosis and calcification of tendons, ligaments, and bony erostoses may occur. *Genu valgun* is an endemic crippling fluorosis seen in parts of India. When toxic levels of fluoride are ingested, metabolic disturbances can occur in both lipid and carbohydrate metabolism, owing to enzyme inhibition by the fluoride anion.

Although several reports have suggested that fluoride is essential for animals, the experimental data for this account remain inconclusive and there is no evidence for a metabolic requirement for fluoride in humans. H. A. Schroeder and co-workers first reported in 1968 that mice given 10 ppm fluoride in drinking water grew better and lived longer than did control animals. During the experimental period, fluoride did not accumulate in soft tissues. In 1972, K. Schwarz and D. Milne reported to have found positive growth responses in rats fed fluoride supplemented up to 7.5 ppm in experimental amino acid diets. The fluoride content of the diet also affected the pigmentation of the rats' incisor teeth. Other data are not supportive of these reported growth effects in animals, and the question of metabolic fluoride essentiality remains open.

Dietary fluoride is rapidly absorbed, probably from the stomach, and is distributed in soft tissues similarly to chloride. Fluoride enters the blood and excess fluoride appears rapidly in urine (Figure 3.58). There are no known proteins or enzymes that contain fluoride.

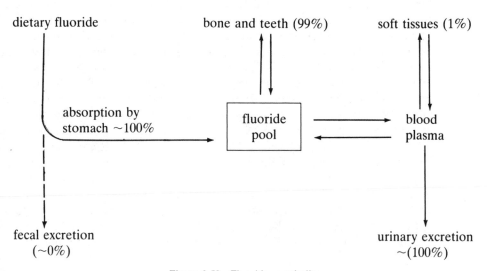

Figure 3.58 Fluoride metabolism.

References

SCHROEDER, H. A., MITCHENER, M., BALASSA, J. J., KANISAWA, M., and NASON, A. P. Zirconium, Niobium, Antimony and Fluorine in Mice; Effects of Growth, Survival and Tissue Levels. *J. Nutr. 95*, 95–101 (1968).

SCHWARZ, K., and MILNE, D. B. Fluorine Requirement for Growth in the Rat. *Bioinorg. Chem. 1*, 331–338 (1972).

Zinc

Date of nutritional recognition:	1934
Relative atomic size:	4.4
Oxidation state:	+2
Recommended dietary allowance:	15 mg
Body burden:	2 g (200 mg)

Zinc is a required trace element for all life forms: bacteria, plants, animals, and humans. The presence of zinc detected in terrestrial plants dates from 1869 and in aquatic plants since 1919. A dietary requirement for zinc in the rat was first reported by W. R. Todd and colleagues in 1934. A. S. Prasad was first to report a zinc deficiency in humans in 1961 among people consuming mostly breads and very little animal protein in Middle-Eastern countries. Parakeratosis, a disease common to swine, was prevalent during the 1940s and early 1950s. This disease was shown in 1955 to be caused by a zinc deficiency and was aggravated by elevated calcium intake. Human parakeratosis, also caused by a zinc deficiency, was reported in 1976. A genetic human disease, acrodermatitis enteropathica, is corrected by additional dietary zinc.

The formal recognition of zinc as an essential nutrient came in 1974, when dietary allowances for the nutrients were made by the National Research Council, Food and Nutrition Board of the National Academy of Science. The RDA for

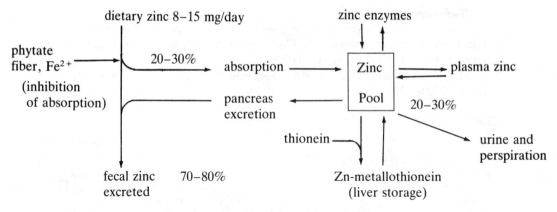

Figure 3.59   Zinc metabolism.

zinc for adults was established at 15 mg.   At the level of this RDA, many adults have marginal zinc intakes.   Zinc absorption is only 20 to 30% of intake, and absorption is reduced further by the dietary presence of phytic acid, fiber, iron II, and various chelates.   Zinc is excreted by the pancreas and a fecal loss of about 1.5 mg of zinc per day is the major excretory route.   Additional losses of zinc occur in urine, 0.5 mg/day, and perspiration, 1 to 5 µg/day (Figure 3.59).

All tissues contain zinc, which functions as a prosthetic moiety or regulator of enzyme activity.   Carbonic anhydrase was the first enzyme to be recognized as a zinc metalloenzyme.   This discovery came in 1940, and by 1960 five more zinc metalloenzymes were known.   Over 200 zinc metalloenzymes are now recognized some of which are listed in Table 3.19.   Zinc is nontoxic when ingested up to 600 mg per day.

TABLE 3.19   ZINC ENZYMES AND PROTEINS

Enzyme/Protein	Zn/molecule
Carbonic anhydrase	1
Carboxypeptidase A and B	1
Liver alcohol dehydrogenase	4
Superoxide dismutase	2
DNA polymerase (*E. coli*)	2
Alkaline phosphatase	2
Leucine aminopeptidase	2
Metallothionine	Many
Glyceraldehyde-3-phosphodehydrogenase	3
Insulin (crystalline)	0.3

References

TODD, W. R., ELVEHJEM, C. A., and HART, E. B.   Zinc in the Nutrition of the Rat.   *Am. J. Physiol. 107*, 126 (1934).

PRASAD, A. S., HALSTED, J. A., and NADIMA, M. Syndrome of Iron Deficiency Anemia, Hepatosplenomegaly, Hypogonadism, Dwarfism and Geophagia. *Am. J. Med. 31*, 532 (1961).

Silicon

Silicon
28
Si
14

Date of nutritional recognition:	1972
Relative atomic size:	3.9
Oxidation state:	$+4, \pm 2$
Requirement:	May be essential
Body burden:	24 mg

Silicon is the most abundant element in the earth's crust after oxygen. Silicon is used by plankton to form shells of silica (SiO_2). The element is concentrated by the ancient plants; bryophytes, ferns, and horsetails. Soil bacteria degrade quartz, synthesize organosilicon compounds, and are even known to be able to replace phosphorus with silicon. Even present-day plants contain a fairly high content of silicon, and some varieties contain 15 to 20% silicon by dry weight. Cereals may contain 30 to 40% of their ash as silicon. People consume 20 to 30 mg/day of SiO_2 and about 1200 mg of total silicon per day, yet silicon is present in animal and human tissues to only a slight extent. The question is, therefore: Is such a ubiquitous element essential to animals and humans? The evidence to date suggests that it is, but the data are not yet conclusive.

Evidence for the essentiality of silicon originates with E. M. Carlisle, who was able to demonstrate that in the actively growing area of bone (osteoblasts), calcium and silicon are present in almost equal concentrations, but as the bone becomes calcified, the silicon is no longer needed and only participates in the calcification "process." These *in vitro* studies and subsequent *in vivo* experiments have demonstrated the apparent need for silicon for proper calcification of growing bone. In rats and in chicks, low-silicon-containing diets contribute to abnormalities in skull and long bone formation, including formational changes in articulating cartilage and bone density.

Silicon is present in animal and human tissues in probably at least three different forms. These forms include water-soluble orthosilicic acid and silicate anions, organosilicon compounds and silicic esters of carbohydrates, and possibly protein. Steroids, choline, lipids, and phospholipids may contain silicon polymers (—O—Si—O—Si—O—) and insoluble oligo- and polysilicates may be absorbed with other organic molecules. While such compounds are suggested to be present based on silicon analysis of animal and human tissue, their presence in these molecules remains to be confirmed. Human tissues containing high silicon concentration include muscle, kidney, and liver. Especially high in silicon content are lymph nodes and lung tissues, the latter concentrated with silicon due to dust and other inhaled abiotic materials.

Dietary silicon is absorbed as silicic acid, silica, and organosilicates by the gastrointestinal tract. Little is known of its metabolism. Silicon is present in blood and urine. Some silica may even be phagostized, the cause of localization of silicon in lymph nodes. From chronic exposure, inhaled silica may lead to silicosis. Some silicates are carcinogenic, as is asbestos, which when inhaled in time may cause mesothelioma of the lung.

References

CARLISLE, E. M. The Nutritional Essentiality of Silicon. *Nutr. Rev. 40*, 193–198 (1982).

CARLISLE, E. M. Silicon: An Essential Element for the Chick. *Science 178*, 619–621 (1972).

SCHWARZ, K., and MILNE, D. B. Growth-Promoting Effects of Silicon in Rats. *Nature 239*, 333–334 (1972).

Selenium

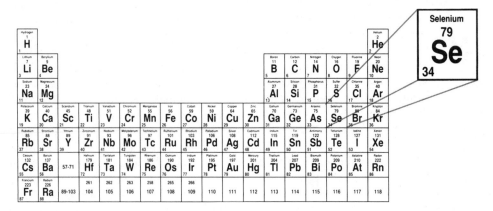

Date of nutritional recognition: 1957

Relative atomic size: 3.9

Oxidation states: $+6, +4, -2$
Recommended dietary allowance: $50-200$ μg
Body burden: 13 mg

In 1817 the Swedish chemist Jon Berzelius discovered the element selenium in association with the element sulfur. Similar in chemical properties to sulfur, selenium remained for many years an unrecognized nutritional factor. Selenium was known first, primarily for its toxicity. In the 1930s it was found to be the causative agent of the toxicity diseases "blind staggers" and "alkali disease" among horses and cattle that consumed seleniferous plants, a discovery made by the research staff at the North Dakota Experiment Station of the U.S. Department of Agriculture.

During the 1950s at the National Institutes of Health, German-born physician Klaus Schwarz discovered that dietary selenium prevented a fatal necrotic liver degeneration in rats fed diets of torula yeast and lacking in vitamin E. This was the first documentation of a biological requirement for selenium in animals, being reported in 1957. This report prompted research that revealed a dietary need for selenium in other animals. More than 40 species of animals are today known to have a biological requirement for selenium. Throughout the 1960s, range animals, cattle and sheep principally, were often found in many parts of the world to have a dietary selenium deficiency. Now, bacteria and algae of several species are also known to need selenium.

In 1973, research at the University of Wisconsin discovered that selenium was an integral part of the active site of a widely dispersed enzyme, glutathione peroxidase. It was found that glutathione peroxidase contained four atoms of selenium, each contained within the amino acid selenocysteine at the active site. With its coenzyme glutathione (GSH), glutathione peroxidase (GSHPx) facilitates the reduction of hydrogen peroxide (H_2O_2) to water and organic hydroperoxides (ROOH) to an alcohol (ROH), as in the following scheme:

Equation 3.24
Glutathione peroxidase.

$$H_2O_2 \text{ (ROOH)} + 2GSH \xrightarrow{\text{GSHPx}} GSSG + H_2O \text{ (ROH)}$$

In this reaction two molecules of glutathione (GSH) are oxidized to GSSG and hydrogen peroxide or ROOH is reduced to water or the alcohol of the organic peroxide. The enzyme helps to keep to very low levels cellular levels of peroxides, which damage cell membranes. GSHPx is presently the only known mammalian enzyme to contain selenium. However, several bacterial enzymes involved in redox reactions also contain selenium. New proteins have been discovered which contain selenium, and their functions are only beginning to become understood (Table 3.20).

In 1979 the first dietary selenium deficiency in people was described to occur in isolated rural populations in the People's Republic of China. The disease,

TABLE 3.20   SELENIUM ENZYMES AND PROTEINS

Enzyme/protein	Se/molecule
Glutathione peroxidase	4/extensive, including humans
Formate dehydrogenase	Bacterial
Glycine reductase	Bacterial
Nicotinic acid hydroxylase	Bacterial
Xanthine dehydrogenase	Bacterial
Thiolase	Bacterial
Hydrogenase	4/bacterial; also contains Ni, Fe
B-Hydroxybutyryl-CoA-dehydrogenase	Bacterial
Spermatozoa protein	1 rat, 1 bull

Keshan disease, named for the county where it was first recognized, is a cardiomyopathy affecting primarily children and young women.   The disease is often fatal, existing in rural populations where the dietary selenium intake is less than 10 μg per day.   A second selenium deficiency, Kashin-Beck disease, known for hundred of years in China along the Sino-Soviet border, became known in 1980. Also known as "big joint disease," this rheumatoid condition affects children extensively in some areas and is permanently crippling in adults.   Both diseases are caused by a primary selenium deficiency of soils or the inability of grains and grasses to assimilate the selenium from soils.

The primary form of food selenium in plants is believed to be L-selenomethionine.   The dietary need for selenium is fulfilled by plant selenium

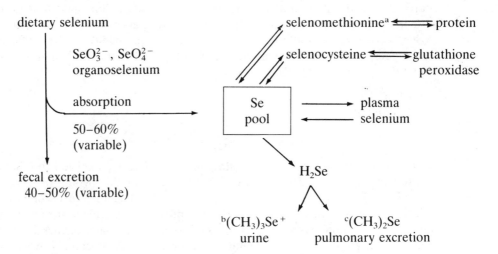

a Not synthesized by animals and humans, dietary source only.

b Major excretory metabolite, trimethylselenonium ion.

c Excretory metabolite with high selenium (toxic?) intake, dimethylselenide.

Figure 3.60   Selenium metabolism.

as well as the two selenium salts, sodium selenite (Na_2SeO_3) and sodium selenate (Na_2SeO_4). A safe and adequate dietary intake of selenium was established by the Food and Nutrition Board in 1980 to be 50 to 200 µg Se per day. The average U.S. diet contains about 80 to 100 µg per day, with dietary intakes being greater for men than for women. A reasonable average absorption of dietary selenium in a mixed diet is 50 to 60%. The metabolism of selenium is generally understood (Figure 3.60). Whereas sulfur compounds undergo general oxidation, selenium compounds follow metabolic pathways of reduction and methylation. The major urinary metabolite is the trimethylselenonium ion. Selenium is an antagonist of mercury, silver, lead, cadmium, and gold, all toxic metals, and the toxic nonmetal arsenic.

Reference

SCHWARZ, K., and FOLTZ, C. M. Selenium as an Integral Part of Factor 3 against Dietary Necrotic Liver Degeneration. *J. Am. Chem. Soc. 79*, 3292 (1957).

Manganese

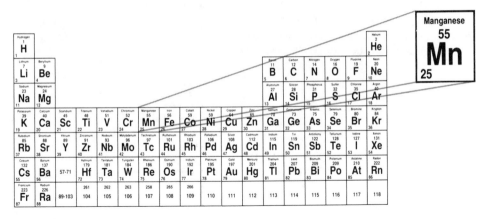

Date of nutritional recognition:	1931
Relative atomic size:	4.6
Oxidation states:	+2, 3, 4, 7
Recommended dietary allowance:	2.5–5.0 mg
Body burden:	12 mg

Manganese was discovered by C. W. Schelle in 1774. By 1913, the presence of manganese in the sera of animals was known. The essentiality of manganese was nutritionally demonstrated for the mouse and rat by A. R. Kemmerer *et al.* and E. R. Orent, and E. V. McCollum in 1931. Manganese deficiency in animals retards growth, impairs lipid metabolism, increases susceptibility to convulsions, increases neonatal mortality and ataxia, and in chickens, specifically, causes what is called "slipped tendon disease." Because manganese affects enzyme activity,

TABLE 3.21 MANGANESE ENZYMES

Enzyme	Mn/molecule
Superoxide dismutase	1
Pyruvate carboxylase	4

it exerts metabolic control over various aspects of metabolism. Manganese is a cofactor of at least two enzymes, superoxide dismutase and pyruvate carboxylase (Table 3.21).

Dietary manganese is poorly absorbed by the gastrointestinal tract with absorption rates being 1 to 4% of dietary intake. Excretion of manganese is almost exclusively via the bile and fecal elimination. Very little manganese appears in urine. Absorption is facilitated by chelating agents, is antagonized by calcium, iron, and phosphorus, and is under some control by ovarian and adrenal corticotrophic hormones (Figure 3.61).

The major depository of manganese is in bone, followed by liver, kidney, and the pituitary gland, with other tissues containing lesser amounts of the mineral. In tissues, subcellular concentration of manganese is in the mitochondrion. Manganese toxicity is rare except for conditions under which the mineral is mined or through other industrial exposure.

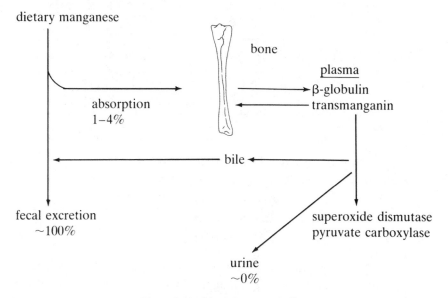

Figure 3.61 Manganese metabolism.

References

BERTRAND, G., and MEDIGRECEANU, M. F. Recherches sur la présence du manganese dans la série animale. *Ann. Inst. Pasteur 27*, 282–288 (1913).

KEMMERER, A. R., ELVEHJEM, C. S., and HART, E. B.   Studies on the Relation of Manganese to the Nutrition of the Mouse.   *J. Biol. Chem. 92*, 623–630 (1931).

ORENT, E. R., and McCOLLUM, E. V.   Effects of Deprivation of Manganese in the Rat.   *J. Biol. Chem. 92*, 651–678 (1931).

Iodine

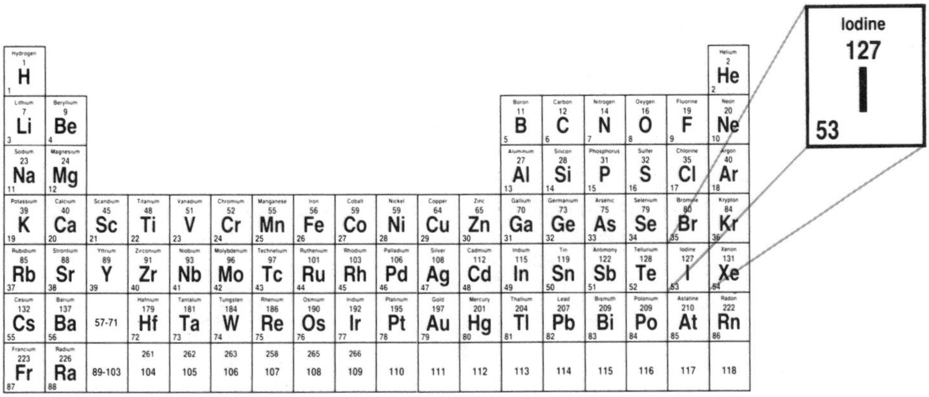

Iodine
127
I
53

Date of nutritional recognition:	1820
Relative atomic size:	4.4
Oxidation state:	-1
Recommended dietary allowance:	150 μg
Body burden:	11 mg

Iodine was discovered in burnt [sic] seaweed by a Napoleonic munitions manufacturer, M. B. Courtois, in 1812 and was so named by the French chemist J. L. Gay-Lussac.   Iodine was found in sponge ash in 1819 by A. Fyfe.   Sponge ash had long been a treatment for goiter.   J. F. Coindet used iodine, believing it to be a drug to treat the disease successfully.   Recognition of iodine as a nutrient is given to C. A. Chatin, a pharmacist and botanist, who attributed traditional goiter to insufficient amounts of iodine in food and water.   Chatin's work was poorly accepted until this century, when human experiments with iodine were concentrated in the United States among schoolchildren beginning in 1912.   Today, goiter is rather a rare disease in developed countries where iodine (as potassium iodide) is added to "iodized salt."   Goiter is a very ancient disease, known to the Chinese, Greeks, and Egyptians.   Marco Polo on his travels to China in 1271 recorded evidence that describes goiter.   Even today in China, as indicated by the following article from the *China Daily*, goiter remains an extensive endemic Chinese disease.

Endemic disease reduced

ZHENGZHOU (Xinhua)—Cases of endemic goiter in Henan Province dropped

TABLE 3.22 IODINE IN SOME
HUMAN TISSUES

Tissue	μg/g wet weight
Thyroid	8000–12,000
Liver	0.20
Ovary	0.07
Lung	0.07
Kidney	0.04
Lymph nodes	0.03
Brain	0.02
Testes	0.02
Muscle	0.01

Reprinted with permission of Dr. E. I. Hamilton.

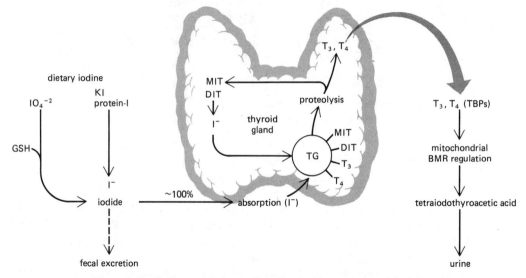

Figure 3.62 Iodine metabolism.   (Reprinted with permission of Dr. E. I. Hamilton.)

from two million in 1980 to 500,000 in 1983, according to Yang Longhe, director of the provincial public health department.

The province has also set up 3,775 stations to inspect the quality of iodated salt and prevent noniodated salt from entering those regions.   In addition, public health departments have injected salt with iodipin in some areas.   At present, 47 of the 66 counties and cities that were affected by the disease have managed to control outbreaks of endemic goiter.

In order to control endemic goiter, Henan has expanded its production of iodated salt by constructing 20 iodated salt plants since 1982, bringing the total to 68.   These plants now produce 155,000 tons of the substance annually, ensuring an adequate supply for all the 20 million people in areas threatened by the disease.*

*CHINA DAILY, Thursday, May 31, 1984, p. 3.

Almost all (80%) dietary iodine is found concentrated in the thyroid gland, where it is sequestered and covalently stored attached to a glycoprotein, thyroglobulin (TG) (Table 3.22). Oxidation of iodine causes it to become covalently attached to tyrosine residues of TG, forming 3-monoiodotyrosine (MIT) and 3,5-diiodotyrosine (DIT) residues (Figure 3.62). Triiodotyrosine, known as T_3, is formed by linkage presumably between MIT and DIT TG residues. Also found within TG is tetraiodothyronine, presumably formed between adjacent DIT residues (Figure 3.54). Upon proteolysis of TG, T_3 and T_4 are secreted into the blood plasma. T_3, and T_4, also known as thyroxine, are the thyroid hormones that circulate attached to TBP (thyroxine binding protein) and serum α-globulin, albumin or prealbumin. The general function of tyroxine is to control basal metabolic rate (BMR) by regulating mitochondrial activity. T_3, arising from the proteolysis of TG or the deiodination of T_4 in the liver or kidney, performs yet unknown functions. Iodine is excreted as reverse T_3 (3',5',3-triiodothyronine) or as tetraiodothyroacetic acid. DIT and MIT released from TG by proteolysis is deiodinated, with the iodide recycled to new TG (Figure 3.63).

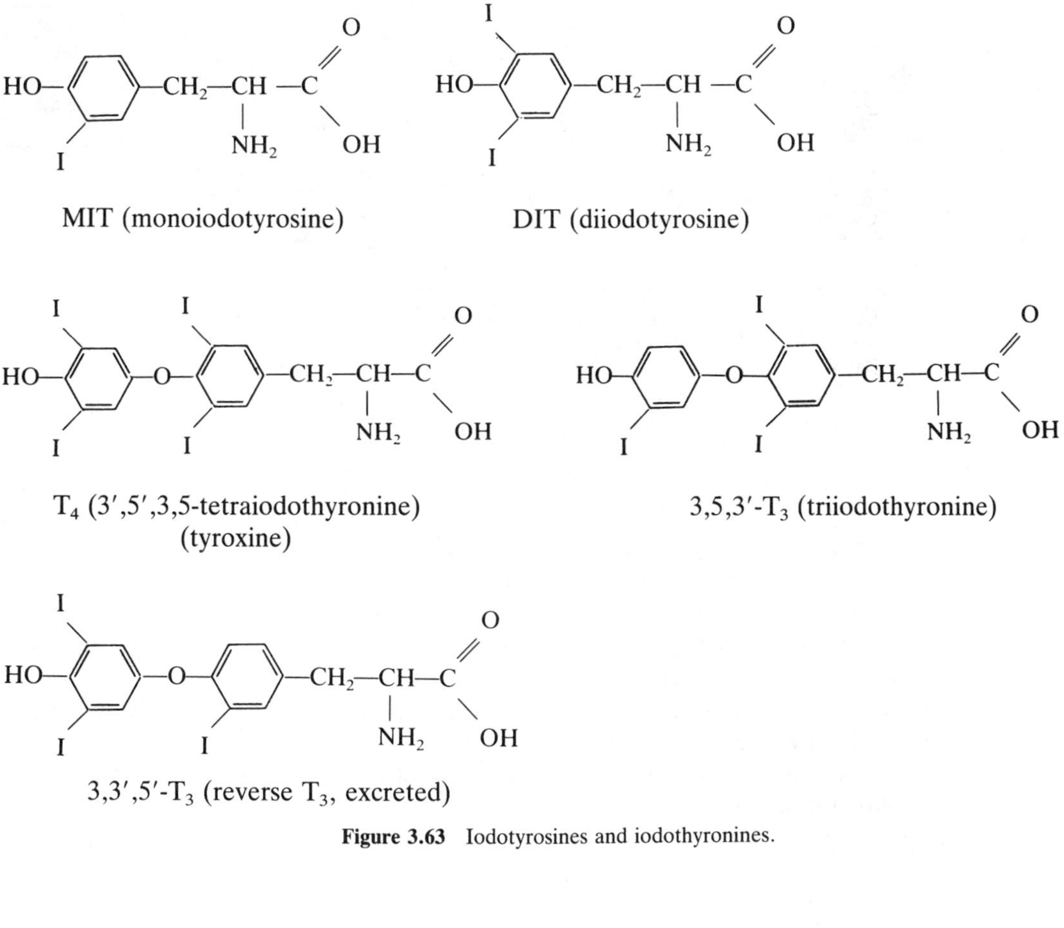

MIT (monoiodotyrosine)   DIT (diiodotyrosine)

T_4 (3',5',3,5-tetraiodothyronine)   3,5,3'-T_3 (triiodothyronine)
(tyroxine)

3,3',5'-T_3 (reverse T_3, excreted)

Figure 3.63 Iodotyrosines and iodothyronines.

Goiter is a direct histological response to the lack of dietary iodine, with a resulting hyperplasia of the thyroid gland (hypothyroidism). Hypothyroidism is prevented by ingestion of 80 μg of iodide daily. The disease may also be aggravated by goitrogens, natural compounds found in the cabbage family of plants, which inhibit iodination of TG. Ions of thiocyanates and perchlorates, in particular, inhibit the uptake of iodide by the thyroid gland. Iodide is moderately toxic, and toxicity can paradoxically produce hypothyroidism.

References

CHATIN, A. Recherche sur l'iode des eaux douces, de la présence de ce corps sur les plantes et les animaux terrestres. *C. R. Acad. Sci. 31*, 280–283 (1850).

CHATIN, A. Recherche de l'iode dans l'air, les eaux, le sol et les produits alimentaires des Alpes de la France et du Piédmont. *C. R. Acad. Sci. 4*, 14–18, 51–54 (1852).

COINDET, J. F. Découverte d'un remède contre la goitre. *Ann. Chim. Phys. 15*, 49–59 (1820).

Copper

																	Copper
																	64
																	Cu
																	29

Date of nutritional recognition: 1928

Relative atomic size: 4.3

Oxidation states: +1, 2

Recommended dietary allowance: 2.0–3.0 mg

Body burden: 10 mg

Located in the eastern Mediterranean is the island of Cyprus, a most important place in the Mycenaean Bronze Age, for it was here that the finest and largest deposits of copper were to be found. Copper from this island was alloyed with tin to form bronze and zinc to form brass.

The use of copper compounds to treat various diseases dates to the time of Hipprocrates. Not until this century, however, was it noticed that animals fed milk diets developed anemia which could not be corrected by dietary iron alone.

TABLE 3.23 COPPER ENZYMES AND PROTEINS

Enzyme/protein	Cu/molecule
Ceruloplasmin	7–8
Superoxide dismutase	2
Lysyl oxidase	?
Tyrosinase	1–4
Cytochrome c oxidase	2
Dopamine β-hydroxylase	4–7
Hemocyanin	20–200
Erythrocuprein	2

In 1928, E. B. Hart and co-workers demonstrated that rats which developed the milk diet anemia required copper along with iron to correct the anemia. Copper is required by plants, bacteria, animals, and humans. It is a constituent of several enzymes and proteins in which the copper participates in various redox reactions (Table 3.23).

Absorption of copper occurs in the upper intestinal tract with about 40% efficiency. Unabsorbed dietary copper and copper excreted into the intestinal lumen in bile are excreted in feces. Lesser amounts of copper are lost through urine, perspiration, and menses. Absorbed copper is transported bound to albumin and stored in part as copper metallothionine in liver (Figure 3.64). In the liver is synthesized ceruloplasmin, a blue-colored copper protein. Ceruloplasmin circulates in the blood plasma and constitutes about 95% of the total plasma copper. The exact function of ceruloplasmin remains unknown, although it probably serves as a copper transport protein and may have a redox function in oxidizing Fe^{2+} to Fe^{3+} for incorporation into transferrin.

Other copper enzymes and proteins also have important physiological and biochemical roles. Copper is a cofactor of superoxide dismutase (see Chapter 12); cytochrome oxidase in electron transport; lysyl oxidase, which oxidatively deaminates lysine and hydroxylysine; and tyrosinase, which converts tyrosine to melanin skin pigments. In crustaceans and some invertebrates the copper protein hemocyanine is the principal carrier of oxygen in blood.

Although human copper deficiency is rare, two diseases of copper metabolism are well known. Wilson's disease is a genetic disease characterized by the accumulation of copper in the liver, brain, and cornea. The disease causes a decrease in serum ceruloplasmin, decreased biliary excretion, and increased urinary copper excretion. Treatment in controlling tissue accumulation of copper is via chelation therapy with D-penicillamine and low-copper diets. A second genetic copper disease is Menke's disease, whose primary manisfestation is reduced copper absorption. The disease may begin *in utero* and takes on characteristics of a dietary copper deficiency. Loss of hair pigmentation, causing "steely hair," is symptomatic of Menke's disease, which is often fatal by the age of about 45.

Copper salts are toxic if ingested in excessive amounts. Copper sulfate has

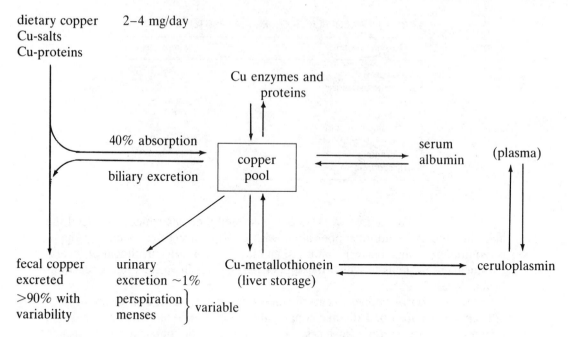

dietary copper   2–4 mg/day
Cu-salts
Cu-proteins

Figure 3.64 Copper metabolism.

long been used as an algicide in aquaria.   Accumulation of copper in Wilson's
disease is the cause of liver cirrhosis and neurological dysfunctions in humans.

Reference

HART, E. B., STEENBOCK, H., WADDEL, J., and ELVEHJEM, C. A.   Iron in Nutrition.
   VII. Copper as a Supplement to Iron for Hemoglobin Building in the Rat.   *J. Biol. Chem.*
   77, 797–812 (1928).

Nickel

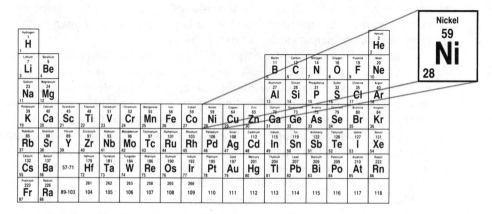

Date of nutritional recognition: 1970
Relative atomic size: 4.2
Oxidation state: +2
Recommended dietary allowance: None
Body burden: 10 mg

The presence of nickel in plants and animals was initially reported by R. Berg in 1925, and G. Bertrand and H. Nakamura made the suggestion in 1936 that nickel might be an essential nutrient. Initial evidence that nickel might be an essential element for the chick was made by Nielson in 1970. Suboptimal growth, reduced hematopoiesis, and changes in the liver content of iron, copper, and zinc have been the generally observed changes in chicks, cows, goats, guinea pigs, sheep, and rats fed low-nickel diets. Nickel appears to interact strongly with iron to affect its absorption from the gastrointestinal tract as measured by reduced hemoglobin, hematocrits, and erythrocyte counts in rats fed a nickel-deficient diet. Nickel deficiency also reduces a number of enzyme activities associated with carbohydrate digestion and metabolism.

In 1980 a nickel metalloenzyme was discovered in the jack bean, *Conavalia ensiformis*. The enzyme was urease (EC 3.5.1.5; Table 3.24), responsible for the hydrolysis of urea to carbon dioxide and ammonia. Ureases from other plants and some bacteria have also been identified as nickel-metalloenzymes. Other bacterial nickel enzymes have now also been identified. No mammalian nickel enzyme, however, has yet been identified.

Many green leafy vegetables contain 1.5 to 3.0 ppm nickel, and the human intake of nickel varies between 170 and 700 μg per day. Dietary nickel appears to be poorly absorbed, with only 1 to 10% being absorbed even at high dietary intakes. The major excretory route for nickel is via the feces, with lesser amounts found in urine and perspiration (Figure 3.65).

Dietary nickel and nickel compounds are normally relatively nontoxic, due in part to poor intestinal absorption. A contact dermatitis to nickel compounds is a common feature of some humans sensitive to nickel. Both the contact dermatitis and a systemic sensitivity to ingested nickel appear possible. Nickel carbonyl, a highly volatile nickel compound, is a known carcinogen.

TABLE 3.24 NICKEL-CONTAINING ENZYMES AND PROTEINS

Enzyme/protein	Ni/molecule
Jack bean urease	2
Nickeloplasmin	1
Factor 430 (F_{430})	1/1500 daltons

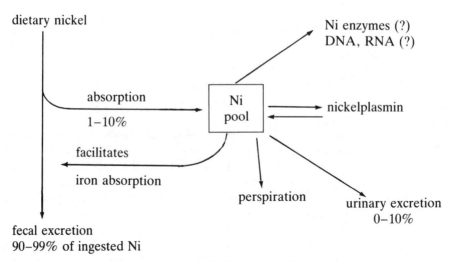

Figure 3.65   Nickel metabolism.

References

BERG, R.   Das Vorkommen seltener Elemente in den Nahrungsmittein und menschlichen Ausscheidungen.   *Biochem. Z. 165*, 461–462 (1925).

BERTRAND G., and MACHEBOEUF, M.   Sur la présence der nickel et du cobalt chez les animaux.   *C. R. Acad. Sci.*   (Paris) *180*, 1380–1383 (1925).

BERTRAND, G., and NAKAMURA, H.   Recherches sur l'importance physiologique du nickel et du cobalt.   *Bull. Soc. Sci. Hyg. Aliment.   24*, 338–343 (1936).

NIELSON, F. H., and SAUBERLICH, H. E.   Evidence of a Possible Requirement for Nickel by the Chick.   *Proc. Soc. Exp. Biol. Med. 134*, 845–849 (1970).

NIELSON, F. H. Evidence of the Essentiality of Arsenic, Nickel and Vanadium and Their Possible Nutritional Significance, in *Advances in Nutritional Research*, Vol. 3, H. H. Draper (ed)., Plenum, New York, pp. 157–172 (1980).

Molybdenum

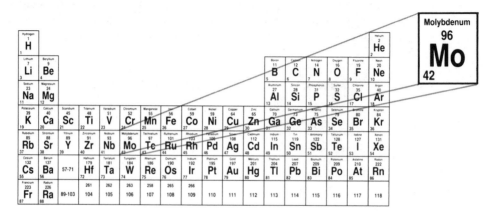

Date of nutritional recognition: 1953
Relative atomic size: 4.5
Oxidation state: +6
Recommended dietary allowance: 0.15–0.50 mg
Body burden: 9 mg

Molybdenum, discovered in 1778 by C. W. Schelle, is today known as an important trace element for bacteria, animals, and humans. Initial nutritional interest focused on molybdenum toxicity in the 1930s, with the recognition that a disease in cattle, locally known as "teart" in England, was molybdenosis. Prevention of teart was possible by administering copper salts or sulfates which interfered with the metabolism and absorption of molybdenum. Thus was established the existence of Mo—Cu and Mo—S antagonisms.

The first indication that molybdenum was an essential nutrient came in 1953, when independently, two research groups, E. C. De Renzo and colleagues and D. A. Richert and W. W. Westerfeld reported that the redox enzymes xanthine oxidase and sulfite oxidase contained molybdenum. A third enzyme containing molybdenum, aldehyde oxidase, was discovered in 1954 (Table 3.25). These enzymes contribute to the oxidation of the nucleic acid bases hypoxanthine and xanthine to uric acid, of sulfites to sulfates, and of aldehydes to ketones. In bacteria, molybdenum is required by nitrogenases and nitrate reductases, which provide plants (legumes) with ammonia from nitrogen (N_2) and nitrates from nitrites which are assimilated into protein.

Molybdenum deficiency in animals can be produced experimentally by feeding low-molybdenum diets and an antagonist, tungsten. Molybdenum deficiency in humans is unknown except for rare cases of malabsorption and the use of total parenteral nutrition for extended periods. Metabolic changes with a molybdenum deficiency include abnormal methionine catabolism and low excretion rates of uric acid and inorganic sulfate. These conditions are corrected by administering molybdenum. In a central valley in China (Henan Province), people naturally consuming low-molybdenum diets have been known to have a high incidence of esophageal cancer. Similar observations for esophageal cancer have been made among the Bantu peoples of the Transki, South Africa.

Molybdenum is effectively absorbed from the gastrointestinal tract, from

TABLE 3.25 MOLYBDENUM ENZYMES

Enzyme	Mo/molecule
Xanthine oxidase	2
Sulfite oxidase	2
Aldehyde oxidase	?
Formate dehydrogenase	?
Nitrogenase	2
Nitrate reductase	1

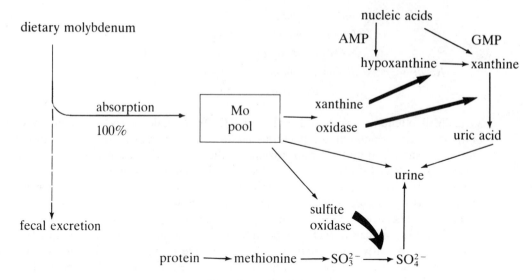

Figure 3.66 Molybdenum metabolism.

which it is incorporated into the molybdenum enzymes (Figure 3.66).   Molybdenum is found in muscle, skin, liver, and spleen as well as other organs.

References

DE RENZO, E. C., KALIETA, E., HEYTLER, P., OLESON, J. J., HUTCHINGS, B. L., and WILLIAMS, J. H.   The Nature of the Xanthine Oxidase Factor.   *J. Am. Chem. Soc. 75*, 753 (1953).

RICHERT, D. A., and WESTERFELD, W. W.   Isolation and Identification of the Xanthine Oxidase Factor as Molybdenum.   *J. Biol. Chem. 203*, 915–923 (1953).

Chromium

Date of nutritional recognition: 1959
Relative atomic size: 4.2
Oxidation states: +2, 3, 6
Recommended dietary allowance: 50—200 μg
Body burden: 6 mg

The discovery of chromium as a nutrient is associated with the discovery that selenium prevented dietary liver necrosis in rats. The rats were found to be hypoglycemic and failed to utilize glucose properly, which was corrected by brewer's yeast or pork kidney powder. The factor preventing the hypoglycemia was independent of the protective effects of selenium against liver necrosis and upon partial purification was eventually found to contain traces of chromium. The discovery that chromium affected glucose metabolism was reported by Klaus Schwarz and Walter Mertz in 1959. Believed to contain chromium in an organic complex named the glucose tolerance factor, or GTF, it has never been isolated or defined chemically from natural sources. Chromium complexes containing nicotinic acid and coordinated amino acids have been synthetically synthesized and isolated from yeast. None has been determined to be the natural GTF. As it may occur naturally, chromium and GTF, as observed by *in vitro* assays, are believed to enhance the behavior of insulin in improving glucose transport across cell membranes.

One of the complications of chromium analysis is the great difficulty with which it is measured accurately. Since 1964, with greater accuracy in chromium analysis, blood levels of chromium reported to be on the order 1000 ng/ml are now known to be less than 1 ng/ml. For this reason, analytical data for chromium prior to 1978 for tissues may not reflect true concentrations of chromium. Chromium is believed to be biologically active in the Cr(III) oxidation state. Dietary chromium intake is quite variable, ranging from 11 to 820 μg/day and averaging about

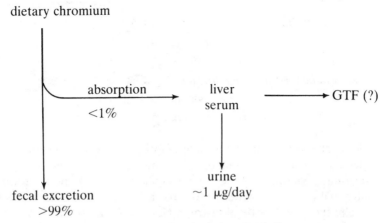

Figure 3.67 Chromium metabolism.

147 μg/day (29 to 455 μg/day); ($N = 25$) for adults. Chromium is poorly absorbed (<1% by the intestinal tract, and urinary excretion of between 1 and 2 μg/day would provide a metabolic balance for an intake of 147 μg per day (Figure 3.67). Urinary excretion of chromium is reported to be about 1 μg per day. At this rate of urinary chromium excretion and with a body burden of approximately 6 mg, it would seem that chromium deficiency for healthy adults would be a rare event. For some people chromium supplementation has been shown to improve glucose tolerance and to reduce cholesterol-HDL ratios, which is an enhanced protective index for the rate of cardiovascular disease. No chromium proteins or enzymes have been specifically identified.

References

SCHWARZ, K., and MERTZ, W.   Chromium (III) and the Glucose Tolerance Factor.   *Arch. Biochem. Biophys. 85*, 292–295 (1959).

Cobalt

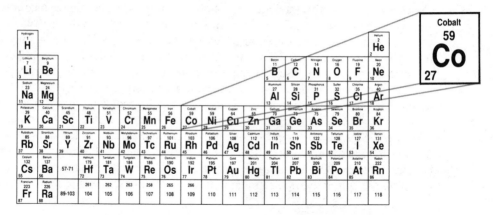

Date of nutritional recognition:	1935
Relative atomic size:	4.2
Oxidation states:	+2, +3
Recommended dietary allowance:	None
Requirement:	As vitamin B_{12}
Body burden:	1.5 mg

The blue glass in the windows of Gothic cathedrals and apothecary jars probably contains cobalt compounds. Nutritionally, cobalt is incorporated into the corrin ring of vitamin B_{12} (see "Cyanocobalamin") by the microflora of the gastrointestinal tract. No other nutritional role for cobalt is known with certainty.

The sheep and cattle industry in New Zealand provided the historical setting for the recognition of the dietary essentiality of cobalt. What has been called "bush sickness" among cattle in New Zealand and "wasting" or "coast disease" in Australia, diseases first attributed to an iron deficiency, were later successfully treated with limonite. Limonite contained nickel, which was ineffective in treating the animals. Further fractionation of limonite revealed traces of cobalt and in 1935, E. J. Underwood and J. F. Filmer reported the effectiveness of cobalt salts in eliminating the anemia. Vitamin B_{12} had at this time not been identified and it was not until 1951 that S. E. Smith showed in ruminants that cobalt deficiency was in effect a vitamin B_{12} deficiency. Humans require dietary vitamin B_{12} since the intestinal flora do not synthesize adequate amounts of the vitamin if given cobalt. For humans, therefore, cobalt per se is not an essential nutrient.

References

SMITH, S. E., KOCK, B. A., and TURK, K. L. The Responses of Cobalt-Deficient Lambs to Liver Extract and Vitamin B_{12}. *J. Nutr. 44*, 455–464 (1951).

UNDERWOOD, E. J. and FILMER, J. F. The Determination of the Biologically Potent Element (Cobalt) in Limonite. *Aust. Vet. J. 11*, 84–92 (1935).

Vanadium

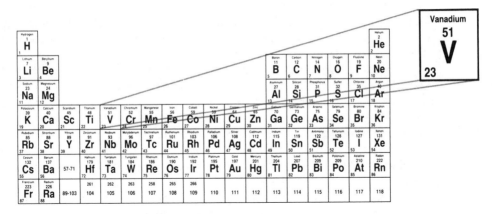

Date of nutritional recognition:	1971
Relative atomic size:	4.4
Oxidation states:	+2, 3, 4, 5
Recommended dietary allowance:	None
Body burden:	100 μg

The element vanadium was discovered and named by Sefström in 1831 after the Scandinavian goddess of beauty, youth, and luster, Vanadis. Vanadium is thought to be essential for the chick and rat, but experimental data have not been conclusive in reaffirming its essentiality. There is no evidence that vanadium is needed by humans even though the daily intake of the element is estimated to be 10 to 60 μg.

In 1971, L. L. Hopkins, Jr. and H. E. Mohr reported that chicks fed diets

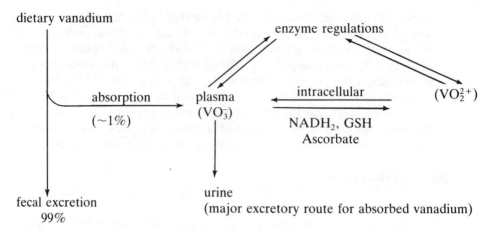

Figure 3.68 Vanadium metabolism.

containing 10 ppb vanadium failed to produce normal wing and tail feathers. In the same year, K. Schwarz and D. Milne reported that rats in all-plastic isolators fed purified amino acid diets failed to grow, but that growth improved when the animals were fed the same diet with 10 μg of vanadium as orthovanadate. C. A. Strasia reported similar findings for the rat.

Vanadium appears to be poorly absorbed by the gastrointestinal tract (Figure 3.68). In rats, using $^{48}VO^{2+}$, only 1% of ingested vanadium was absorbed. The principal form of intracellular vanadium *in vivo* appears to exist as the vanadyl $[VO^{2+}(IV)]$ ion maintained by glutathione, $NADH_2$, and perhaps ascorbic acid in the reduced state bound to phosphates. In plasma, vanadium exists as the vanadate $[VO_3^-(V)]$ ion. Vanadium therefore can act as a redox ion and has been reported to facilitate the binding of oxygen to the heme proteins hemoglobin and myoglobin *in vivo*.

Vanadium is a cofactor of only one known protein, hemovanadin (Table 3.26), found in ascidian worms. This protein may function in analogous fashion to hemoglobin, as an oxygen carrier in the ascidians. Vanadium as vanadate is an inhibitor and perhaps a regulator of Na^+—K^+ ATPase, ribonuclease, and other enzymes. Vanadium also has varied physiological effects on the kidney, liver, eye, heart, and nervous system. Because vanadium is so poorly absorbed, most vanadium compounds are not very toxic.

TABLE 3.26 PROTEINS AND ENZYMES CONTAINING VANADIUM

Enzyme/protein	V/molecule
Hemovanadin	?
Numerous enzymes inhibited or activated by vanadyl or vanadate ions	

References

HOPKINS, L. L., JR., and MOHR, H. E.   The Biological Essentiality of Vanadium, in *Newer Trace Elements in Nutrition*, W. Mertz and W. E. Cornatzer, Eds.   Marcel Dekker, New York, pp. 195–213 (1971).

SCHWARZ, K., and MILNE, D. B.   Growth Effects of Vanadium in the Rat.   *Science 174*, 426–428 (1971).

STRASIA, C. A.   Vanadium Essentiality and Toxicity in the Laboratory Rat.   Ph.D. Dissertation.   University Microfilms, Ann Arbor, Mich. (1971).

WATER

Name:	Hydrogen oxide
Molecular weight:	18
Specific gravity:	1.0
Melting point:	0°C
Boiling point:	100°C

No other compound is more essential to life than water, for without it there would be no life of any kind.   Bacteria, plants, animals, and humans all require exogenous water.   Different life forms contain different anatomical proportions of water. Wheat and corn, properly dried, contain only a small amount of water.   Fresh fruits and vegetables may be 80 to 90% water.   The water content of foods as discussed in Chapter 7 (see Table 7.5) is an important factor as it affects caloric density.

The water content in humans varies according to age, sex, bone density, and gross body weight.   It usually varies between 45 and 65% of total body weight, with the water content generally higher in the young, in men, and in lean people. Most water is localized in cells (55%), with the remaining extracellular water (45%) being contributed by interstitial fluids and blood.   Smaller amounts of water are to be found in bone, the gallbladder (as bile), secretory glands, and spinal, synovial, vitreous, and aqueous fluids.

Water is biologically important because of its many unusual physical and chemical properties.   It has been called the universal solvent, for it is capable of dissolving not only polar molecules and inorganic salts, but also large organic molecules which may be either polar or contain hydrophobic components.   Water has a high specific heat (1 cal/g) and a high heat of vaporization (80 cal/g).   These physical properties of water help to prevent rapid fluctuations in body temperature, either hot or cold, and permit small amounts of water (perspiration and transpiration) to remove large amounts of body heat during exercise.   Water's large dielectric constant and extensive intermolecular hydrogen bonding (Chapter 1) relative to other organic liquids (e.g., alcohols) are factors contributing to its special properties.

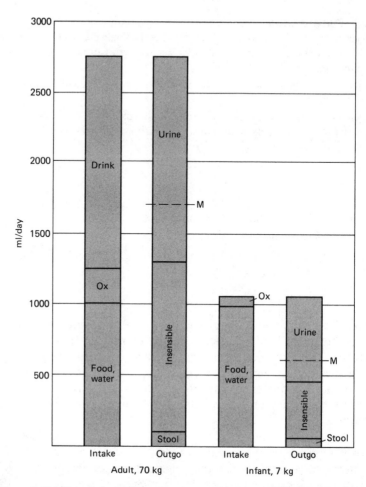

Figure 3.69 Water balance. Routes and approximate magnitude of water intake and outgo without sweating. M is minimal urine volume at maximal solute concentration. Ox is water of oxidation, "metabolic water." [From *Recommended Dietary Allowances*, 9th rev. ed., National Academy of Sciences, New York (1980).]

Other characteristics that make water physiologically important include its low viscosity and moderate surface tension, permitting blood flow and lubrication for eyelids, articulating joints, and for peristalsis.   Water also permits transmission of light (eye) and sound (ear).

While the primary function of water remains as a solvent for the myriads of biochemical reactions in cells and blood, water also enters directly into some biochemical reactions.   Molecular water is consumed during the hydrolysis of proteins, lipids, and carbohydrates undergoing digestion and metabolism.   It is also consumed during hydroxylation reactions and photosynthesis and is produced as the terminal product of oxidative phosphorylation.   Water produced in this manner is often referred to as "metabolic water."   About 10% of our daily water need is fulfilled by the formation of metabolic water. The remaining 90% of our daily water requirement is ingested in foods and as various liquids (Figure 3.69).

Water is eliminated from the body primarily as urine or an insensible perspiration via epidermal and pulmonary evaporation. About 5% of the total elimination of body water is contained in feces, providing lubrication and a soft stool. Urinary water provides the solvent for the elimination of water-soluble vitamins, minerals, and other metabolites. Insensible perspiration of skin provides for elimination of some body salts, and insensible perspiration of both skin and lungs carries away body heat by way of evaporation.

4

Nutrient Digestion and Absorption

A vigorous and healthy man has just eaten a good meal; in the midst of this feeling of well-being the foods that are at the moment carried to the various parts of the organism are energetically digested, and the digestive juices dissolve them easily and quickly. Should this man receive bad news, or should sad and baneful passions suddenly arise in his soul, his stomach and intestines will immediately cease to act on the foods contained in them. The very juices in which the foods are already almost entirely dissolved will remain as though struck by a moral stupor, and . . . digestion ceases entirely. . . . Pierre Jean Georges Cabanis, 1802. From Stewart Wolf, The Stomach's Link to the Brain. *Fed. Proc. 44*, 2889–2893 (1985).

THE DIGESTIVE PROCESS

All forms of life must assimilate from their environment, a continuous supply of nutrients (Table 2.2) and energy. Among higher life forms (e.g., animals and humans) nutrients and energy are heterogeneously supplied from a diet containing a great diversity of foods. Digestion constitutes the physical, chemical, and microbiological process, which begins in the mouth with the mastication of food and ceases with the absorption of individual nutrients across the microvilli of the intestinal mucosa. Digestion of food is foremost a chemical process under physiologic and hormonal controls initiated by the senses: sight and smell. It is a process whereby macromolecules—starch, proteins, and triglycerides and other smaller molecules—undergo hydrolysis and reduction primarily to their monomeric constituent components in preparation for absorption. Other nutrients, vitamins, and

144

minerals, and also drugs, undergo either minor or no chemical change prior to absorption.

Digestion begins in the mouth but may be facilitated by pretreatment of some foods with enzymes, microbiological fermentations, or cooking. Once ingested, foods at various stages of digestion pass through the various anatomical components comprising the gastrointestinal (GI) tract (Figure 4.1). The GI tract is lined with tissues of ectodermal origin and lies outside the body proper. For descriptive purposes, digestion of food beginning in the oral cavity and terminating with the anal sphincter, and the absorption of nutrients, are separately detailed by the major anatomical components of the GI system: the mouth, stomach, and intestinal tract.

Mouth

Admittance of food into the buccal cavity (ingestion) invites a series of complex physiological and hormonal events in preparation for the digestion of food. The presence of food in the mouth stimulates the secretion of saliva from the bilateral sets of three salivary glands (buccal, lingual, and parotid). Secreted saliva is mixed during mastication and provides lubrication for swallowing the bolus of food. During mastication, the teeth assist with the mechanical degradation of the food, increasing its surface area. The maintenance of adequate dentition for mastication is most important for proper eating and digestion. Loss of dentition among the elderly often leads to changes in life-long dietary practices, loss of weight from reduction in caloric ingestion, and marginal or severe vitamin and mineral deficiencies. Loss of teeth due to abrasion from dirt and grit in the processed flours of ancient peoples probably contributed to nutritional deficiencies and early death.

Secreted saliva, in addition to providing lubrication for swallowing, contains the enzyme salivary α-amylase or ptyalin. Enzymatically active in the mouth at neutral to slightly acidic conditions, α-amylase [α-(1→4)-glucan-4-glucanohydrolase; Figure 4.2] hydrolyzes the α-(1→4) glycosides of glycogen and starch, giving rise to maltose, isomaltose, and oligosaccharides. As the bolus of food enters the stomach, hydrolysis of starch continues until the fall in pH and proteolytic enzymes of the stomach inactivate α-amylase, with cessation of carbohydrate degradation.

Hydrolysis of disaccharides, proteins, or triglycerides does not transpire in the buccal cavity. No proteolytic enzymes are present in saliva, and the presence of a buccal lipase becomes active only under the acidic conditions of the stomach.

Stomach

Concurrent with the ingestion of food, the stomach responds to various stimuli by secreting gastric juice, consisting of mucus secretions, hydrochloric acid (HCl) from the gastric glands, a glycoprotein, the intrinsic factor (IF) for the intestinal absorption of vitamin B_{12}, and pepsinogen, the zymogen precursor of pepsin. The stomach is the first organ encountered for protein and triglyceride hydrolysis. The

Human Digestive System

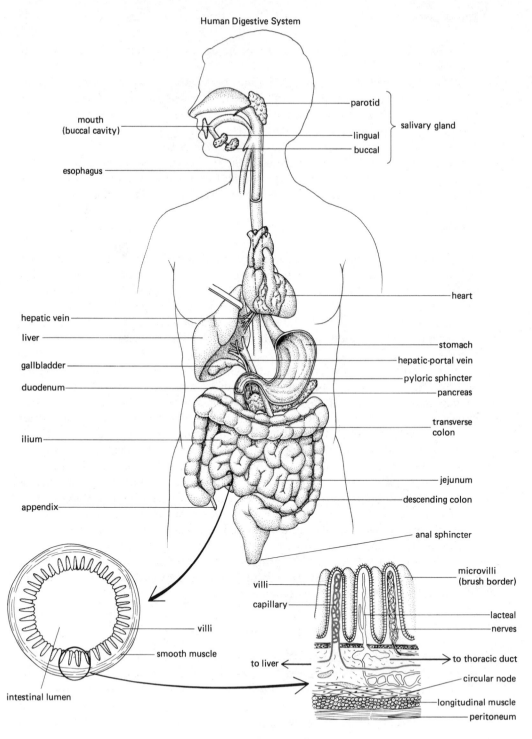

parotid

mouth
(buccal cavity)

lingual

salivary gland

buccal

esophagus

heart

hepatic vein

liver

stomach

hepatic-portal vein

gallbladder

pyloric sphincter

duodenum

pancreas

transverse
colon

ilium

jejunum

descending colon

appendix

anal sphincter

microvilli
(brush border)

villi

capillary

lacteal

nerves

villi

to liver

to thoracic duct

smooth muscle

circular node

intestinal lumen

longitudinal muscle

peritoneum

Figure 4.1

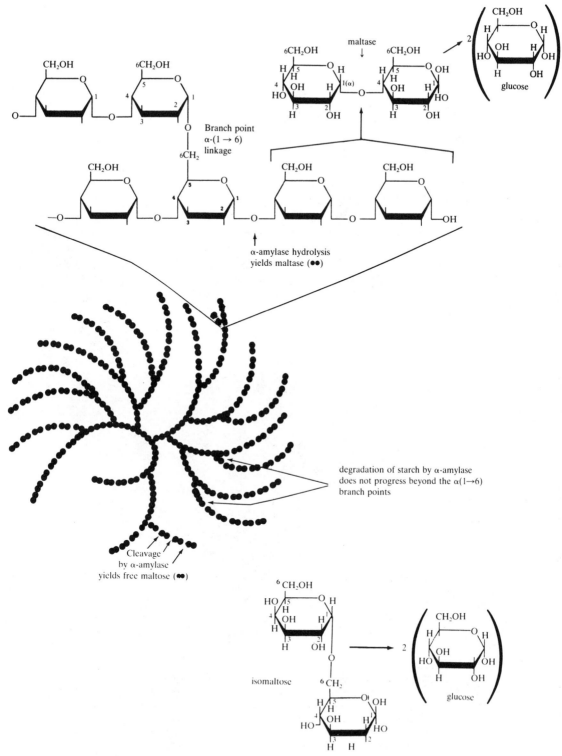

Figure 4.2 Hydrolysis of starch by α-amylase, isomaltase, and maltase.

stomach is the major site for protein digestion following the conversion of the enzymatically inactive pepsinogen to the enzymatically active pepsin by HCl and then by pepsin autocatalytically. The pepsin of the stomach rapidly degrades proteins to polypeptides, oligopeptides and small, limited amounts of amino acids. Proteins are degraded by pepsin primarily by hydrolysis of the peptide bonds of phenylalanine, tyrosine, and tryptophan, and secondarily by bonds of aspartic acid, glutamic acid, and leucine residues. The lipase entering the stomach from the mouth in the bolus of food becomes enzymatically active as the pH falls to between 4.5 and 5.4. As the pH of the food in the stomach continues to fall to approximately pH 2 to 3, which is optimum for the proteolytic activity of pepsin, lipase activity lasts only briefly and triglyceride hydrolysis is restricted. The digestive products from the stomach enter the upper small intestine through the pyloric sphincter as chyme. It is the duodenum that is the major site of lipid digestion and where final degradation of dietary proteins and carbohydrates is completed prior to absorption by cells of the intestinal mucosa. Absorption of most nutrients is limited primarily to the duodenum and jejunum.

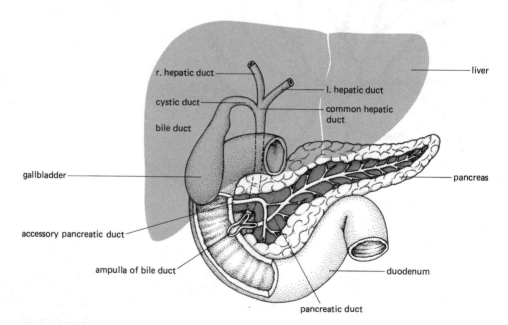

Figure 4.3 Pancreas, gallbladder, and duodenum. Connections of the liver, gallbladder, and pancreas with the duodenum. The anatomical arrangement of the entry of the pancreatic duct and the bile duct is not always as shown here; they enter the duodenum separately in 29% of persons. [From G. H. Bell, J. N. Davidson, and H. Scarborough, *Textbook of Physiology and Biochemistry*, Chapter 17, Williams & Wilkins Company, Baltimore, Md. (1961).]

Upper Small Intestinal (Duodenum) Lumen

Entering the upper small intestine, or duodenum, from the stomach, the chyme (pH 2 to 3) is rapidly neutralized (pH 6 to 7) by the secretions of the pancreas and gallbladder (Figure 4.3). Entering the duodenum through the pancreatic duct are the enzymes for the continuing degradation of carbohydrates, proteins, lipids, and nucleic acids (Table 4.1). Produced by the cells of the pancreas for the secretion into the duodenum is an α-amylase similar in function to salivary amylase for continued hydrolysis of α-(1→4) glycosides. Glucose, maltose, isomaltose, and mixed oligosaccharides are produced by the pancreatic amylase activity from the remaining starches and glycogen.

In addition to secreting an α-amylase, the pancreas synthesizes and secretes several zymogens. These zymogens secreted into the duodenum include two proteolytic zymogens, trypsinogen and chymotrypsinogen, and a peptidylzymogen, procarboxypeptidase. Conversion of these zymogens into the active enzymes is initiated by an enteropeptidase synthesized and secreted by cells of the gastrointestinal mucosa. The enteropeptidase hydrolyzes a polypeptide, converting trypsinogen to trypsin. Thereafter, trypsin converts the remaining zymogens to active

TABLE 4.1 PANCREATIC AND INTESTINAL ENZYMES AND ZYMOGENS

Proteolytic zymogens	Proteolytic enzymes	Carbohydrate enzymes
Trypsinogen	Trypsin	α-Amylase
Chymotrypsinogen	Chymotrypsin	Sucrase
Procarboxypeptidase	Aminopeptidase	Maltase
	Carboxypeptidase	Lactase
		Isomaltase
Lipid enzymes	Other enzymes	
α-Lipase	Endonucleases	
Retinyl esterase		
Tocopheryl esterase		
Cholesterol esterase		

Secreted intraintestinal enzymes
Aminopeptidases
Dipeptidases
Maltase
Sucrase
Lactase
β-Lipase
Esterases
Nucleases
Nucleotidases
Phosphatases
Enterokinases
Nucleosidases
Enteropeptidases

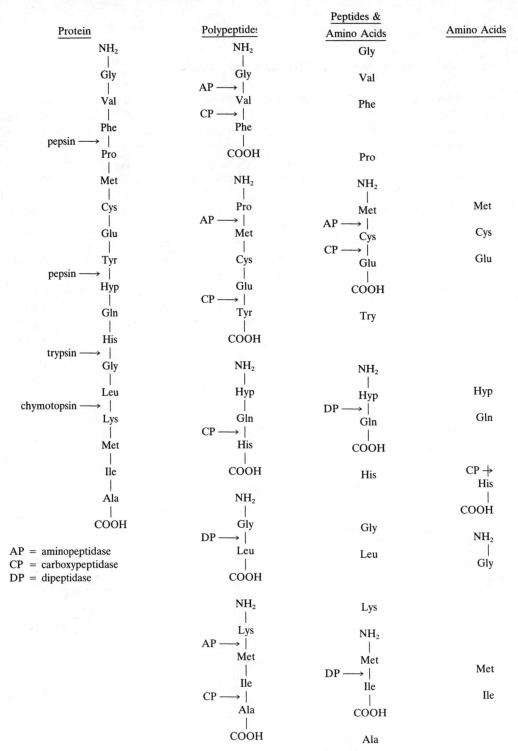

Figure 4.4 Hydrolysis of proteins.

enzymes.   Like pepsin, trypsin and chymotrypsin are proteolytic endopeptidases cleaving proteins inside their amino acid extremities (Figure 4.4).   Trypsin hydrolyzes peptide bonds adjacent to lysyl or hystidyl residues, while chymotrypsin hydrolyzes peptide bonds adjacent to phenylalanyl, tyrosyl, or tryptophanyl residues.   Trypsin and chymotrypsin are able to degrade proteins and large polypeptides not hydrolyzed by pepsin to even smaller polypeptides, dipeptides, and possibly some free amino acids.   Having been activated by trypsin, the procarboxypeptidase hydrolyzes amino acids from terminal carboxyl residues of polypeptides.   Enzymes that hydrolyze terminal amino or carboxyl residues of polypeptides are classified as exopeptidases.   A third class of digestive enzymes secreted in pancreatic juice are the pancreatic esterases, pancreatic lipases, cholesterol, and retinyl esterases.   Pancreatic lipase, in the presence of liver bile acids, hydrolyzes emulsified fats and oils, triacylglycerols, principally at the α and α' esters of the triglyceride.   The luminal products of pancreatic lipase activity are free fatty acids from the α- and α'-glycerol esters and a monoglyceride, 2-monoacylglyceride (Figure 4.5).   Cholesterol and retinyl esterases hydrolyze the fatty acid esters attached to cholesterol and vitamin A (Figure 4.6).

Bile Acids and Bile Salts

The bile acids are formed by the liver as terminal metabolites of cholesterol metabolism.   They are stored in the gallbladder (when anatomically present) and enter the duodenum through the bile duct in the presence of chyme from the stomach, possibly by hormonal action.   The major human bile acid is cholic acid. The other, less abundant bile acids are formed by the addition of the amino acids glycine or taurine to choloyl-CoA, forming the bile acids, glycocholic and taurocholic acid (Figure 4.7).   The other bile acids are deoxycholic and lithocholic acid. In the intestinal tract, the bile salts (Na^+, K^+) are amphipathic and function to emulsify the luminal lipids, the triacylglycerols, cholesterol, acylcholesterol, phospholipids, and lipid-soluble vitamins.   Emulsification of lipids by the bile salts results in the formation of micelles, very small lipid droplets in an aqueous environment similar to formation of a colloid.   The result of emulsification is a large expansion of the total lipid surface area exposed to lipase activity.   Micellar lipids are then rapidly hydrolyzed to free fatty acids, glycerides, glycerol, free cholesterol, and vitamin A.

   The bile salts, having facilitated the digestion and absorption of lipids, may pass through the remainder of the GI tract and be excreted in the feces (ca. 10%) or they may be reabsorbed (ca. 90%) by the ileum.   Reabsorbed bile salts are returned to the liver by the enterohepatic circulation (Figure 4.8) and are again stored in the gallbladder to repeat their function in lipid digestion.   Thirty grams of bile salts may be recycled in this manner each day through this enterohepatic circulation.   Cholestyramine, a strong anion-exchange resin, is sometimes used medically to bind intestinal bile salts, breaking the chain of absorption and enterohepatic circulation, facilitating the excretion of additional bile salts.   In this man-

lipase (esterase)

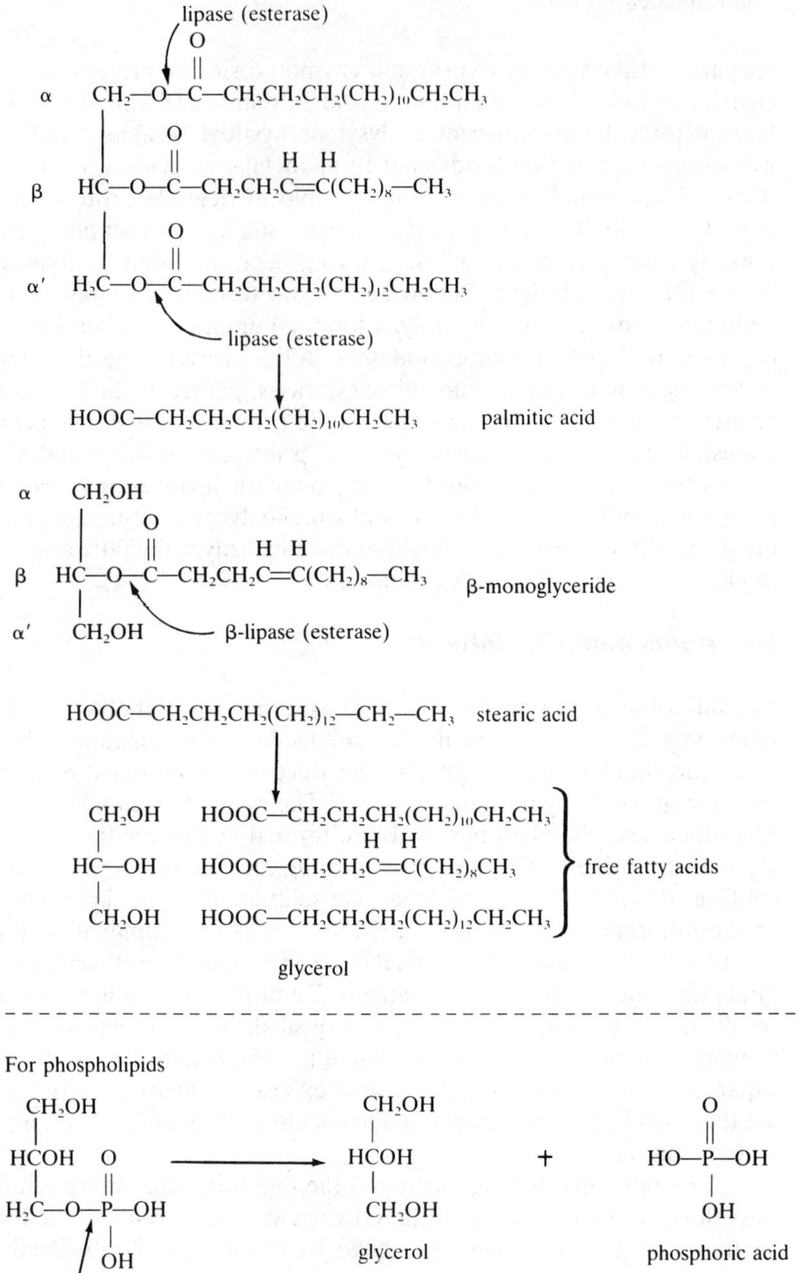

$$\alpha \quad CH_2-O-\overset{\overset{\displaystyle O}{\|}}{C}-CH_2CH_2CH_2(CH_2)_{10}CH_2CH_3$$

$$\beta \quad HC-O-\overset{\overset{\displaystyle O}{\|}}{C}-CH_2CH_2\overset{H}{C}=\overset{H}{C}(CH_2)_8-CH_3$$

$$\alpha' \quad H_2C-O-\overset{\overset{\displaystyle O}{\|}}{C}-CH_2CH_2CH_2(CH_2)_{12}CH_2CH_3$$

lipase (esterase)

$$HOOC-CH_2CH_2CH_2(CH_2)_{10}CH_2CH_3 \quad \text{palmitic acid}$$

$$\alpha \quad CH_2OH$$
$$\beta \quad HC-O-\overset{\overset{\displaystyle O}{\|}}{C}-CH_2CH_2\overset{H}{C}=\overset{H}{C}(CH_2)_8-CH_3 \quad \beta\text{-monoglyceride}$$
$$\alpha' \quad CH_2OH \quad \beta\text{-lipase (esterase)}$$

$$HOOC-CH_2CH_2CH_2(CH_2)_{12}-CH_2-CH_3 \quad \text{stearic acid}$$

$$\begin{array}{ll}
CH_2OH & HOOC-CH_2CH_2CH_2(CH_2)_{10}CH_2CH_3 \\
| & \qquad\qquad\quad H\ \ H \\
HC-OH & HOOC-CH_2CH_2C=C(CH_2)_8CH_3 \\
| & \\
CH_2OH & HOOC-CH_2CH_2CH_2(CH_2)_{12}CH_2CH_3
\end{array} \right\} \text{free fatty acids}$$

glycerol

- -

For phospholipids

$$\begin{array}{l}
CH_2OH \\
| \\
HCOH \quad O \\
| \quad\ \ \| \\
H_2C-O-P-OH \\
\qquad\quad | \\
\qquad\quad OH
\end{array} \longrightarrow
\begin{array}{l}
CH_2OH \\
| \\
HCOH \\
| \\
CH_2OH \\
\text{glycerol}
\end{array} +
\begin{array}{l}
\quad O \\
\quad \| \\
HO-P-OH \\
\quad | \\
\quad OH \\
\text{phosphoric acid}
\end{array}$$

phosphatase

Figure 4.5 Hydrolysis of triglycerides.

152

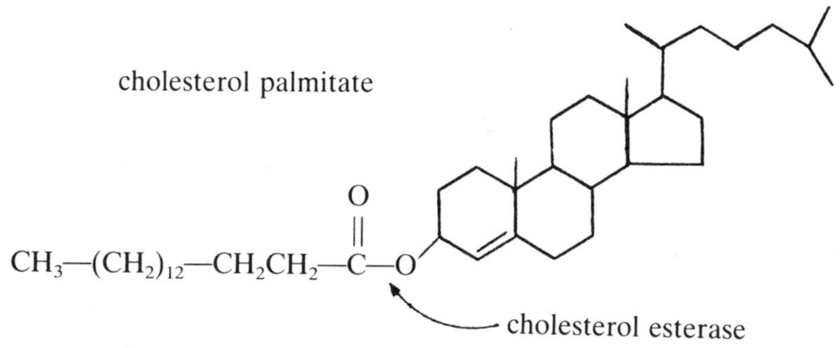

cholesterol palmitate

$$CH_3-(CH_2)_{12}-CH_2CH_2-\overset{\overset{O}{\|}}{C}-O$$

cholesterol esterase

Hydrolysis by cholesterol esterase yields free cholesterol and palmitic acid

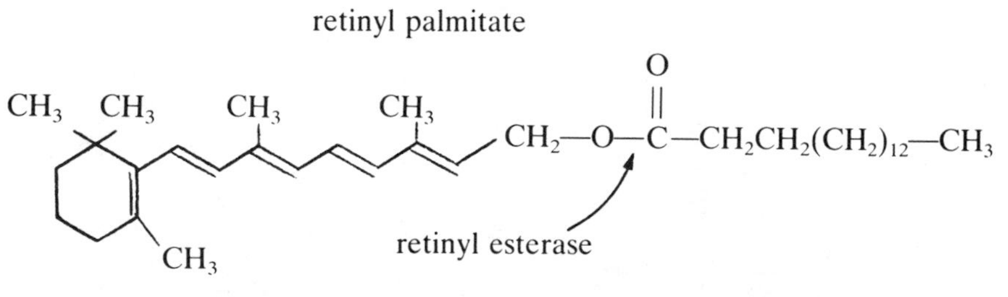

retinyl palmitate

$$CH_2-O-\overset{\overset{O}{\|}}{C}-CH_2CH_2(CH_2)_{12}-CH_3$$

retinyl esterase

Hydrolysis by retinyl esterase yields retinol and palmitic acid

Figure 4.6 Hydrolysis of cholesterol and retinyl esters.

ner, cholestyramine effectively reduces circulating serum cholesterol by accelerating the excretion of its metabolites.

Intestinal Mucosa

The intestinal mucosa, lining the approximately 18 feet of small intestine, is entirely covered with conical-shaped projections known as villi.   There are 20 to 40 villi per square millimeter of intestinal area.   Each villus is covered by microvilli (1.0 $\times$ 0.1 μm), the brush border, which dramatically raises the surface area for nutrient absorption from approximately 10 m^2 to 300 m^2.   Each villus contains an arteriole and venule and a blind lymphatic duct (lacteal; Figure 4.9).   Nutrients absorbed by the arteriole or venule are transported to the liver by the hepatic portal system of the general blood circulation.   Nutrients absorbed by lacteals transgress the lymphatic system and enter the circulatory system via the thoracic duct at the left subclavian vein present under the sternum (Figure 4.12).

In addition to providing the great surface area for nutrient absorption, villi secrete a mucus that protects their columnar epithelial cells and provides for peristaltic lubrication of the small intestine.   The columnar epithelia of the microvilli

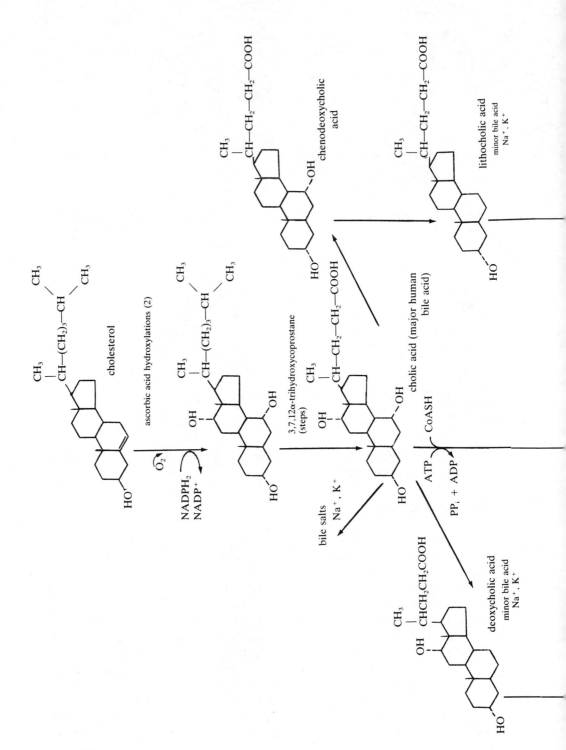

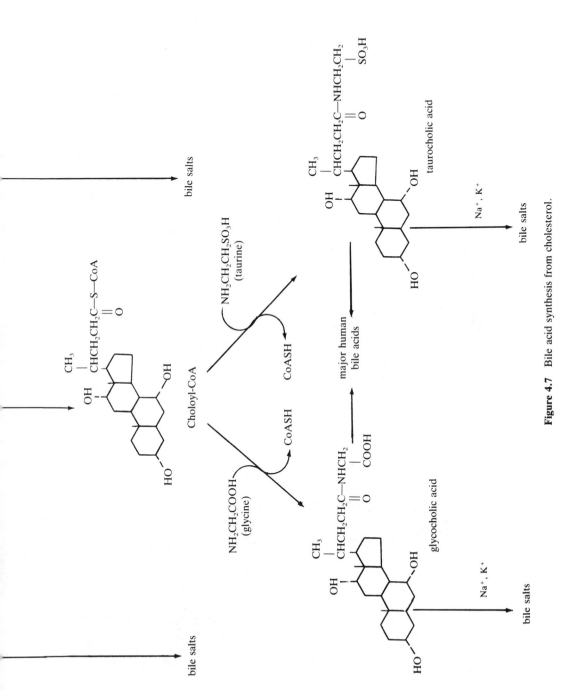

Figure 4.7 Bile acid synthesis from cholesterol.

155

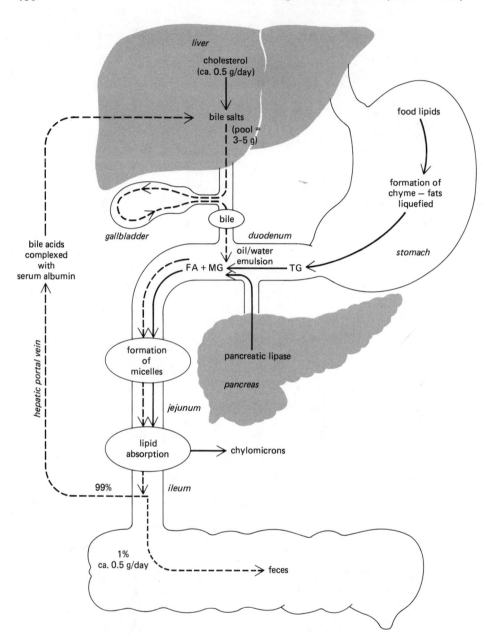

Figure 4.8 Enterohepatic circulation of bile salts and digestion of lipids. Dashes (----) indicate enterohepatic circulation of bile salts. (TG, triacylglycerol; MG, monoacylglycerol; FA, long-chain fatty acids.) [From *Harper's Review of Biochemistry*, 19th ed., Long Medical Publications, Los Altos, Calif. (1983).]

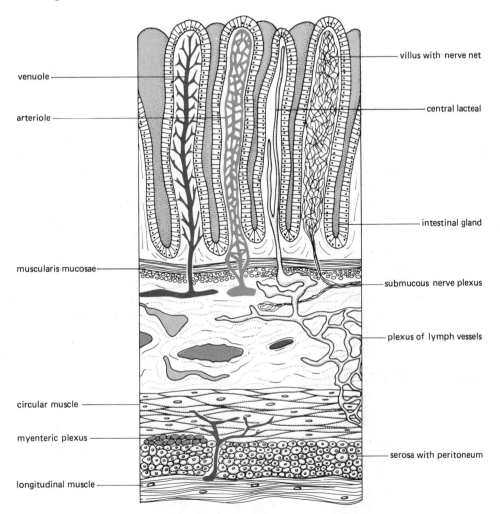

venuole

arteriole

muscularis mucosae

circular muscle

myenteric plexus

longitudinal muscle

villus with nerve net

central lacteal

intestinal gland

submucous nerve plexus

plexus of lymph vessels

serosa with peritoneum

Figure 4.9 Intestinal mucosa. Diagram of a cross section through the human small intestine. The villus on the extreme left shows the venous drainage and the adjacent villus shows the arterial supply. The third villus shows the central lateral of the lymphatic system. [From G. H. Bell, J. N. Davidson, and H. Scarborough, *Textbook of Physiology and Biochemistry*, Chapter 17, Williams & Wilkins Company, Baltimore, Md. (1961).]

or brush border is the final barrier to nutrient absorption and is the demarcation line as to "outside" and "inside" the body.

The intestinal mucosa facilitates the entry of nutrients from the "outside" by secreting into the intestinal lumen from between the villi enzymes that complete the digestive process. Secreted by the crypts of Lieberkühn are maltase, lactase, and sucrase. These enzymes promote the hydrolysis of the disaccharides to their constituent monosaccharides. Aminopeptidases and dipeptidases also secreted by cells of the intestinal mucosa complete the degradation of polypeptides and most dipeptides to amino acids (Figure 4.4). An intestinal β-lipase (Figure 4.5) completes the hydrolysis of most monoglycerides to a free fatty acid and glycerol. Intestinal nucleases, nucleotidases, and intracellular nucleosidases degrade the nucleic acids, DNA and RNA.

Digestion of Vitamins and Minerals

Unlike the major components of the diet, carbohydrates, proteins, and lipids, which comprise the majority of caloric intake and dietary bulk and undergo extensive chemical degradations, vitamins and minerals are subjected to only minor chemical changes. Vitamins such as riboflavin and biotin, which may be covalently attached to protein, may be hydrolyzed but otherwise are not degraded further. Folic acid, which may contain from two to six additional glutamic acid residues (polyglutamate) is absorbed as the monoglutamyl folate following hydrolysis (see "Folic Acid" Chapter 3). Minerals, either ionically or coordinate covalently bonded to proteins or carbohydrates, may be disassociated from proteins or carbohydrates during digestion. Some minerals will undergo redox reactions in the stomach and intestines due to changes in pH as in the case with Fe^{3+} reduction by dietary ascorbic acid, or have their oxidation state changed by other dietary components prior to absorption.

ABSORPTION OF NUTRIENTS

The principal end products of digestion—glucose, amino acids, fatty acids, monoglycerides, glycerol, nucleic acids, cholesterol, vitamins, and minerals—present in the intestinal lumen are absorbed by the cells of the intestinal mucosa and enter the general circulatory system by way of the capillary beds or lacteals of the villi. Absorption of the nutrients is a process of great complexity, often involving the participation of intracellular enzymes, transport proteins, and ion pumps. Despite the great complexity in each nutrient's individual absorption, absorption of all nutrients can be classified as occurring by either passive diffusion or by an active transport process requiring an expenditure of energy (Figure 4.10).

Passive diffusion from the intestinal lumen across the mucosal cell occurs only for some nutrients and drugs. This process is akin to that of osmosis, whereby selected nutrients move from an area of high concentration (the intestinal lumen) into a lower nutrient concentration in the capillary bed or lacteal, through the semipermeable membrane of the mucosal cells of the intestine. Most nutrients, however, move across the intestinal mucosal cells with great selectivity and expenditure of energy (ATP) despite an often favorable concentration gradient of nutrient for passive absorption. Here in the mucosal cell, a change in nutrient composition may take place prior to entry into the capillary bed or lymph system. A list of some nutrients and their manner of known absorption is given in Table 4.2.

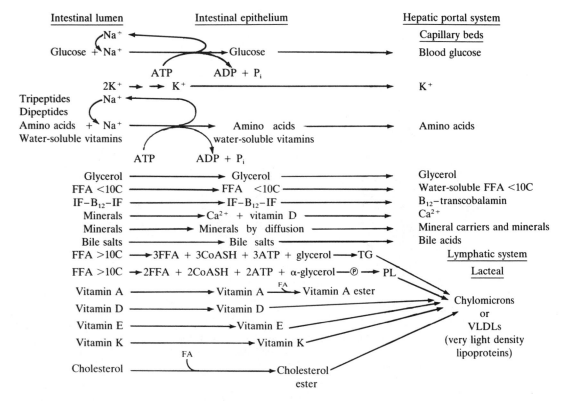

Figure 4.10 Absorption of nutrients.

Absorption of Carbohydrates

For most people, carbohydrates in the diet provide the largest contribution of total caloric need and singularly account for the largest nutrient mass ingested. Glucose is the most abundant dietary monosaccharide, present in mixed diets as a component of disaccharides, oligo- and polysaccharides. Lesser amounts of fructose, galactose, mannose, and other monosaccharides are to be found in the intestinal lumen. The absorption of glucose and most monosaccharides from the intestinal lumen of the duodenum across the microvilli to the capillary bed is by an active transport process requiring ATP and a sodium (Na^+) ion gradient.

Fiber

One of the largest components of the bulk diet of humans and certainly for animals with a rumen or cecum is cellulose. Like starch and glycogen, cellulose, the major structural component of the cell wall of plants, is a polysaccharide composed of glucose. Cellulose, however, remains indigestible by humans and monogastric

TABLE 4.2 NUTRIENT ABSORPTION[a]

Passive diffusion	Active transport
Fructose	Glucose
Mannose	Galactose
Xylose	Fatty acids (long chain)
Fatty acids (short chain)	Bile acids
Monoglycerides	Cholesterol
Nucleic acids	Amino acids
Ascorbic acid (high concentration)	Ascorbic acid
Niacin (high concentration)	Thiamin
Pyridoxine	Riboflavin
Vitamin A	Niacin
Vitamin D	Folate
Vitamin E	Vitamin B_{12} (intrinsic factor)
Vitamin K	Ca^{2+}
Cholesterol	Fe^{2+}
Bile salts	Zn^{2+}
Water	Na^+
Ca^{2+}	
Cu^+	
K^+	
Cl^-	

[a]Most nutrients are absorbed in the duodenum and ileum. Lipids, subject to the critical micelle formation in the presence of bile salts, are absorbed in the jejunal region.

animals who lack the enzyme β-(1→4) glycosidase, necessary for the hydrolysis of the β-(1→4) glycosides of cellulose. Ruminants and animals with a cecum have a digestive system populated with a microflora that synthesizes and secretes the β-(1→4) glycosidase and are thus able to hydrolyze the cellulose and absorb the glucose. In humans cellulose remains mostly nondigestible, is not absorbed, and has little or no caloric dietary value. Cellulose and other nondigestible components of the diet—hemicelluloses, pectin, lignin, gums, mucilages, algal polysaccharides, and others—constitute what has become collectively known as dietary fiber. There is no consensus on a specific definition of dietary fiber. This is because fiber has a diverse chemical composition and some fiber components, such as pectins and gums, are fermentable, yielding absorptive acids, aldehydes, and ketones. Some estimates from animals and human experimentation suggest that 50% of dietary fiber is degradable by bacterial enzymes and may be absorbed. For this reason the author's preferred definition of dietary fiber is "those carbohydrates and lignin remaining for excretion following digestion and absorption."

Dietary fiber has gained a reputation as a significant contributor to healthful dietary practices. Its additional inclusion to the diet is reported to assist constipation, appendicitis, diverticulitis, hemorrhoids, polyps, ulcers, cancer, and metabolic diseases. Added dietary fiber helps constipation and probably diverticulitis. Other health claims for fiber do not seem to be substantiated. One real beneficial effect of fiber added to the diet is the reduction in caloric density of the diet being consumed (see Chapter 9).

Absorption of Protein as Amino Acids, Di- and Tripeptides

Gastrointestinal proteins are hydrolyzed to their constituent amino acids, di- and tripeptides. Soluble proteins and proteins that have been denatured are most readily hydrolyzed. All of the digestive enzymes, components of the pancreas, mucosal secretions, and exfoliated tissues of the intestinal lumen are subject to digestion right along with dietary protein. The amino acids di- and tripeptide released from all these sources are absorbed by an active-transport (ATP) sodium (Na^+)-ion-dependent system. Passing through the microvilli, the di- and tripeptides undergo intracellular hydrolysis, and with the remaining amino acids they enter the capillary bed of the villi. Each amino acid shares its transport system through the microvilli with other amino acids, based on similarity in structural and chemical characteristics. Only a small number of basic transport systems are needed for the absorption of both the D- and L-isomers of the amino acids. Small peptides and, to a very small extent, proteins may be absorbed. Proteins, as immunoglobulins, may be absorbed from maternal milk colostrum following birth, and protein absorption may be the cause of some food allergies.

Absorption of Lipids

The absorption of lipids and the products of lipid digestion from the intestinal lumen is complex, owing to the variety of lipids in the diet, the participation of the bile salts in micelle formation, and the intracellular synthesis of triglycerides within the microvilli (Figure 4.11).

Dietary lipids and the products of lipid digestion, free fatty acids, monoglycerides, cholesterol, phospholipids, and the lipid-soluble vitamins, combine with the bile salts synthesized in the liver to form round microdroplets approximately 50 Å in diameter. These microdroplets, called micelles, are formed by the dietary lipids and bile salts in preparation for absorption by the microvilli. Micelles contain all the products of lipid digestion, with the exclusion of the shorter-chain free fatty acids (FFAs) and glycerol, both of which are water soluble. Free fatty acids of 10 or less carbons $(<C_{10})$ and glycerol may pass directly through the microvilli and into the capillary bed of the villus entering the general hepatic portal circulation.

Monoglycerides and free fatty acids $(>C_{10})$ entering the microvilli are reassembled into triglycerides. For the synthesis of triglycerides, free fatty acids are activated by the formation of a fatty acid acetylcoenzyme A (FA-CoA). The formation of each FA-CoA requires activation by ATP. This reaction predominates for the long-chain free fatty acids, which are then esterified with a β-monoglyceride, forming newly synthesized triacylglycerides.

Free intracellular glycerol may also be esterified with activated (FA-CoA)

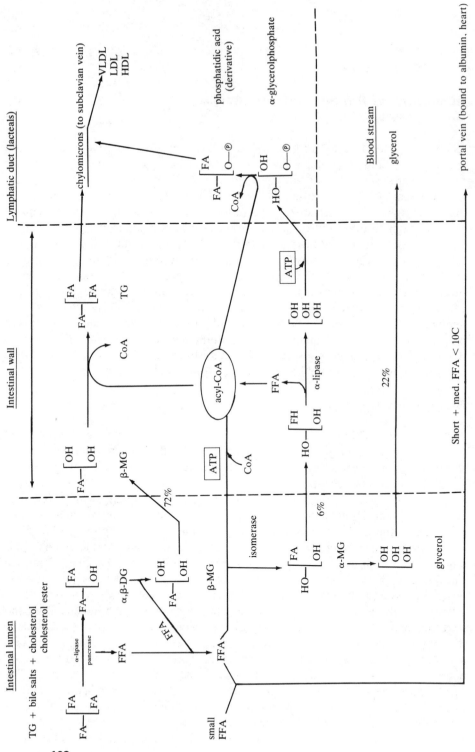

Figure 4.11 Absorption of lipids. Modified from F. H. Mattson and R. A. Volpenheim. The Digestion and Absorption of Triglycerides, *J. Biological Chemistry 239*, 2722 (1964); and F. J. Stare, Ed., *Atherosclerosis*, Medcom, Inc., New York (1974).

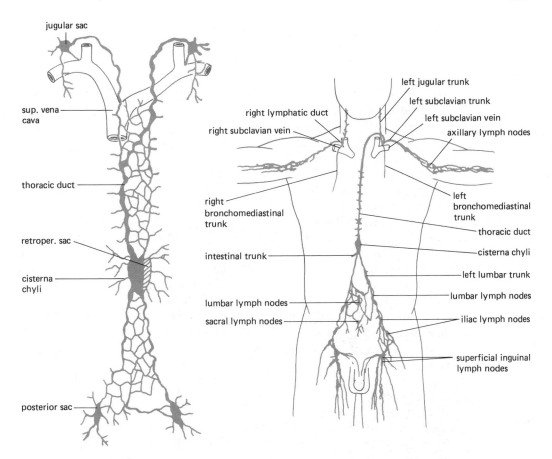

Figure 4.12 Primary lymphatic vessels in humans. (Left) Diagram of the definitive thoracic duct emerging from a lymphatic plexus. From L. B. Arey, Developmental Anatomy, 7th ed., W. B. Saunders Company, Philadelphia, Pa. (1965). (Right) Diagram of the larger lymphatic ducts of the body, showing entry into the subclavian vein. (Reprinted, by permission, from Benninghoff and Goerttler, *Lehrbuch der Anatomie des Menschen*, 10th ed., © 1975, Urban & Schwarzenberg, Baltimore-Munich.) Lipids absorbed by the intestinal villi traverse the lymphatic system and thoracic duct and reenter the circulatory system via the left subclavian vein.

fatty acids. In this pathway, glycerol is phosphorylated by ATP, forming α-glycerolphosphates. Two FA-CoAs are esterified with α-glycerolphosphate, forming α-phosphatidic acid. Dephosphorylation and reaction with an additional FA-CoA completes the synthesis of a triglyceride. Triglycerides assembled within the microvilli enter the lacteal of the villi as chylomicrons and lipoprotein complexes: the very light density lipoprotein (VLDL). From the lacteals the chylomicrons and VLDLs transverse the lymphatic system to the thoracic duct, in which lymph and lipids enter the general systemic circulation through the left subclavian vein (Figure 4.12).

Absorption of the Lipid-Soluble Vitamins

Vitamins A, D, E, and K, being hydrophobic, are absorbed predominately in association with micelles. Micelles formed in the presence of the bile salts, phospholipids, monoglycerides, free fatty acids, and cholesterol also include in their composition the lipid-soluble vitamins and previtamin A, β-carotene. Carried by the chylomicrons, the fat-soluble vitamins enter the lymphatic system and after joining the circulatory system, they are deposited in the liver.

Vitamin A is freed of its esterified fatty acid by retinyl esterase (Figure 4.6) before its inclusion in micellar formation. After entering the microvilli, free vitamin A is reesterified by FA-CoA, forming a new retinyl ester, generally palmitate, and is then included in the chylomicron for lymphatic transport. Approximately 80 to 90% of dietary vitamin A is absorbed in the small intestine, and 75% is reesterified in the mucosal cells. The chylomicrons also carry the remaining 25% unesterified retinol. β-Carotene is absorbed with approximately 50 to 60% efficiency in the intestinal mucosa, where it is symmetrically cleaved by a dioxygenase (Figure 3.23). The two molecules of retinol formed are reduced to retinal by an $NADH_2$ or $NADPH_2$ reductase upon which it is then esterified. Uncleaved β-carotene also enters the chylomicron and the lymphatic system. Vitamin D is absorbed from the intestinal lumen with approximately 50% efficiency. It is incorporated unchanged into the chylomicron prior to entering the lacteal of the lymphatic system.

Vitamin E esters and their isomers (tocopheryls) are hydrolyzed by an esterase, producing free succinic or acetic acids and vitamin E prior to absorption by micelles. About 30% of the free tocopheryls are absorbed and they are not reesterified prior to chylomicron formation.

Like the other lipid-soluble vitamins, vitamin K is absorbed into the mixed micelle. About 50% of the exogenous vitamin K from dietary sources and vitamin K synthesized endogenously by the intestinal microflora is absorbed. Absorption rates and mode of absorption vary considerably depending on the chemistry of the vitamin K analog. Vitamin K is also transported in the lymph by the chylomicron.

Absorption of Cholesterol

The dietary intake of cholesterol varies considerably between individuals, but averages about 600 mg per day, consisting of free cholesterol and cholesterol esters. In the presence of liver bile and a pancreatic esterase, cholesterol esters are hydrolyzed, producing free cholesterol and a single fatty acid. The free cholesterol is incorporated within the mixed-lipid micelles and is absorbed by passive diffusion into the microvilli. About one-half of all dietary cholesterol is absorbed in this manner. The remaining cholesterol is excreted through the feces. Prior to excretion, cholesterol may undergo bacterial reduction to coprostanol and cholestanol neutral sterol isomers (Figure 4.13). The free fatty acid may reappear as

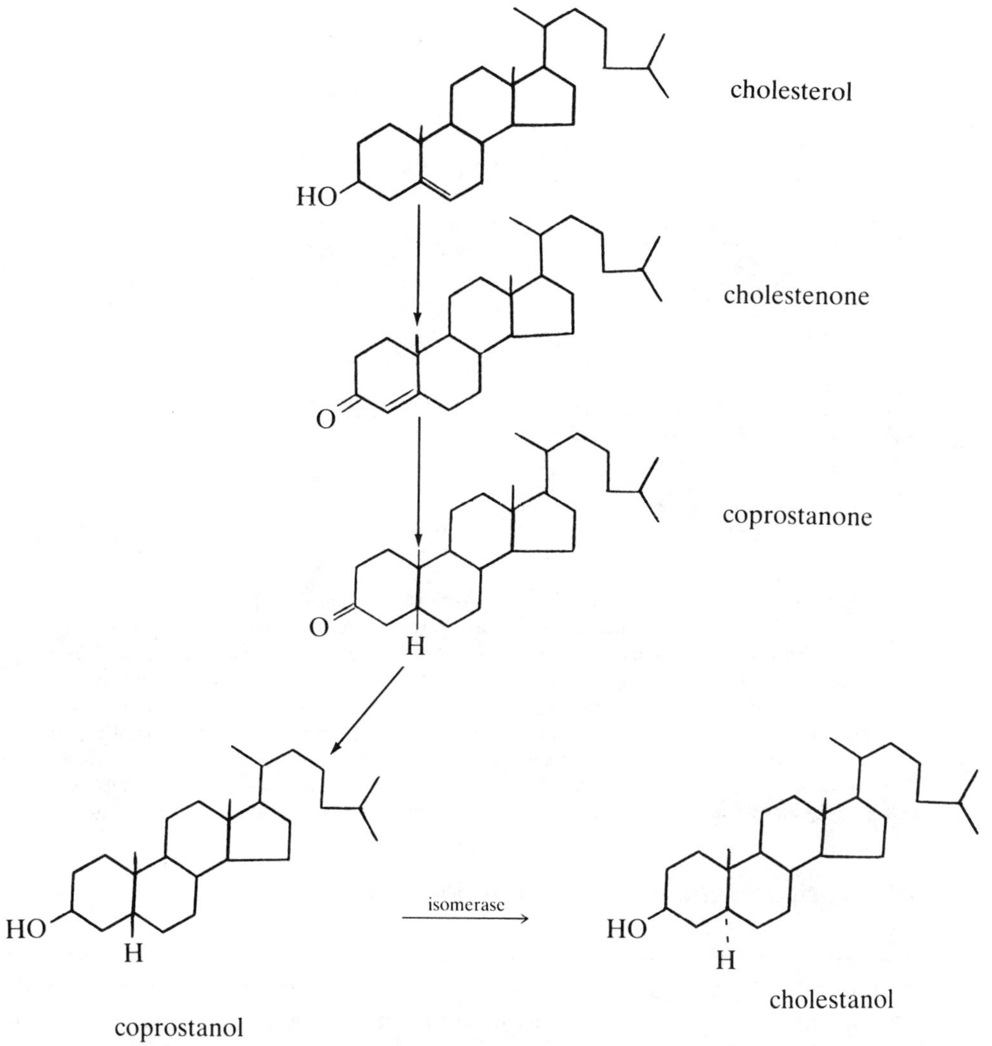

Figure 4.13 Excretory cholesterol metabolites of the intestinal microflora. Coprostanol and cholestanol are the excretory metabolites, accounting for ca. 1% of ingested cholesterol.

part of a newly synthesized triglyceride or be reesterified to cholesterol within the microvilli.

Cholesterol esters resynthesized within the microvilli are incorporated into the chylomicrons, and VLDLs and enter the lacteals as described previously. Chylomicrons are comprised of 2 to 7% cholesterol and VLDLs contain 6 to 12% cholesterol. Approximately 11 g of cholesterol circulates within the lipoproteins found in blood (Table 4.3, Figure 4.14).

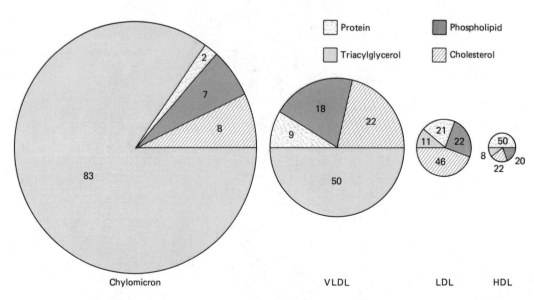

Figure 4.14 Composition of the lipoproteins. The chemical composition and size ranges of the different classes of human serum lipoproteins. As the particle size decreases, the ratio of protein to fat increases and the density also increases. Chylomicrons are the carriers of absorbed dietary fat and are synthesized in the intestine. Very low-density lipoproteins (VLDLs) originate mainly in the liver and carry fats synthesized there from carbohydrates. Low-density lipoproteins (LDLs) are the main carriers of cholesterol to peripheral tissues. High-density lipoproteins (HDLs) carry cholesterol to the liver for degradation. (Reproduced from *Lipid Biochemistry: An Introduction*, by M. I. Ginn and A. T. James, 1980, with permission of Chapman & Hall, Publishers, London, England.)

Absorption of the Water-Soluble Vitamins

The water-soluble vitamins, vitamin C and the vitamin B-complex, are efficiently absorbed by the normal gastrointestinal tract. When present in normal physiological concentrations, most B vitamins and vitamin C appear to be efficiently and predominantly absorbed by an active-transport sodium (Na$^+$)-ion-dependent ATPase system. When present in excessive dietary (pharmacologic) amounts, the vitamin carrier systems appear to become saturated, and absorption is increased by passive diffusion. Under such conditions absorption efficiency is generally decreased but total absorption of vitamins is enhanced.

Vitamin C is actively transported by a Na$^+$-dependent ATP system. With dietary intakes of less than 180 mg per day, about 80% of vitamin C is absorbed. When 1 g or more of vitamin C is found in the daily diet, absorption is reduced to 50%.

Thiamin, vitamin B$_1$, is probably absorbed at physiological concentrations via an ATP sodium (Na$^+$)-ion transport system. Absorbed as free thiamin, it is

TABLE 4.3   COMPOSITION OF THE LIPOPROTEINS[a]

Lipoprotein	Sedimentation density[b]	Diameter (nm)	Triglyceride	Composition (%) phospholipid	Cholesterol	Protein
Chylomicron	0.95	100	80–95	7	8	1–2
Very light density (VLDL)	1.00	55	50–80	15–18	10–22	9–10
Low density (LDL)	1.05	22	7–8	18–22	46	21–25
High density (HDL)	1.18	15	2–3	30	20	45–50

[a]Values for sedimentation densities and diameters are approximate averages. Note the relationship of lipoproteins between sedimentation density and diameter; density and triglyceride content (see also Figure 4.14). Data compiled from various references showing ranges.
[b]H_2O = 1.0 g/cc.

phosphorylated en route into the epithelial mucosa of the microvilli, appearing as thiamin pyrophosphate (TPP). A pyrophosphatase produces free thiamin again for entry into the hepatic portal circulation.

Riboflavin, vitamin B_2, present in FMN or FAD in the intestinal lumen, must be freed by enzymatic hydrolysis prior to absorption. In the microvilli, absorbed free riboflavin is phosphorylated by ATP, forming FMN just prior to entering the hepatic portal circulation.

Niacin and NAD^+, vitamin B_6, biotin, and pantothenic acid appear to easily enter the microvilli and hepatic portal circulation system by passive diffusion. An active transport mechanism, however, could be operative for these vitamins at very low vitamin concentrations.

Folic acid absorption is by an active transport process at low luminal concentrations. Prior to absorption by the microvilli, folic acid is present in the intestinal lumen as dietary pteroylpolyglutamic acid. Folate polyglutamate (containing several glutamic acid residues in peptide linkage) must be hydrolyzed to a folate monoglutamate prior to absorption. Folic acid (5-methyltetrahydropteroylglutamate) in the reduced form (5-methyl-THFA) is released into and circulates in blood plasma.

Vitamin B_{12}, cyanocobalamin, absorption is unique among the water-soluble vitamins in that active transport requires a glycoprotein (MW 50,000) to bind vitamin B_{12} (intrinsic factor, IF) and absorption occurs in the ileum, whereas all other vitamins are absorbed predominantly in the duodenum and jejunum. Absorption of vitamin B_{12} may occur by diffusion if luminal concentrations are high. Prior to combining with IF, vitamin B_{12} is hydrolyzed from its attachment to protein. The binding of vitamin B_{12} to IF and its dimethylation renders the vitamin B_{12}–IF complex resistant to proteolytic enzymes. With the assistance of Ca^{2+}, the vitamin

B_{12}–IF complex binds to ileal receptors and vitamin B_{12} enters the microvilli. Vitamin B_{12} transverses the microvilli and then enters the plasma of the hepatic portal system, where it circulates bound to specific proteins, the transcobalamins.

Absorption of Minerals

Minerals are absorbed by either passive or active transport systems through the intestinal mucosa often using specialized transport proteins, as in the case for Fe^{3+}-ferritin and the hormonal control of Ca^{2+} absorption by vitamin D. Absorption of various metal ions is often competitive, as they compete for transport ligands (Table 3.13). Such is the case for zinc and copper, whose absorption is mediated by a primary intestinal metallothionin protein. Absorption of minerals is also affected by a variety of antagonisms: ionic state, organic molecules, and fiber. For additional information on mineral absorption, the reader is referred to sections on the various nutrients in Chapter 3.

5

Mammalian and Plant Cells

THE MAMMALIAN CELL

The products of animal and human digestion are required for the synthesis of new biomolecules, the replacement of excreted essential nutrients, and the energy (calories) for all cellular and organ functions. The nutrients encounter their final barrier, the cell plasma membrane, prior to entering major metabolic pathways. The variety and function of cells within the human body is extensive, with most cells highly specialized to perform specific functions. Each cell has its specific metabolic activity for its own specialized function. There is no cell that performs all metabolic processes. The human liver cell, however, performs a great many metabolic functions and contains the major metabolic pathways for the synthesis and degradation of carbohydrates, protein, fats, and nucleic acids. The liver degrades heme and metabolizes cholesterol, synthesizing the bile acids, which become bile salts. It converts ammonia to urea and detoxifies drugs. The liver, in addition to its other specialized metabolic functions, stores nutrients such as glycogen, vitamins A and D, and iron. Better than any other cell, the liver cell typifies a general metabolic cell.

Figure 5.1 is a representation of a general mammalian metabolic cell, such as a hepatocyte, which would contain the major cellular organelles and metabolic pathways. Each cell is surrounded by a plasma membrane, the final barrier to the nutrients prior to their metabolism. The plasma membrane is a lipid bilayer with the inclusion of proteins and enzymes. Proteins, carbohydrates, and metals comprise and serve as membrane receptors for hormones, nutrients, and metabolites. Like the plasma membrane of the microvilli of the small intestine, nutrients

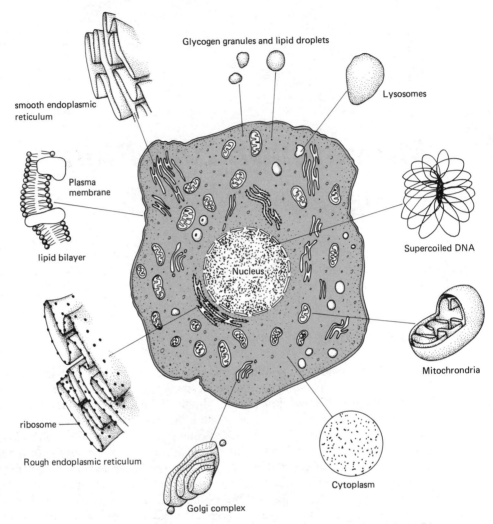

Glycogen granules and lipid droplets

Lysosomes

smooth endoplasmic
reticulum

Plasma
membrane

Supercoiled DNA

lipid bilayer

Nucleus

Mitochrondria

ribosome

Rough endoplasmic reticulum

Cytoplasm

Golgi complex

Figure 5.1 Microanatomy of a typical mammalian cell. (Adapted from *Bio-chemistry*, 2nd ed., A. L. Lehninger, Worth Publishers, Inc., 1975, reprinted with permission.)

and metabolites move into and out of metabolic cells by passive and facilitative diffusion or an active transport system requiring ATP. In maintaining electrical neutrality, ions, particularly Na^+, K^+, and Cl^-, are moved in and out of the cell, sometimes with an expenditure of energy from ATP.

Organelles, components of the cell that comprise the microanatomy, carry out the specialized functions within the cell. All of the organelles bathe in the fluid portion of the cell, the cytoplasm. Contained in the cytoplasm are the aqueous nutrients, ions, and enzymes of glycolysis and the gluconeogenic pathway, the hexosemonophosphate shunt, and the enzymes for the synthesis of fatty acids from acetyl-CoA. The enzymes of the citric acid cycle, β-oxidation, faty acid elongation, and electron transport system are located within the mitochondrion. It is within mitochondria that most ATP is synthesized. Mitochondria are abundant and metabolically active in cells requiring ATP and are few in number in metabolically less active cells.

Both the smooth and rough endoplasmic reticula of cells are metabolically active. Within the channels of the smooth endoplasmic reticulum are synthesized lipids: cholesterol and steroids. The rough endoplasmic reticulum is recognizable by the presence of ribosomes. Here in the ribosomes are assembled the proteins from amino acids.

The Golgi complex of the cell appears to "package" enzymes and zymogens for secretion and is highly concentrated in specialized secretory cells. The Golgi inclusions are often associated with the rough endoplasmic reticulum "packaging" and modify proteins by the addition of lipids (lipoproteins) and carbohydrates (glycoproteins) prior to secretion. In addition, the Golgi apparatus may assist in the synthesis and formation of new plasma membrane.

Some cells may contain lysosomes. Lysosomes contain lysozyme and other degradative enzymes. The function of lysosomes is the digestion of foreign debris that may be engulfed by the cell during phagocytosis. Lysosomes have been called "suicide sacs," for upon cell death, lysosomal enzymes are released and autodegradation of cell material ensues.

Governing the totality of cellular activity is the cell's nucleus. Isolated from the cytoplasm by its nuclear membrane, the nucleus contains all the genetic material, deoxyribonucleic acid (DNA), except for a small amount found in mitochondria. Within the nucleus, replication and transcription take place. Replication of DNA takes place during cell division, and transcription yields ribonucleic acids (RNA) for protein synthesis. Also located within the cytoplasm are storage depots of energy which are mobilized as required. Glycogen granules and droplets of lipids, triglycerides, are present in highly active mammalian metabolic cells.

THE PLANT CELL

There also exists no one typical plant cell, yet there is less diversity and specialization of cell function within plants than within the cells and organs of the animal kingdom. Plants generally possess much of the same metabolism that many animal cells perform and do so with an architectural array of similar organelles. Figure 5.2 is representative of a typical plant cell from a soybean leaf. The plant cell contains organelles similar to the mammalian cell, including cytoplasm, mitochondrion, rough endoplasmic reticulum, Golgi complex, and nucleus. The plant cell may also contain inclusions of lipid droplets and carbohydrate (starch) granules. The plant cell is not equivalent to any mammalian cell and differs by synthesizing specialized pigments, plant hormones, metabolites, and macromolecules.

Structurally, the plant cell is different from mammalian cells in possessing a rigid cell wall, glyoxysomes, vacuoles, and chloroplasts. The plant's cell wall is rigid, to withstand the hydrostatic pressures of turgor. Much of the plant's cell wall is comprised of cellulose, the most abundant biomolecule. Much of the remaining structural content of the mature plant cell wall is lignin, a major component of wood. Pectins, methylated polymers of glucuronic acid and galacturonic acid, and hemicelluloses, polymers of arabinose, galactose, mannose, and xylose, comprise the cell walls. These components of the cell wall, it may be recalled, constitute dietary fiber (see Chapter 9).

The glyoxysome is a plant organelle not found in mammalian cells. When found in plant cells, the glyoxysome contains the enzymes of the glyoxylate cycle, which converts fatty acids into acetate and oxaloacetate by β-oxidation. Oxaloacetate is then converted to phosphoenolpyruvate, which leads to glucose (gluconeogenesis).

The predominant feature of plant cells that sets them apart from mammalian cells is the presence of cellular chloroplasts, the synthesis of photoreceptive pigments, and direct utilization of light energy for the synthesis of ATP. The chloroplast is an assembly of photoreceptive stacks, or grana, composed of thylakoid discs (Figure 6.4). The stacked thylakoids contain chlorophyl, the primary photoreceptive pigment, secondary photoreceptive pigments, and the components and enzymes of cyclic phosphorylation. Acyclic phosphorylation is thought to be located on the lamellae between thylakoids. The chloroplasts of algae and plants and the mitochondria of plants, animals, and humans are functionally alike in their synthesis of ATP, and function differently only with respect to their source of energy for phosphorylation.

ANIMAL AND PLANT METABOLISM

The sum of all chemical events within a living animal or plant cell is what is referred to as metabolism. Cellular metabolism has the purpose of maintaining the homeostasis of the cell within a population of other cells. Metabolism occurs in a freely open system with an active exchange of energy, essential nutrients, metabolites, and metabolic waste materials between the cell and its environment.

Metabolism can generally be subdivided into anabolic and catabolic metabolism. Anabolic metabolism, anabolism, is the building up of macromolecules e.g., protein synthesis from amino acids. Anabolic metabolism generally requires an expenditure of energy (ATP), which results in increased cellular organization and a decline in internal entropy (S). Catabolic metabolism, catabolism, is the degradation of large and small biomolecules e.g., proteins to amino acids. Catabolic metabolism generally results in the cellular synthesis of ATP and an increase in the entropy (S) of the molecules that are undergoing catabolism.

Anabolic and catabolic metabolic pathways are generally determined by their

TABLE 5.1 MAJOR METABOLIC PATHWAYS OF PLANTS AND ANIMALS AND THEIR RELATIONSHIP TO ENERGY, ENTROPY, AND REDUCTIVE CAPACITY

Pathway	ATP	S (internal) cell	S (environment)[a]	NADPH + H+[b]	NADH + H+, FADH$_2$ FMNH$_2$[b]
Anabolic					
Glycogenesis	Consumed[c]	−	+	Used	
Gluconeogenesis	Consumed[c]	−	+	Used	
Fatty acid synthesis	Consumed[c]	−	+	Used	
Protein biosynthesis	Consumed[c]	−	+	Used	
Sterol biosynthesis	Consumed[c]	−	+	Used	
Cyclic phosphorylation	Generated[c,d]	−	+	Produced	
Noncyclic phosphorylation	Generated[c,d]	−	+	Produced	
Calvin cycle	Consumed[c]	−	+	Used	
Catabolic					
Glycogenolysis	Generated[e]	+	+		Produced
Glycolysis	Generated[e]	+	+		Produced
β-Oxidation	Generated[e]	+	+		Produced
Oxidative deaminations	Generated[e]	+	+		Produced
Citric acid cycle	Generated[e]	+	+		Produced
Electron transport	Generated[e]	+	+		Produced

[a]$NADPH + H^+ \rightarrow NADP^+$.

[b]$NAD^+ + 2H \rightarrow NADH + H^+$; $FAD + 2H \rightarrow FADH_2$; $FMN + 2H \rightarrow FMNH_2$.

[c]$ATP \rightarrow ADP + P_i$.

[d]Cyclic and noncyclic phosphorylation is anabolic at the expense of solar energy and increased solar entropy.

[e]$ADP + P_i \rightarrow ATP$.

biosynthetic or degradative activity and whether ATP is consumed or generated in the process. As a general condition, anabolic processes require energy (ATP) and catabolic processes yield energy (ATP). The names of the major anabolic and catabolic metabolic pathways and the relationships between oxidation, reduction, energy utilization, and entropy is shown in Table 5.1.

Anabolic pathways generally consume ATP and contribute to a decreased net cellular entropy at the expense of an increase in environmental (external) entropy, and such chemical processes utilize and consume $NADPH + H^+$. Anabolic pathways are generally pathways of reduction. Quantitatively, the largest reductive pathway is the reduction of carbon dioxide by the Calvin cycle in photosynthesis, described in Chapter 6. For plants, ATP synthesis can be considered anabolic, for the energy for most of plant ATP synthesis originates with the solar energy falling on plant leaves.

Catabolic pathways in both plants and animals yield a net synthesis of ATP at the expense of an increase in the internal cellular entropy and in total environmental entropy. Major catabolic pathways produce $NADH + H^+$, $FADH_2$, or $FMNH_2$ from the oxidation of substrates, generally carbohydrates and amino and fatty acids. For the biological world as a whole, the overall process of photosynthesis is shown in Equation 5.1.

Equation 5.1
General photosynthesis/energy equation.

$$6CO_2 + 6H_2O + (N) + \text{solar energy } (h\nu) + ATP$$

$$\rightarrow C_6H_{12}O_6 \text{ (proteins (N); lipids)} + 6O_2 \uparrow + ADP + P_i$$

Photosynthesis may be viewed as *the* major anabolic process whereby CO_2 is reduced by $NADPH + H^+$ to form carbohydrates, to be followed by the synthesis of proteins and lipids. This process is carried out only by phototrophs and is accomplished extensively by algae, plankton, and higher plants.

Animals and humans, the chemotrophs, utilize the energy stored in plants— carbohydrates, protein, and lipids—by oxidizing these organic compounds, with the concurrent release of energy, which is partially conserved and transferred to ATP.

Equation 5.2
General oxidation/energy equation.

$$C_6H_{12}O_6 \text{ (proteins:lipids)} + O_2 + ADP + P_i \rightarrow 6CO_2 \uparrow$$

$$+ H_2O + (N) + ATP + \text{heat}$$

The oxidation of carbohydrates, protein, and lipids in Equation 5.2 is a summation of the respiratory process of either plants, animals, or humans. Respiration and oxidative phosphorylation is the metabolic opposite of photosynthesis and reduction

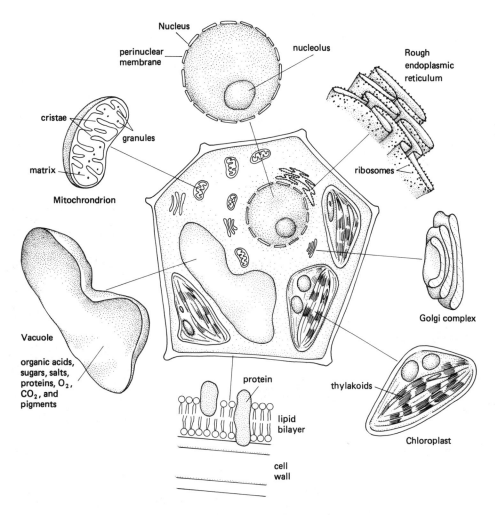

Figure 5.2 Microanatomy of a typical plant cell.   Adapted from *Biochemistry*,
2nd ed., A. L. Lehninger, Worth Publishers, Inc., 1975, reprinted with permission.

of CO_2 by plants.   The only thermodynamic difference between photosynthesis
and respiration is the liberation of heat in Equation 5.2.   Heat is liberated because
respiration and oxidation phosphorylation is not 100% efficient in converting food
energy into ATP energy.   The summation of energy on both sides of Equations
5.1 and 5.2 is, however, equal.   The metabolic and energy relationships between
phototrophs (plants) and organic chemotrophs (humans) are shown in Figure 5.3.

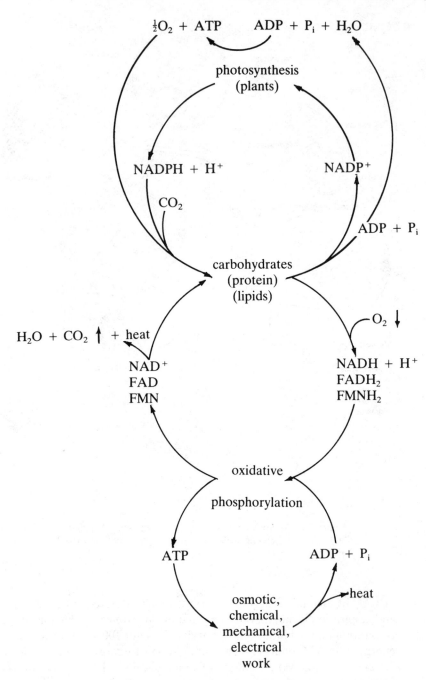

Figure 5.3 Interrelationship of photosynthesis with animal/human respiration.

METABOLIC MAPS

Highway maps produced by cartographers are necessary when driving into unfamiliar country. National maps show the federal interstate highway system and its interchanges at major cities, and state highway maps reveal only a state's portion of the interstate highway system. You do see on state highway maps detail of primary and secondary state roads, and additionally, smaller cities and towns are located on these maps. Maps of cities, both large and small, provide detailed information on local travel and often provide the names of individual streets. Metabolic charts, which are hung on office walls in nutrition and biochemistry departments, are cellular road maps. They show us where metabolic trips begin and end. They take us through both the major and less important metabolic cities. They show metabolic crossroads and side trips to be taken, and major routes may have to be examined carefully to be navigated successfully. Like real highways, some metabolic roads have hills which require energy to overcome and which we can coast down later. Some metabolic roads even have two-way traffic, properly separated, of course.

In the following chapters, I hope you will view the metabolic pathways as highway maps. Major cities on our map are glucose, triglyceride, ribulose-5-phosphate, the amino acid cities (i.e., valine, tyrosine, lysine, etc.), α-ketoglutarate, cholesterol, oxaloacetate, the tri-city ketones, and glycerol, among others. These metabolic cities are found on the major metabolic highways: glycolysis, β-oxidation, Calvin and citric acid cycles, sterol synthesis, electron transport, and so on. Metabolic highways are serviced by ATP, $NAD^+/NADH_2$, $NADP^+/NADPH_2$, vitamins B_6 and B_{12}, and so on. Major interchanges are to be also found, and none is more important on our metabolic map than acetyl coenzyme A. Happy metabolic motoring!

6

Photosynthesis

ENERGY TRANSFER

Located just 93×10^6 miles (150×10^6 km) from Earth (next door by astronomical distances) is a middle-aged star, our sun. Driven by hydrogen fusion ($1H^4 \rightarrow {}_2He^4 + 2e^-$) the sun's surface temperature is raised to about 10,800°F (6000°C). From its surface is emitted a continuous flow of thermal, ultraviolet, and visible energy in discrete energy packets called quanta. Calculations estimate that the emission of all forms of solar energy is equivalent to 7.2×10^{31} cal per day. Each day Earth receives about $5 \times 10^{-13}\%$ of the total emitted solar energy. The land area of Earth receives approximately 30% of each day's allocation of solar energy, equivalent to 1.1×10^{21} cal. More than 99.9% of all this solar energy received on Earth is either absorbed as heat, reflected back into space, or is used to drive our weather systems, consisting of evaporation, precipitation, and the convection currents of air and oceans. Of the remaining 0.1% of solar energy, 0.00005% is captured, stored, and utilized by algae and higher plants in a metabolic process called photosynthesis. All biologically useful energy enters and begins its journey through food chains by the photosynthetic process. With the exception of direct energy solar power conversion, nuclear power, wind power, tidal power, hydro-electromechanical power, and gravitational attraction, all other energy is supplied from the fossil fuels: oil, natural gas, and coal. These hydrocarbon energy sources are the remnants of the photosynthetic plants and animals (?) existing millions of years ago. Energy derived from these fossil fuels are irreplaceable; once used, they are gone forever. By contrast, energy sources derived from photosynthesis— foods, nonfossil fuels, and fiber—are forever renewable on a seasonal or annual

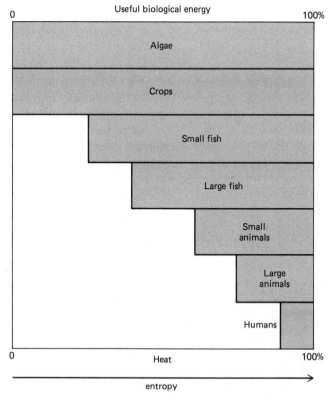

Figure 6.1 Energy transfer within a food chain.

basis. Energy trapped by algae and higher plants by photosynthesis may enter a complex food web of nature or an agricultural food chain devised by humans. Energy transfer through a food chain from algae and crop plants to humans is shown in Figure 6.1. In this hypothetical food chain, energy stored by photosynthesis by algae and cereal grains would be 100% transferable if eaten by humans. Energy transferred between levels of a food chain, between the primary energy producers (plants) and humans may result in a 60% loss of the energy stored in each preceding level of organization. Such organization of food chains makes it clear that a large agricultural base must be sustained and remain productive to supply energy to an ever-growing human population.

PHOTOSYNTHESIS PROCESS

Plants, in the presence of sunlight, with adequate carbon dioxide and water, initially photosynthesize carbohydrates and can then use this carbohydrate energy to synthesize proteins and lipids. Photosynthesis is generally expressed by Equation 6.1.

Equation 6.1
Equation of photosynthesis.

$$6CO_2 + 6H_2O \xrightarrow{h\nu} C_6H_{12}O_6 + 6O_2 \uparrow$$

In this equation the organic product is glucose and the oxygen gas evolved is derived from water. Nearly all atmospheric oxygen is produced by plants from water by photosynthesis. The carbon dioxide is provided to the plants by the atmosphere from oxidations and animal and human respiration. Water is absorbed in higher plants from the soil by roots. Light ($h\nu$) energy is provided by the sun in quanta, discrete units of light energy sufficient to excite electrons. Photosynthesis is a dynamic process of plants which is affected by light intensity, temperature, and availability of carbon dioxide. For descriptive purposes the photosynthetic process is often divided into two major sets of chemical equations: (1) the light reactions and (2) the dark reactions. In plants, both light and dark reactions are operative in the presence of light, but in the absence of sufficient light only the dark reactions are operative.

Light Reactions

The light reactions are the "photo" half of photosynthesis in plants and are shown in Figure 6.2. Light energy ($h\nu$) falling on a plant's cellular surface is absorbed by the plant and converted to chemical (ATP) energy. The selective absorption of light energy of the wavelengths 400 to 525 nm and 600 to 680 nm are accomplished by the primary photosensitive pigments, chlorophylls a and b, and accessory pigments, the carotenoids (β-carotene) and the xanthophylls (Figure 6.3). Absorbed light energy is transferred within the plant's thylakoid and chloroplast (Figure 6.4) at photoreactive center I to an electron (e^-). The light energy transferred to e^- causes it to be excited, and it is raised to a higher energy level and a primary electron acceptor, PEA. This process is equivalent to using a large rubber mallet at the county fair (light) to raise the ringer (e^-) to the bell (PEA). With the potential energy raised, the e^- travels through a series of electron carriers, cytochromes, to which is coupled the enzymatic capacity for the synthesis of ATP from ADP and P_i. As a result of this process, called *cyclic phosphorylation*, some of the light energy transferred to the e^- is captured, stored, and retained by the chloroplast as molecules of ATP. To the extent that it occurs within the thylakoids in plants, cyclic phosphorylation requires only photocenter I and its accompaniment of enzymes and electron carriers.

Synthesis of ATP by *noncyclic phosphorylation* requires the integration of both photoreactive centers I and II (Figure 6.2). In noncyclic phosphorylation, photoreactive center II, found in the intergranal lamella, absorbs light, and an excited electron is (e^-) raised to a higher potential energy level. This e^- cascades through a portion of the same electron carrier system as that responsible for the synthesis of ATP by cyclic phosphorylation, terminating in an electron void left by

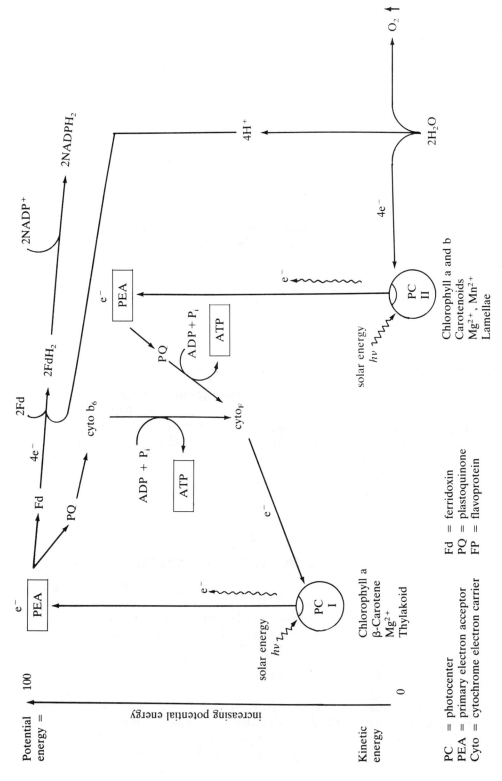

Figure 6.2 Light reactions of photosynthesis (schematically simplified).

PC = photocenter
PEA = primary electron acceptor
Cyto = cytochrome electron carrier

Fd = ferridoxin
PQ = plastoquinone
FP = flavoprotein

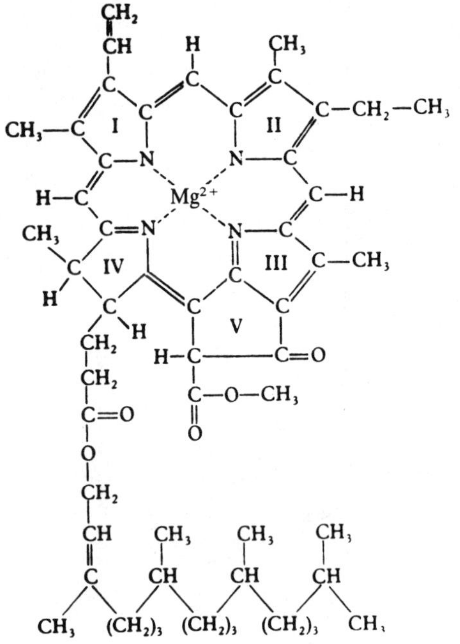

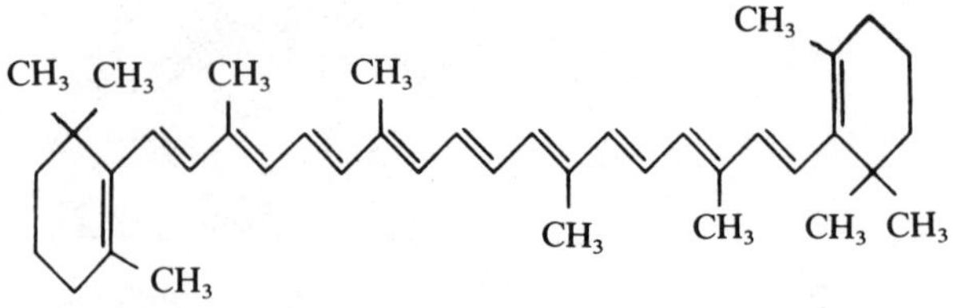

β-Carotene

Responsible for autumn folage color and precursor to vitamin A. β-Carotene, a carotenoid, absorbs light energy with transference to chlorophyll.

Chlorophyll a

Chlorophyll a is the major photoreceptive pigment in plants and is responsible for our green world. Replacement of —CH$_3$ in ring II by —CHO produces chlorophyll b. The chlorophylls are a major source of dietary magnesium.

Note: The extensive use of isoprene, a five-carbon monomeric unit (see Chapter 3), is demonstrated here in the side chain of chlorophyll, β-carotene, and spiralloxanthin.

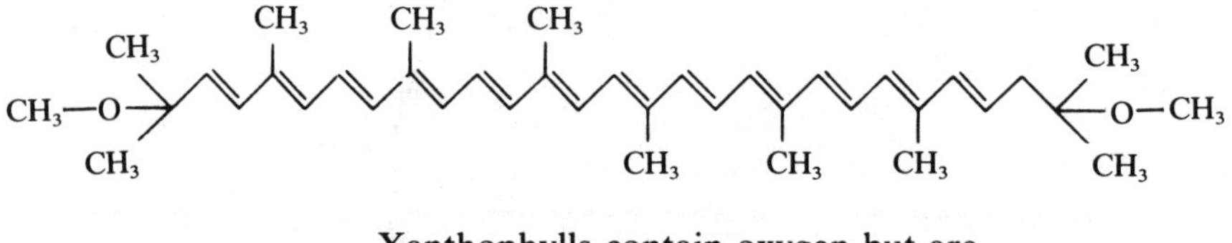

Xanthophylls contain oxygen but are otherwise similar to the carotenoids. This xanthophyll is spirilloxanthin.

Figure 6.3 Chlorophyll and the secondary light-absorbing pigments.

the excitation of an e$^-$ from photoreactive center I. In this process ATP is synthesized from ADP and P$_i$ and chemical energy is now transferable.

Electrons from photoreactive center I have an alternative chemical pathway from the primary electron acceptor for cyclic (ATP) phosphorylation. These elec-

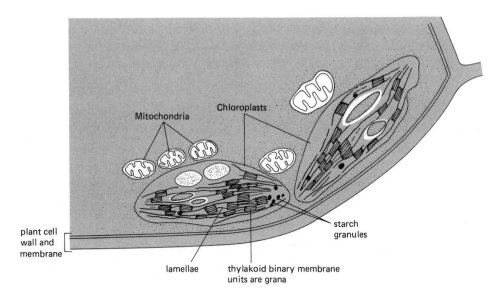

Figure 6.4 Plant chloroplasts. Drawn from an electron micrograph of a soybean plant cell. (Courtesy of Dr. John Burke, Plant Stress and Water Conservation Laboratory, U.S. Department of Agriculture.)

trons may alternatively reduce $NADP^+$ formed from the oxidation of $NADPH_2$ during the synthesis of glucose (see "Dark Reactions"). In this reaction $NADP^+$ is reduced by a flavoprotein. The protons of hydrogen (H^+) and electrons needed to form $NADPH_2$ for further biosynthesis of glucose are provided to $NADP^+$ by the splitting (oxidation) of water by the plant. Assisted by Mn^{2+}, the water split by the plant provides for the evolution of oxygen ($O_2 \uparrow$) gas, electrons for photocenter II for noncyclic phosphorylation, and electrons and hydrogen for reduction of $NADP^+$ to $NADPH^+ + H^+$. This entire process is energetically driven by sunlight, from which it derives its name, the light reactions. A chemical summation of noncyclic phosphorylation events and $NADP^+$ reduction is given in Equation 6.2.

Equation 6.2
Equation of noncyclic phosphorylation.

$$2H_2O + ADP + P_i + 2NADP^+ \rightarrow ATP + 2NADPH + 2H^+ + O_2 \uparrow + H_2O$$

The electrons and hydrogen for $NADPH + H^+$ in the equation 6.2 are derived from the first water molecule. The second water molecule is derived from the condensation of ADP and P_i in the synthesis of ATP.

The important products of the light reactions are the synthesis of ATP and $NADPH + H^+$, for both are used in the dark reactions of photosynthesis. The oxygen produced during the light reactions by higher plants is important to animals, humans, and even for plant life.

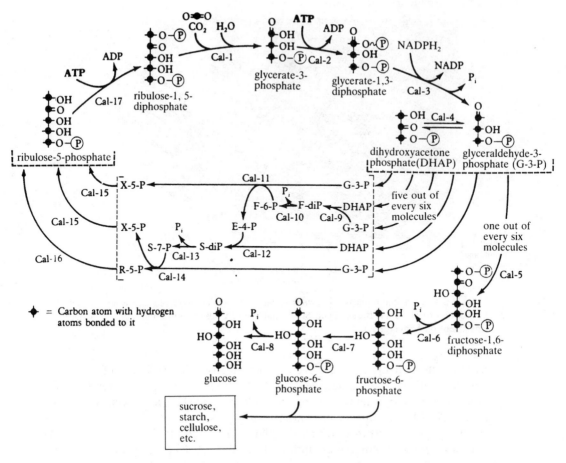

Figure 6.5 Calvin cycle (for the reduction of CO_2 and the synthesis of carbohydrates). Carbon carbohydrates as CO_2 is fixed into organic form, then reduced to the oxidation level characteristic of carbon in sugar molecules. For net synthesis of one glucose molecule, six molecules of CO_2 must be fixed, resulting in the formation of 12 molecules of glyceraldehyde-3-phosphate (G-3-P). Only one out of every six molecules of G-3-P (two per glucose synthesized) is actually used for sugar synthesis, since the other five out of every six molecules (10 per glucose) are reutilized within the cycle to regenerate the initial five-carbon acceptor molecule, ribulose-1,5-diphosphate. Abbreviations used in the regeneration sequence shown in brackets are as follows: G, glyceraldehyde; DHAP, dihydroxyacetone phosphate; F, fructose; E, erythrose; S, sedoheptulose; X, xylulose; and R, ribose. (Modified from W. M. Becker, *Energy of the Living Cell*, Harper & Row, 1977, with permission of the author.)

Dark Reactions

The dark reactions are the "synthetic" half of photosynthesis. In the chloroplast, ATP and $NADPH^+ + H^+$ synthesized in the light reactions are consumed in the reduction and conversion of CO_2 to glucose and other carbohydrates. The chemical details of the reduction of CO_2 to glucose became possible when the radioisotope, $^{14}CO_2$, was made available toward the end of World War II. Melvin Calvin and his associates of the University of California at Berkeley are responsible for providing much of the information on how CO_2 is incorporated into glucose. For this work, Calvin received the Nobel Prize in Chemistry in 1961 and the chemical cycle for the photosynthetic reduction of CO_2 bears his name, the Calvin cycle (Figure 6.5).

The Calvin Cycle

The Calvin cycle (Figure 6.5) is thermodynamically driven by the ATP and NADPH + H⁺ synthesized by the light reactions. No light or other external energy is needed beyond the ATP requirement; thus CO_2 reduction may occur in the presence or absence of light. The first two reactions of the Calvin cycle are the most important, as they use the ATP and NADPH + H⁺ produced by the light reactions for CO_2 fixation. The first reaction (Equation 6.3) is the carboxylation of ribulose-1,5-diphosphate (a five-carbon sugar), forming two molecules of a three-carbon carbohydrate, 3-phosphoglycerate (six carbons total).

Equation 6.3
Carbon dioxide formation by plants.

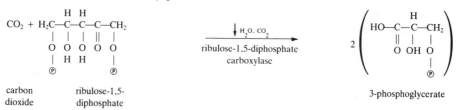

The ATP and NADPH + H⁺ produced in the light reactions is used in the second chemical reaction of the cycle (Equation 6.4).

Equation 6.4
Reduction of 3-phosphoglycerate.

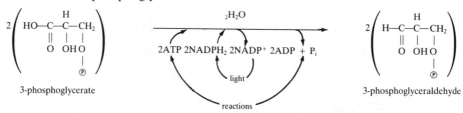

Equation 6.4 is the reverse of the glycolysis reaction (see Chapter 7), in which 3-phosphoglyceraldehyde is converted to 3-phosphoglycerate with the accompanying synthesis of ATP and NADH + H⁺. Equation 6.4 is thermodynamically very much "uphill," requiring the expenditure of two molecules of ATP to assure the reaction's completion.

In the remaining reactions of the Calvin cycle (Figure 6.5), isomerization of one of the molecules of 3-phosphoglyceraldehyde to dihydroxyacetonephosphate and its condensation with another molecule of 3-phosphoglyceraldehyde yields the hexose, 1,6-diphosphofructose. 1,6-diphosphofructose loses P_i, yielding 6-phosphofructose, which can isomerize to glucose-6-phosphate. Glucose (six carbons) may then polymerize, becoming cellulose [β-(1→4) glycosides] or starch [α-(1→4)-glycosides], or dimerize with fructose to become sucrose. To this point the cycle has added only the one carbon atom from CO_2. To complete the cycle, ribulose-1,5-diphosphate must be regenerated. This is accomplished by the condensation of fructose-6-phosphate with glyceraldehyde-3-phosphate (nine carbons) in lieu of glucose synthesis, which yields a four-carbon carbohydrate, erythrose-4-phosphate, and a five-carbon carbohydrate, xylulose-5-phosphate. Ribulose-1-5-diphosphate is then regenerated in two possible ways. Xylulose-5-phosphate is epimerized to ribulose-5-phosphate, which is phosphorylated by ATP to ribulose-1,5-diphosphate or sedhepulose-7-phosphate (seven carbons). Sedhepulose-7-phosphate combines with 3-phosphoglycerate (three carbons) to yield two molecules of ribulose-5-phosphate, which phosphorylated with two ATP molecules (one ATP each), completing the cycle. One complete turn of the Calvin cycle for each added CO_2 can be summarized as shown in Equation 6.5.

Equation 6.5
Chemical summary of the Calvin cycle.

$$\text{ribulose-1,5-diphosphate} + CO_2 + 3ATP + 2NADPH + 2H^+ + 2H_2O \xrightarrow{\text{one turn}}$$

$$\text{ribulose-1,5-diphosphate (regenerated)} + \tfrac{1}{6}(C_6H_{12}O_6) + 3P_i + 3ADP + 2NADP^+$$

To complete the synthesis of one completely new glucose molecule, six turns of the cycle are necessary. Three molecules of ATP are used in reducing one molecule of CO_2, and 18 molecules of ATP are expended in the synthesis of one molecule of glucose. With this information and knowing the $\Delta G^{\circ\prime}$ energy value for ATP and the caloric value of glucose, an estimate of the efficiency for the Calvin cycle can be made (Figure 6.6).

The calculated value of efficiency for the Calvin cycle, 81%, demonstrates

$\Delta G^{\circ\prime}$ of hydrolysis for ATP $\quad = -7.3$ kcal/mol

Glucose (caloric value) $\quad\quad\quad = 686$ kcal/mol

ATP consumed $(-7.3 \text{ kcal} \times 18) = 131$ kcal

$\dfrac{131 \text{ kcal}}{686 \text{ kcal}} \times 100 = 19\%$

$100\% - 19\% = 81\%$ efficiency for the conversion of "ATP energy" into "glucose energy"

Figure 6.6 Energy efficiency of the Calvin cycle.

TABLE 6.1 ANNUAL PRODUCTION OF GRAINS AND MEATS
(10^6 Metric Tons)

Grains					
Wheat	360	Millet	45	<15	Cabbage
Rice	320	Banana	35		Onions
Corn	300	Tomato	35		Beans
Potato	300	Sugarbeet	30		Peas
Barley	170	Rye	30		Sunflower seeds
Sweet potato	130	Oranges	30		Mango
Cassava	100	Coconut	30		
Grapes	60	Cottonseed oil	25		
Soybeans	60	Apples	20		
Oats	50	Yams	20		
Sorghum	50	Peanuts	20		
Sugarcane	50	Watermelon	20		

Meats	
Pork	43
Beef	42
Poultry	21
Lamb	5
Goat	1.5
Buffalo	1
Horse	0.7

Source: Jack R. Harlan, "The Plants and Animals That Nourish Man,"
in *Human Nutrition*, Chapter 6, Scientific American Press, New York
(1978).

the metabolic conservation of energy for this single pathway. Overall thermodynamic efficiency of plants, however, is much, much lower. Taking into consideration the needed quantum light energy capable of synthesizing sufficient ATP to
make a mole of glucose, plant thermodynamic efficiency drops to about 35%.
When thermodynamic calculations consider the entire solar energy falling on the
surface of a plant's leaf, conservation of solar energy for cultivated crops is around
1%, and much less than 1% of total solar energy is stored by plants for use as
food, fuels, and fiber. Every year, however, 10^6 metric tons of CO_2 is converted
by plants into organic matter by photosynthesis, dwarfing any other single annual
human effort. Table 6.1 provides recent estimates of annual grain production and
compares the photosynthetic event to annual meat production.

PLANT RESPIRATION

As described above, plants produced ATP and $NADPH_2$ in the light reactions for
the fixation and reduction of CO_2 in the dark reactions. Plants continue to undergo
metabolism and growth in the absence of light and without the synthesis of ATP

and $NADPH_2$ by noncyclic phosphorylation.   Continuation of plant metabolism in the dark is possible because of respiration.   Like animals (Chapter 7) plants metabolize their own carbohydrates from photosynthesis, producing $NADPH_2$ by the hexose monophosphate shunt, and plants possess mitochondria, which synthesize ATP by oxidative phosphorylation.   During respiration, plants, like animals, produce CO_2 and consume O_2.

7

Metabolism and Energy Utilization

Energy stored by plants by the reduction of CO_2 in the Calvin cycle is transferred to animals and humans as carbohydrates, lipids, and proteins. Carbohydrates in the typical American diet contribute 48% of the total dietary calories consumed; lipids, typically fats and oils, contribute 40% of total calories; and protein contributes the remaining 12% of calories consumed. In our "Western" American diet, much of the carbohydrate is refined sugars, lipids are animal fats and refined vegetable oils, and protein is usually of high quality, derived principally from animal sources. Throughout much of the world, human diets are much different from the Western diet. In the diets of people from the developing countries, most calories are supplied by naturally occurring sugars and complex carbohydrates. Calories supplied by animal fat and refined oils are greatly reduced. Calories from protein is lessened and the quality of the protein consumed is often much lower.

It makes little difference, calorically speaking, whether dietary energy is obtained from high- or low-carbohydrate diets, from plant oils or animal fats, from high- or low-quality proteins. The need for energy is constant for all living beings, and people require 1200 to 4000 calories per day, which varies from person to person depending primarily on age and level of physical activity. This chapter examines the major catabolic pathways, with a primary focus on the conversion of food energy into ATP and the synthesis of $NADPH + H^+$. The major anabolic pathways are then examined from the viewpoint of $NADH + H^+$, ATP utilization, and ATP's ability to both receive and transfer energy. We also examine why lipids possess a greater number of calories on an anhydrous basis than do either carbohydrates or proteins. Such insight should prove valuable in understanding the caloric density of foods.

CATABOLIC PATHWAYS OF CARBOHYDRATES

Glycolysis

For many animals, especially the herbivores and many people in developing countries, carbohydrates supply the majority of caloric needs. Glucose, the end product
of cellulose digestion in some animals and starch digestion in humans, is stored in
muscle, heart, or liver as the polysaccharide glycogen. Glycogen is a ready store
of energy and it or glucose can be rapidly degraded to either pyruvate or lactate
by the enzymes of the cytoplasm with the concomitant synthesis of ATP. The
glycolytic or Embden–Meyerhof pathway is shown in Figure 7.1. Glycolysis occurs

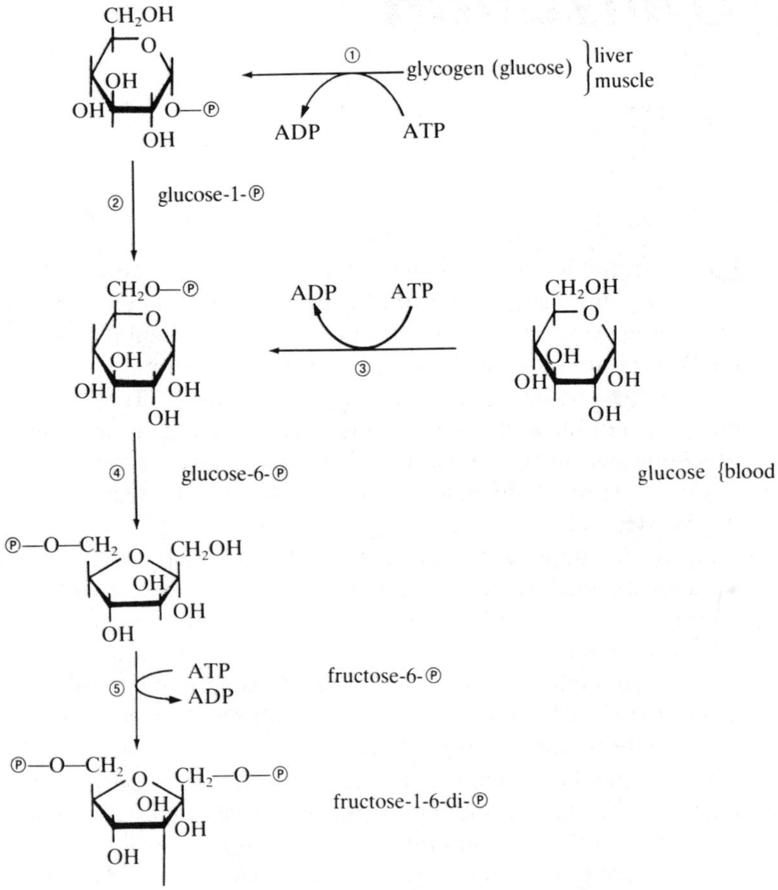

Figure 7.1 Glycolytic pathway. 1. Phosphorylase b   2. Phosphoglucomutase
3. Glucokinase 4. Phosphoglucoisomerase 5. Phosphofructokinase 6. Aldolase
7. Glyceraldehyde-3-phosphodehydrogenase   8. Phosphoglycerolkinase
9. Phosphoglycerolmutase   10. Enolase   11. Pyruvate   kinase   12. Pyruvate
decarboxylase

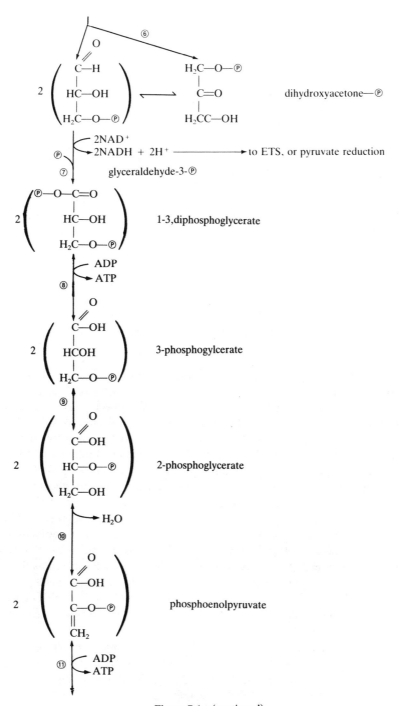

Figure 7.1 (continued)

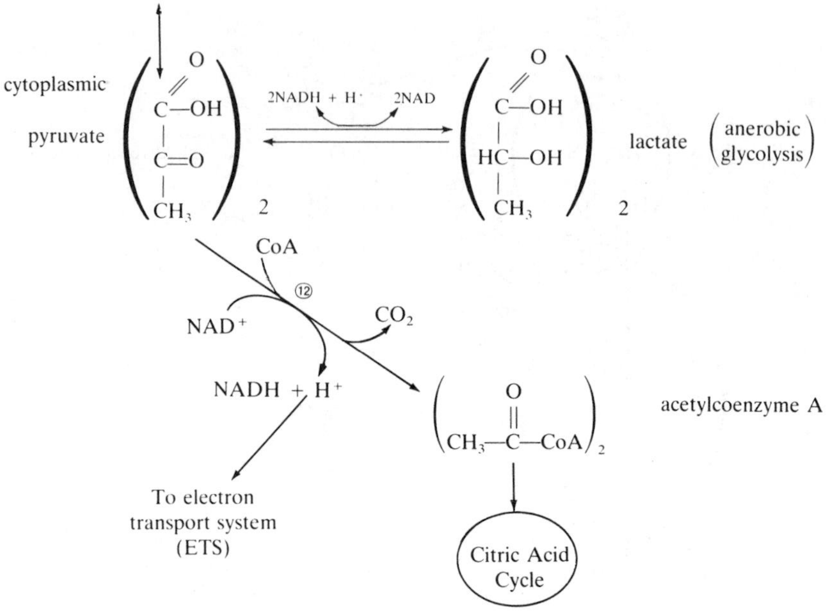

Figure 7.1   (continued)

in vivo under either aerobic or anaerobic conditions.   Aerobic glycolysis, beginning with the phosphorylation of glucose by ATP, activates glucose as either glucose-1-$\circledP$ (from glycogen) or glucose-6-$\circledP$ (from blood).   This six-carbon molecule is isomerized and phosphorylated with a second molecule of ATP to form fructose-1,6-di-$\circledP$.   This hexose is then divided into two three-carbon molecules—dihydroxyacetone-$\circledP$ and glyceraldehyde-3-$\circledP$—by an aldolase.   Both three-carbon molecules transverse the remaining intermediate steps of glycolysis, being transformed into pyruvic acid.   Conversion of 1,3-diphosphoglycerate to 3-phosphoglycerate and phosphoenolpyruvate to pyruvate (one-half of the glucose) yields one molecule each of ATP.   These steps are repeated for the remaining one-half of the original glucose molecule, yielding two more ATP molecules.   Thus it is observed that phosphorylation of one molecule of glucose by ATP, forming glucose-6-$\circledP$ or glucose-1-$\circledP$, results in a net yield of two ATP molecules during glycolysis in the conversion of glucose to two molecules of pyruvate.   Such phosphorylations are called substrate-level phosphorylations (SLPs) because ATP is synthesized from phosphorylated metabolites and ADP.   The net yield of ATP is shown in Equation 7.1.

   Under anaerobic conditions, the two molecules of reduced NADH + H$^+$ (produced by the oxidation of glyceraldehyde-3-$\circledP$) are used to reduce two molecules of pyruvate to lactate.   This happens in muscle tissue when muscular contractions are rapid and pyruvate cannot enter the citric acid cycle (Figure 7.2)

Equation 7.1
Net yield of ATP by substrate-level phosphorylation in glycolysis.

1. Phosphorylation of glucose $= -1$ ATP

2. Phosphorylation of fructose-6-Ⓟ $= -1$ ATP

3. 1,3-Diphosphoglycerate $\times$ 2 (SLP) $= +2$ ATP

4. <u>Phosphoenolpyruvate $\times$ 2 (SLP)</u> $= +2$ ATP

   Net yield of ATP from SLP $= +2$ ATP

because of a deficiency of oxaloacetate.   Such events cause lactic acid to accumulate and produce a respiratory oxygen debt.

   With purely aerobic conditions, pyruvate is oxidatively decarboxylated and transformed into acetylcoenzyme A, the most important metabolic intermediate common to the catabolism of carbohydrates, fatty acids, and amino acids. (Details of the oxidative decarboxylation of pyruvate is described in the section "Thiamin," Chapter 3.)   Acetyl coenzyme A condenses with oxaloacetate, forming citric acid in the initial metabolic step of the citric acid cycle, whereby the catabolism of glucose is continued.

The Citric Acid Cycle

From glycolysis, two molecules of pyruvate are decarboxylated and are condensed with coenzyme A, forming two molecules of acetylcoenzyme A.   In this reaction the carboxylic moiety of pyruvate is lost as respiratory CO_2 and the remaining acetyl, a two-carbon unit, is metabolized through the citric acid cycle.

   The citric acid cycle (CAC), or tricarboxylic acid cycle (TCH), is also known as the Krebs cycle, bearing the name of Sir Hans Krebs, who elucidated the details of this metabolic pathway within the mitochondrion.   For this remarkable accomplishment, Krebs received the Nobel Prize in Medicine in 1953.

   Acetylcoenzyme A (acetyl-CoA), in the first reaction of the CAC, condenses with oxaloacetate, a four-carbon dicarboxylic acid, forming the six-carbon tricarboxylic acid, citric acid (Equation 7.2).   The complete CAC is shown in Figure 7.2.

Equation 7.2
Condensation reaction.

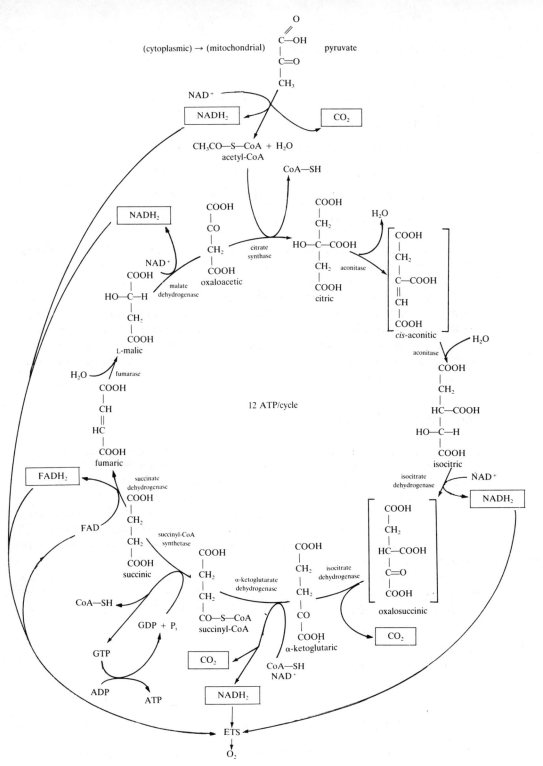

Figure 7.2 Citric acid cycle.

The six-carbon atoms of citric acid then pass through a series of CAC metabolic intermediates. Four of citric acid's six carbons are retained throughout the CAC and reappear as oxaloacetate, completing one turn of the cycle. The two carbon atoms unaccounted for are lost in thiamin-mediated oxidative decarboxylations of the CAC intermediates, oxalosuccinate and α-ketoglutarate. During each turn of the CAC, one ATP equivalent is made in a substrate-level phosphorylation (SLP) of GDP $\rightarrow$ GTP, guanosine diphosphate to guanosine triphosphate. While glycolysis yields four equivalent ATPs from substrate-level phosphorylations of glucose metabolites, the CAC yields only two equivalent ATPs through the synthesis of GTP. The net reactions of one turn of the CAC can be summarized as in Equation 7.3.

Equation 7.3
Chemical summary of the citric acid cycle.

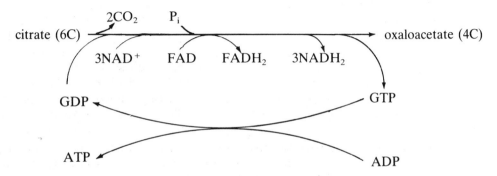

Two turns of the CAC are necessary to fully oxidize the equivalent of one molecule of glucose (6C). The equivalent of these six-carbon atoms are lost as CO_2; two are lost in the oxidative decarboxylations of pyruvate and its conversion to acetyl CoA, and four are lost in the oxidative decarboxylations during two turns of the CAC.

Oxidation of one molecule of glucose has now been followed through glycolysis and the CAC. Six molecules of CO_2, equivalent to all the carbon atoms of one glucose molecule, have been lost along with the oxygen atoms of glucose. What remains metabolically unaccounted for in the glucose molecule ($C_6H_{12}O_6$) are the atoms of hydrogen. These hydrogen atoms in glucose were used to reduce NAD^+ and FAD to $NADH + H^+$ and $FADH_2$, forming reduced niacinamide and flavin coenzymes. These reduced coenzymes are then oxidized in the mitochondrial electron transport system. The electron transport system (ETS) is the fixed common pathway for the oxidation of reduced coenzymes formed in the catabolic pathways of carbohydrates, fatty acid, and amino acid degradation. The ETS provides the majority of newly synthesized cellular ATP by the oxidative phosphorylation of ADP.

The Electron Transport System and Oxidative Phosphorylation

The ETS is found, along with the CAC, within the mitochondrion. The ETS is composed of a sequential series of enzymes and membrane-bound proteins, the cytochromes, arranged for the enzymatic coupling of P_i to ADP, forming ATP, and for the reduction of oxygen, forming metabolic water. The ETS, the formation of ATP and metabolic water, is shown in Figure 7.3.

In the first reaction of the ETS, $NADH_2$ formed from the oxidation of glucose, fatty acids, and CAC metabolites is oxidized by FAD, forming $FADH_2$ with the concurrent synthesis of one ATP molecule from ADP and P_i. $FADH_2$ is then oxidized by coenzyme Q (CoQ), also known as ubiquinone. $CoQ \cdot H_2$ gives up two protons ($2H^+$) to the mitochondrial matrix and transfers two electrons ($2e^-$) from the two hydrogen atoms to oxidized cytochrome b (Fe^{3+}). The two electrons, one at a time, are sequentially passed along to each oxidized Fe^{3+} form of the succeeding cytochrome. The final acceptor of the pair of elections is oxygen ($\frac{1}{2}O_2$). Oxygen (O^{2-}) returns the pair of electrons to the two protons discharged from coenzyme Q in combining to form a molecule of water. It is this water that is called metabolic water, for it is formed as a result of metabolism.

In the cascade of the pair of electrons from the discharge of the two protons by coenzyme Q through the sequential array of cytochromes, two molecules of ATP are synthesized from $2ADP + 2P_i$. ATP is synthesized, resulting from the coupling of cytochromes b and c_1 and cytochromes a and a_3 with oxygen. From $NADH_2$, arising from the catabolic pathways, hydrogen and electrons flow through the ETS, with the resulting synthesis of ATP. Each $NADH_2$ gives rise to the synthesis of three ATPs in the ETS by oxidative phosphorylation, sometimes referred to as a P/O ratio equal to 3 (ATP formed/oxygen consumed). While $NADH_2$ produces P/O ratios of 3, $FADH_2$ produces a P/O ratio equal to 2. Why this happens can be seen in Figure 7.3. $FADH_2/FMNH_2$ derived from the β-oxidation of fatty acids, CAC intermediate succinate, or other metabolic oxidations bypasses the synthesis of the first ATP in the ETS and therefore yields only two ATPs synthesized by the enzymes of cytochromes b and c_1, a and a_3. The net reactions of the ETS from $NADH_2$ and $FADH_2/FMNH_2$ can thus be summarized as in Equation 7.4.

Equation 7.4
Chemical summary of the electron transport system.

$$NADH_2 + 3ADP + 3P_i + \tfrac{1}{2}O_2 \longrightarrow NAD^+ + 3ATP + H_2O \qquad \text{P/O} = 3$$

$$FADH_2/FMNH_2 + 2ADP + 2P_i + \tfrac{1}{2}O_2 \longrightarrow FAD/FMN + 2ATP + H_2O \qquad \text{P/O} = 2$$

Close examination of glycolysis and the CAC reveals that the metabolism of glucose yields a considerable amount of collective reduced coenzymes, $NADH_2$ and $FADH_2$, which are oxidized by the ETS, producing ATP. From a single

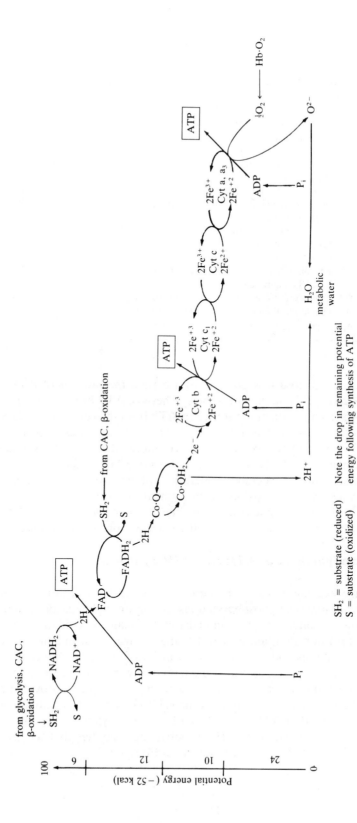

Figure 7.3 Electron transport system and oxidative phosphorylation.

SH_2 = substrate (reduced)
S = substrate (oxidized)

Note the drop in remaining potential energy following synthesis of ATP

TABLE 7.1 SEQUENTIAL SUMMARY OF ATP SYNTHESIS FROM THE
CATABOLISM OF GLUCOSE

1. Phosphorylation of glucose: from glycogen -1 ATP or from glucose -2 ATP	-1ATP
2. Phosphorylation of fructose-6-℗	-1 ATP
3. Oxidation of 2 glutaraldehyde-3-℗ by 2NAD$^+$ (NADH$_2$)	$+6$ ATP by ETS
4. Phosphorylation by 2 1,3-diphosphoglycerates	$+2$ ATP by SLP
5. Phosphorylation by 2 phosphoenolpyruvates	$+2$ ATP by SLP
6. Oxidation of 2 pyruvates by 2NAD$^+$ (NADH$_2$)	$+6$ ATP by ETS
7. Oxidation of 2 isocitrates by 2NAD$^+$ (NADH$_2$)	$+6$ ATP by ETS
8. Oxidation of 2 α-ketoglutarates by 2NAD$^+$ (NADH$_2$)	$+6$ ATP by ETS
9. Phosphorylation of 2GDP by succinyl-CoA (2ATP equivalents)	$+2$ ATP by SLP
10. Oxidation of 2 succinates by 2FAD (FADH$_2$)	$+4$ ATP by ETS
11. Oxidation of 2 malates by 2NAD$^+$ (NADH$_2$)	$+6$ ATP by ETS
Net ATPs from glycolysis and CAC via ETS	$+38$ ATP

molecule of glucose it is possible to ascertain the number of ATPs theoretically synthesized.   This summary for the synthesis of ATP from glucose is given in Table 7.1.   An examination of the source of ATP from the complete oxidation of glucose reveals that most of the net yield of the 38 ATPs arises from the NADH$_2$ and FADH$_2$ formed by the oxidation of CAC intermediates and the single SLP initiated by succinyl-CoA.   Fully 24, or 63%, of the net ATPs synthesized from the oxidation of glucose is from the metabolic operations of the CAC.   When reduced coenzymes are included from the oxidation of pyruvate to acetyl-CoA, 79% of the ATP is formed.   Under aerobic conditions, glycolysis accounts for just 21% of the ATP formed by the oxidation of reduced coenzymes produced in this pathway.

Thermodynamics of ATP and ATP Synthesis

We have examined how and where ATP is synthesized in plant chloroplasts by cyclic and noncyclic phosphorylations during the light reactions and in the mitochondria of plants, bacteria, animals, and humans by oxidative phosphorylation. Let us turn our attention now to the thermodynamics; the energy considerations of ATP synthesis and the metabolic transfer of energy within cells.

In Chapter 1 we described the laws of thermodynamics and the relationships between energy, work, and ATP.   In addition, Chapter 1 provided a brief explanation of how energy is "stored" by the ATP molecule.   Recapitulating, the amount of energy stored in ATP is equal to a free-energy yield of $\Delta G^{\circ\prime} = -7.3$ kcal/mol under standard conditions.   The negative sign signifies that the energy "stored" in ATP is released upon hydrolysis as in Equation 7.5.

Equation 7.5
Hydrolysis of ATP.

$$\text{ATP} \xrightarrow{\text{Mg2+-ATPase}} \text{ADP} + P_i + (-7.3 \text{ kcal/mol})$$

The reaction in Equation 7.5 can be diagrammed showing the approximate energy content of the reactant (ATP) and products (ADP + P_i) (Figure 7.4). In order to "store" the -7.3 kcal/mol of hydrolysis in ATP, the drop in potential energy across the point of ATP synthesis (ADP + $P_i \rightarrow$ ATP) in the chloroplast from the light reaction in substrate-level phosphorylation, and in the mitochondrion in the ETS must be greater than -7.3 kcal/mol. In the ETS, the potential drop in energy across all the electron carriers from $NADH_2$ to O_2 is approximately 52 kcal per electron pair. Figure 7.4 demonstrates that approximately 12 kcal of potential energy is used in the synthesis of the first ATP, 10 kcal is used in the synthesis of the second ATP, and 24 kcal is expended in the synthesis of the third and final ATP. The total amount of energy "stored" by oxidative phosphorylation of ADP per $NADH_2$ is 21.9 kcal. From this value an estimate of overall thermodynamic efficiency can be calculated for a P/O ratio of 3. This efficiency is 21.9 kcal/52 kcal $\times$ 100, or 42%. The ETS is therefore 42% efficient in conserving total potential electron energy as ATP.

Why, one may ask, is ATP synthesized and so important as a carrier of free energy? ATP is an unusual carrier of free energy for anabolic reactions, for its $\Delta G^{\circ\prime}$ of hydrolysis is of intermediate value among a variety of energetically active compounds. Table 7.2 provides a list of energy-containing compounds ranging

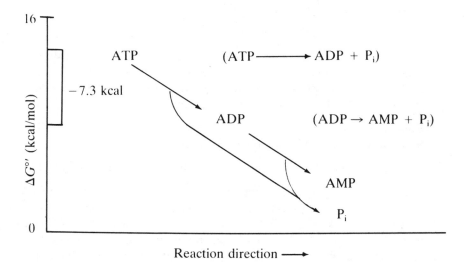

Figure 7.4 Free energy of hydrolysis of ATP and ADP.

TABLE 7.2 FREE ENERGY OF HYDROLYSIS OF ENERGY-CONTAINING COMPOUNDS

Name	$\Delta G^{\circ\prime}$ (kcal/mol)	Direction of phosphate or energy transfer
Phosphoenolpyruvate	−14.8	
α-Glycerol phosphate	−11.8	
Creatine phosphate	−10.3	
Acetylphosphate	−10.1	
ATP (→ AMP + PP$_i$)	−8.6	
Acetyl-CoA	−8.2	
ATP (→ ADP + P$_i$)	−7.3	
Aminoacetyl AMP	−7.0	
PP$_i$ (→ 2P$_i$)	−6.7	
Glucose-1-phosphate	−5.0	
Fructose-6-phosphate	−3.8	
Glucose-6-phosphate	−3.3	
3-Phosphoglycerate	−3.1	
Glycerol-1-phosphate	−2.2	

from $\Delta G^{\circ\prime}$ = −14.8 kcal/mol to −2.2 kcal/mol. The free energy of hydrolysis for the reaction ATP → ADP + P$_i$ (−7.3 kcal/mol) is intermediate among these compounds. Compounds with $\Delta G^{\circ\prime}$ less than ATP can be phosphorylated by ATP as in Equation 7.6.

Equation 7.6
Phosphorylation of glucose by ATP.

$$\text{ATP + glucose} \longrightarrow \text{ADP + glucose-1-}\textcircled{P}$$

In this equation ATP transferred −5.0 kcal/mol of its −7.3 kcal/mol to glucose. This reaction energy transfer was 68% efficient. It may be recalled from glycolysis that conversion of phosphoenolpyruvate to pyruvate is a substrate-level phosphorylation (SLP) which yields ATP (Equation 7.7).

Equation 7.7
Phosphorylation of ADP by phosphoenolpyruvate.

$$\text{phosphoenolpyruvate + ADP} \longrightarrow \text{ATP + pyruvate}$$

In this reaction phosphoenolpyruvate has a $\Delta G^{\circ\prime}$ of −14.8 kcal/mol and transfers its phosphate to ADP, yielding ATP with a $\Delta G^{\circ\prime}$ of −7.3 kcal/mol. This phosphate transfer shows how ATP is formed only by molecules with a higher $\Delta G^{\circ\prime}$ of hydrolysis than that of ATP. This reaction energy transfer is about 50% efficient.

Creatine phosphate ($\Delta G^{\circ\prime}$ = −10.3 kcal/mol) is a high-energy compound found in muscle used in the phosphorylation of ADP for muscular contraction (Equation 7.8).

Equation 7.8
Phosphorylation of ADP by creatine phosphate.

$$\text{creatine phosphate} + \text{ADP} \longrightarrow \text{ATP} + \text{creatine}$$

This equation is thermodynamically permissible. During muscular rest, creatine is phosphorylated by ATP, forming creatine phosphate, which seemingly is thermodynamically impossible.

The reaction proceeds, however, by expending the energy of two molecules of ATP (Equation 7.9).

Equation 7.9
Phosphorylation of creatine by ATP.

$$\text{creatine} + 2\text{ATP} \longrightarrow \text{creatine phosphate} + 2\text{ADP} + P_i$$

In this equation, the $\Delta G^{\circ\prime}$ of creatine phosphate is restored in a reaction energy transfer that is 70% efficient. These examples of energy transfer between molecules which have both greater and lesser $\Delta G^{\circ\prime}$ than ATP should serve to emphasize why coupling energies for the synthesis of ATP in the light reactions (plants) and oxidation phosphorylation (plants, animals, and humans) must be larger than $+7.3$ kcal/mol $+$ ATP.

CATABOLIC PATHWAYS OF LIPIDS

Lipids, triglycerides principally, provide about 40% of American dietary requirements for calories. Lipids as adipose tissue are also the major store of body energy and possess more than twice the caloric density (9 kcal/g) of carbohydrates or protein (4 kcal/g). In this section we examine the oxidation of triglycerides.

Triglycerides, in comparison to equal anhydrous weights of carbohydrate and protein, contain more calories because they have a higher proportion of total hydrocarbon (see Figure 7.8). Body stores of triglycerides are mobilized in response to low blood glucose and insulin levels by the release of free fatty acids (FFAs) from triglycerides into the blood stream. Bound to serum albumin, FFAs are taken up by the cell's cytoplasm. These cytosolic FFAs undergo an enzymatic activation by ATP and are transferred to carnitine (a molecule similar in structure to lecithin), which acts as a mitochondrial membrane shuttle moving FFAs from the cytoplasm into the mitochondrial matrix, as shown in Equations 7.10 and 7.11.

Equation 7.10
Activation of cytoplasmic fatty acids.

(1) $CH_3CH_2(CH_2)_n COOH$

$$+ \text{ATP} \xrightarrow{\text{CoASH (cytoplasmic)}} CH_3CH_2(CH_2)_n - \overset{\overset{\displaystyle O}{\displaystyle \|}}{C} - S - CoA + AMP + PP_i$$

Transfer of Activated Fatty Acid to Carnitine

$$\text{(2)} \quad CH_3CH_2(CH_2)_n\overset{\overset{\displaystyle O}{\|}}{-}C-CoA \; + \; HOOC-CH_2-\underset{\underset{\displaystyle OH}{|}}{\overset{\overset{\displaystyle Carnitine}{}}{C}}H-CH_2-\overset{+}{N}(CH_3)_3 \longrightarrow$$

$$HOOC-CH_2-\underset{\underset{\underset{\displaystyle O=C-(CH_2)_nCH_2CH_3}{|}}{\overset{|}{O}}}{C}H-CH_2-\overset{+}{N}(CH_3)_3 \; + \; CoASH \;\text{(cytoplasmic)}$$

Once transferred by carnitine into the intramitochondrial matrix, the fatty acid is reesterified with coenzyme A. This coenzyme A, however, is of mitochondrial origin (Equation 7.11)

Equation 7.11
Transfer of acylcarnitine to mitochondrial coenzyme A.

$$HOOC-CH_2-\underset{\underset{\underset{\displaystyle O=C-(CH_2)nCH_2CH_3}{|}}{\overset{|}{O}}}{C}-CH_2-\overset{+}{N}(CH_3)_3 \; + \; CoASH \underset{\text{mitochondrial}}{\longrightarrow}$$

$$CH_3CH_2(CH_2)_n\overset{\overset{\displaystyle O}{\|}}{-}C-S-CoA \; + \; \text{carnitine}$$

and provides an activated free fatty acid for β-oxidation.

β-*Oxidation*

The oxidation of fatty acids was first described by F. Knoop, a German biochemist, in 1904. Oxidation of fatty acids and cleavage of the thioester occurs at the third or β-carbon of the fatty acid, and the cyclic process of fatty acid dehydration bears the name β-oxidation. β-Oxidation, it may be remembered, is initiated by activation of a cytoplasmic free fatty acid by ATP and it exists as a thioester (Figure 7.5). Equation (1) of Figure 7.5 is the dehydrogenation of the activated fatty acid by a flavoprotein containing oxidized FAD, yielding an unsaturated C:2,3 activated fatty acid. Hydration of either a cis or trans fatty acid [equation (2) or (2′)] produces a stereoisomer which upon dehydrogenation by NAD⁺ [equation (3)] produces a (C:3)β-ketoacetyl-CoA fatty acid and NADH₂. The β-ketoacetyl-CoA

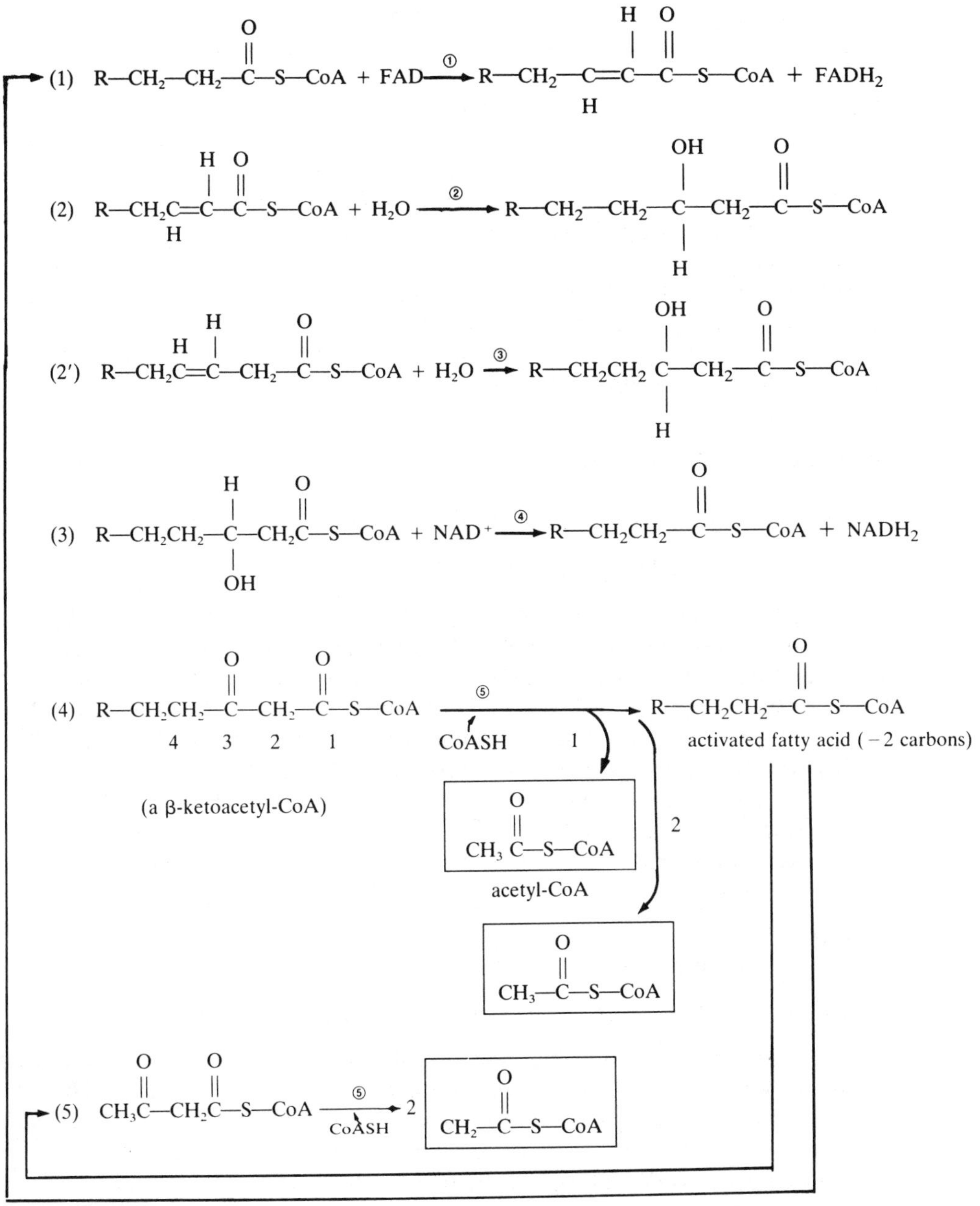

(1) $R-CH_2-CH_2-C(=O)-S-CoA + FAD \xrightarrow{①} R-CH_2-CH=CH-C(=O)-S-CoA + FADH_2$

(2) $R-CH_2CH=CH-C(=O)-S-CoA + H_2O \xrightarrow{②} R-CH_2-CH_2-CH(OH)-CH_2-C(=O)-S-CoA$

(2') $R-CH_2CH=CH-CH_2-C(=O)-S-CoA + H_2O \xrightarrow{③} R-CH_2CH_2-CH(OH)-CH_2-C(=O)-S-CoA$

(3) $R-CH_2CH_2-CH(OH)-CH_2C(=O)-S-CoA + NAD^+ \xrightarrow{④} R-CH_2CH_2-C(=O)-S-CoA + NADH_2$

(4) $R-CH_2CH_2-C(=O)-CH_2-C(=O)-S-CoA$ ... $\xrightarrow{⑤}$ ... $R-CH_2CH_2-C(=O)-S-CoA$

4 3 2 1   CoASH   1   activated fatty acid (-2 carbons)

(a β-ketoacetyl-CoA)

$CH_3\,C(=O)-S-CoA$

acetyl-CoA

$CH_3-C(=O)-S-CoA$

(5) $CH_3C(=O)-CH_2C(=O)-S-CoA \xrightarrow[CoASH]{⑤} 2\ CH_2-C(=O)-S-CoA$

Figure 7.5 β-Oxidation of fatty acids. 1. Acyl-CoA dehydrogenase 2. Enoyl-CoA hydratase (trans fatty acid) 3. Enoyl-CoA hydratase (cis fatty acid) 4. β-Hydroxyacyl dehydrogenase 5. Thiolase.

fatty acid is cleaved between C:2 and 3, producing acetylcoenzyme A. The remaining fatty acid fragment, shortened by the loss of two carbon atoms, condenses with another molecule of coenzyme A. This activated free fatty acid [equation (4)] recycles to equation (1) for repetition of the cyclic process. In each repetitive cycle of β-oxidation, the activated fatty acid is shortened by two carbon atoms until buteryl-CoA is cycled. In the final cycle of β-oxidation, this four-carbon fatty acid is symmetrically cleaved to yield two acetyl-CoAs [equation (5)].

Inspection of the β-oxidation of fatty acids reveals that any fatty acid of even carbon number $n = 6$ or greater undergoes $(n/2) - 1$ cycles, producing $(n/2) - 1$ molecules of $FADH_2$ and $n/2$ molecules of acetyl-CoA. β-Oxidation of stearic acid, a saturated C_{18} fatty acid, would go through eight cycles, producing eight molecules of $FADH_2$ and $NADH_2$ and nine molecules of acetyl-CoA. These reactions can be summarized as in Equation 7.12.

Equation 7.12
β-Oxidation of stearic acid.

$$\text{stearic acid} + \text{ATP} + 9\text{CoASH} + 8\text{FAD} + 8\text{NAD}^+ + 8H_2O \xrightarrow{\text{8 cycles}} 9\,\text{acetyl-CoA}$$

$$+ 8\text{FADH}_2 + 8\text{NADH}_2 + \text{AMP} + \text{PP}_i$$

All the acetyl-CoA produced by β-oxidation of fatty acids enters the citric acid cycle. It may be recalled that each turn of the CAC results in the oxidation of two atoms of carbon and the synthesis of reduced coenzymes and GTP equivalent to 12 ATPs per cycle. It should be apparent, therefore, that β-oxidation of cytoplasmic long-chain fatty acids, activated by two ATPs, generates large quantities of $FADH_2$ and $NADH_2$ for ATP synthesis from the electron transport chain and oxidative phosphorylation of ADP. Complete oxidation of the C_{18} fatty acid, stearic acid, by β-oxidation nets 146 ATPs or 1066 kcal/mol of stearic acid (calculations shown in Table 7.3). The number of kcal/mol for the complete oxidation of stearic acid by O_2 is shown in Equation 7.13.

Equation 7.13
Complete oxidation of stearic acid by oxygen.

$$\text{stearic acid} + 27O_2 \longrightarrow 18CO_2 + 18H_2O + (-2596 \text{ kcal/mol})$$

β-Oxidation of stearic acid results in the conservation of 41% of the total energy of stearic acid, preserved and transferred as ATP equivalents. The efficiency of recovered energy as ATP is reduced for shorter-chain fatty acids, as each requires activation by the equivalent of two ATPs, and short-chain fatty acids contain proportionately less oxidizable hydrocarbon.

Even-carbon-numbered unsaturated fatty acids are metabolized in the same general way as even-numbered saturated fatty acids. Polyunsaturated fatty acids (PUFA) pose some metabolic problems because of the multiple unsaturated double bonds and their location. Nevertheless, these problems are surmounted by enzymes present in the mitochondrial matrix, and polyunsaturated fatty acids also

TABLE 7.3 ENERGY YIELD AND EFFICIENCY OF THE COMPLETE
OXIDATION OF STEARIC ACID (C_{18}:O) BY β-OXIDATION AND THE
CITRIC ACID CYCLE THROUGH ELECTRON TRANSPORT

		P/O ratio	Total ATP
From β-oxidation	8 FADH$_2$	× 2 =	16
of stearic acid	8 NADH$_2$	× 3 =	24
	From β-oxidation	=	40 ATP
From CAC	9 GTP	× — =	9
	9 FADH$_2$	× 2 =	18
	27 NADH$_2$	× 3 =	81
		=	108 ATP
	Gross		
	−(activation) 2ATP		148 ATP
	Net yield		146 ATP

β-oxidation of stearic acid $\Delta G^{\circ\prime} = -7.3 \times 146 = 1066$ kcal/mol
Complete oxidation of stearic acid $\Delta G^{\circ\prime}$ by $O_2 = 2596$ kcal/mol

$$\frac{1066}{2596} \times 100 = 41\% \text{ efficient}$$

follow the same general pathway of β-oxidation. Monounsaturated and PUFA
have a slightly lower caloric value than do saturated fatty acids of similar carbon
number, as unsaturation results in the reduction of the amount of reduced coenzymes formed and hydrogen traversing the electron transport chain for ATP synthesis. Odd-carbon-numbered fatty acids (C:15, 17, 19, etc.) are oxidized in the
usual β-oxidation pathway until the three-carbon unit proprionyl-CoA (instead of
buteryl-CoA) is reached. Propionyl-CoA is then carboxylated (carboxybiotin) and
enters the CAC as succinyl-CoA or succinate.

CATABOLIC PATHWAYS OF PROTEINS

Protein provides about 12% of the average American's dietary requirement for
calories. Protein metabolism is continuous and constant in the normal and ade-
quately nourished adult and can be biochemically assessed by measurement of
nitrogen balance (nitrogen consumed, nitrogen excreted). In the absence of food
(calories) for an extended period, carbohydrates stored as muscle, heart, and liver
glycogen are rapidly depleted. This loss of carbohydrate is followed by the hydrolysis of triglycerides, the mobilization of body depot fat, and the oxidation of
fatty acids by β-oxidation. In the advent of extended starvation and catexia,
massive amounts of the body's protein stores (e.g., muscle tissue) are mobilized
for the body's energy requirements. Such events are serious when they occur and
may result in extreme negative nitrogen balance.

Metabolically, proteins are enzymatically converted intracellularly to amino acids. Each of the 20 commonly found amino acids in protein follows catabolic routes after either transamination or deamination. Transamination from one amino acid leads to the synthesis of another amino acid, with the concurrent generation of new α-keto acid [See "Pyridoxal (B$_6$)," Chapter 3]. In transamination reactions, nitrogen is not lost, only transferred from one amino acid in the synthesis of another amino acid. In deamination reactions, however, the loss of the amino moiety results in the production of ammonia (NH$_3$) as ammonium ions (NH$_4^+$), and as in transamination reactions, the synthesis of an α-keto acid. A deamination reaction requiring vitamin B$_6$ is the initial metabolic reaction common to the elimination of nitrogen from amino acids. Deamination is shown in Equation 7.14 for phenylalanine.

Equation 7.14
Deamination of phenylalanine.

phenylpyruvic acid,
an α-ketocarboxylic acid

The metabolism of the hydrocarbon portion of each of the deaminated amino acids is different and for many amino acids, quite complex. Their ultimate oxidation, however, follows the established final common pathways of the citric acid cycle and the electron transport system. The hydrocarbon portion of all 20 amino acids commonly found in protein enters catabolic pathways as either pyruvate, acetyl-CoA, α-ketoglutarate, succinyl-CoA, fumarate, or oxaloacetate. With the exception of pyruvate, these metabolites are all associated with the citric acid cycle. The hydrocarbon portions of all deaminated amino acids therefore enter common catabolic pathways as either pyruvate or intermediates of the citric acid cycle. Points of entry of the hydrocarbon portions of the amino acids into the citric acid cycle are shown in Figure 7.6.

It may be apparent from Figure 7.6 that the caloric value and yield of ATP from each amino acid can be somewhat different depending on the point of entry of its hydrocarbon skeleton into the citric acid cycle. Alanine, glycine, lysine, and so on, whose hydrocarbon skeletons become pyruvate, will yield more ATP than will the hydrocarbons of other amino acids, whose entry to the CAC occurs later. The size of the hydrocarbon portion of the amino acid also has a bearing on caloric yield. For example, phenylalanine and tyrosine, larger-molecular-weight amino acids, are divided and enter the CAC as two hydrocarbon fragments, acetyl-CoA and fumarate. Such variations in amino acid metabolism contribute to the average caloric value of proteins (ca. 4 kcal/g).

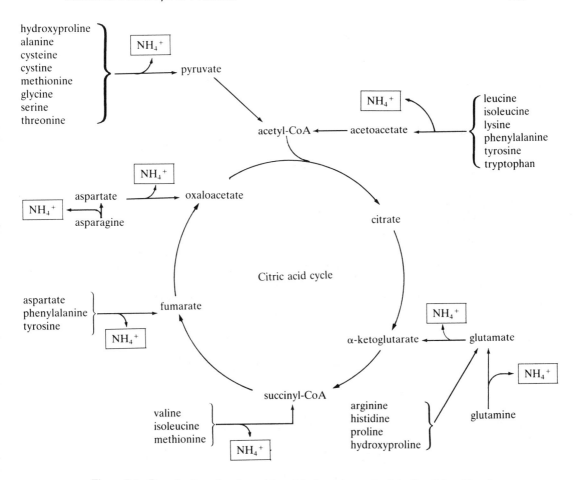

Figure 7.6 Deamination of amino acids and hydrocarbon entry into the citric acid cycle.

Elimination of Ammonia: The Urea Cycle

Ammonia produced from the deamination of amino acids and other amines is strongly basic and very toxic. Cells of the liver and to a lesser degree, the kidney and brain, detoxify ammonia by its conversion to the less toxic and water-soluble compound, urea. The conversion of ammonia to urea from amino acids proceeds in the liver, kidney, and brain, predominately through a single common pathway of a glutamic acid transamination–deamination and the urea cycle. Ammonia arising from deamination reactions in tissues other than the liver, kidney, or brain is coupled to the amino acid glutamate and is carried in the blood plasma to the liver or kidney as the basic amino acid glutamine (Equation 7.15).

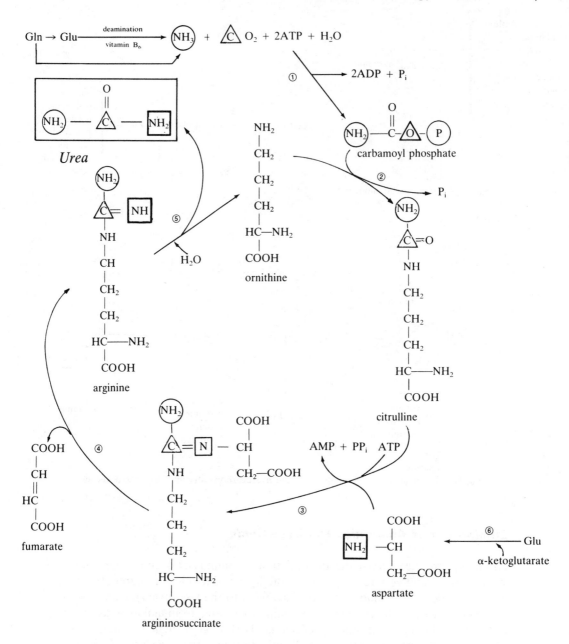

Figure 7.7 Urea cycle. 1. Carbamoyl phosphate synthetase 2. Ornithine-carbamoyl transferase 3. Argininosuccinate synthetase 4. Argininosuccinate lyase 5. Arginase 6. Transaminase (vitamin B_6).

Equation 7.15
Conversion of ammonia to glutamine.

$$NH_3 + HOOC\!-\!\underset{\underset{H}{|}}{\overset{\overset{NH_2}{|}}{C}}\!-\!CH_2CH_2\!-\!COOH \xrightarrow[\text{ATP} \; \text{ADP} + \text{Pi}]{} HOOC\!-\!\underset{\underset{H}{|}}{\overset{\overset{NH_2}{|}}{C}}\!-\!CH_2CH_2\!-\!\overset{\overset{O}{\|}}{C}\!-\!NH_2 + H_2O$$

glutamic acid   glutamine

The formation of glutamine in Equation 7.15 requires ATP and results from the ammonia being coupled to glutamate. Glutamine, via a deamination reaction in liver or kidney, yields ammonia, which is converted into carbamoyl phosphate, the first reaction of the urea cycle (Figure 7.7). This reaction requires two molecules of ATP and carboxybiotin. The remaining amine of glutamic acid enters the urea cycle either through carbamoyl phosphate or via a transamination from glutamic acid to aspartic acid, which then enters the urea cycle via coupling to citrulline in the formation of arginosuccinic acid. The latter reaction also requires an energy expenditure of one molecule of ATP for completion. The urea cycle, beginning with the synthesis of carbamoyl phosphate and ending with urea and the regeneration of ornithine, requires the expenditure of three molecules of ATP per molecule of urea generated. The derived ammonia (amino groups from glutamine, glutamate, and aspartate) in urea is contributed equally from a molecule of carbamoyl phosphate and aspartic acid. The ketone moiety of urea is from CO_2 (C) and water (O).

Energy, ATP, and the Catabolic Pathways

We have examined how the caloric energy of food (starch → glucose; fats and oils → fatty acids and glycerol; proteins → amino acids) is converted in the catabolic pathways to a more useful form of metabolic energy, ATP. The unanswered question throughout this discussion of energy transfer is: Where was the energy in the organic nutrients that was transferred and conserved as ATP? The energy transferred from the organic nutrients to ATP in the catabolic pathways was originally stored by plants during photosynthesis and was retained in the covalent bonds of the starch, lipids, proteins, and other organic molecules. Table 7.4 lists some representative bond energies that are present in organic nutrients. Examination of this table reveals that the organic nutrients of foods, which contain predominately C—C, C—H, C—S, C—N, and C—O bonds, contain a great deal of stored energy expressed as kcal/mol.

The caloric value of food—carbohydrates, lipids, and proteins—is the amount of potential energy stored in the molecule's covalent bonds. During catabolic metabolism, the potential energy available for release and transfer to ATP is related to the total amount of hydrocarbon within molecules. The hydrocarbon content (—CH$_2$—) of the organic nutrients determines the caloric value of foods. The

TABLE 7.4 REPRESENTATIVE BOND
ENERGIES THAT ARE PRESENT IN
NUTRIENTS AND IMPORTANT
BIOMOLECULES

Bond	kcal/mol
H—C	81
C—C	144
C—S	175
C—N	174
C—O	257
H_2N—H	103
HOH_2C—H	92
HC—H	108
HO—H	119
OC=O	128
O—O	119
O—P	144
S—S	102
N≡N	226

lipids, i.e., fats and oils, contain 9 kcal/g, more than twice the caloric value of carbohydrates and protein (4 kcal/g) because they proportionately contain about twice the amount of hydrocarbon. Figure 7.8 demonstrates the approximate 2.25:1:1 caloric ratios for lipids, carbohydrates, and protein represented by the fatty acids hexonic and palmitic acids, glucose and the dipeptide glutamylglycine. These molecules approximate the elemental composition of dietary fats, starch, and protein. Figure 7.8 shows the hydrocarbon ratios of palmitic acid, glucose, and glutamylglycine to be 1.98:1:1.2, which approaches the average caloric ratio of 2.25:1:1 for lipids, carbohydrates, and protein. When hexonic acid, with the same number of carbons (six) as glucose, and glutamylglycine are used in such calculations, the energy ratios go down because of a higher percentage of oxygen in hexanoic acid (27.6%) than palmitic acid (13.3%), which does not contribute to caloric value, yet hexanoic acid (MW 116) still has nearly 72% hydrocarbon. As Figure 7.8 indicates, as the molecular weight of fatty acids increases, the percentage of hydrocarbon, and hence calories, also increases.

Caloric Density of Foods

The proportion of hydrocarbon in molecular structure is but one factor that contributes to the caloric value of foods. The second factor contributing to the caloric value of foods is the proportionate content of water. These two predominant factors then contribute to the caloric density of foods. Foods containing a high proportion of water (also fiber) possess a lower caloric density than that of foods low in moisture and with a proportionately higher content of either fats or oils.

Representative of nutrient carbon

Elemental composition

CH₂OH

H—O H
H
OH H
HO OH
H OH

glucose
(MW 180)
($C_6H_{12}O_6$)

	%	
Carbon	40	
Hydrogen	7	47% hydrocarbon
Oxygen	53	

$CH_3CH_2CH_2CH_2CH_2COOH$
hexanoic acid
(MW 116)
($C_6H_{12}O_2$)

	%	
Carbon	62	
Hydrogen	10	72% hydrocarbon
Oxygen	28	

$CH_3(CH_2)_{14}COOH$
palmitic acid
($C_{16}H_{32}O_2$)
(MW 240)

	%	
Carbon	80	
Hydrogen	13	93% hydrocarbon
Oxygen	7	

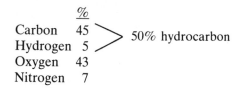

glutamylglycine
($C_7H_{10}O_5N$)
(MW 188)

	%	
Carbon	45	
Hydrogen	5	50% hydrocarbon
Oxygen	43	
Nitrogen	7	

Figure 7.8 Hydrocarbon content of organic nutrients.

Table 7.5 CALORIC DENSITY OF SELECTED FOODS

Food/nutrient	Percent water (approx.)	Caloric density (cal/g)
Water	100	0
Fiber	Varied	0
Diet soda	100	0
Lettuce (iceburg)	96	0.13
Tomato	94	0.20
Orange	86	0.36
Apple	84	0.39
Potato	75	0.76
Egg	75	1.48
Fish (salmon)	71	1.41
Chicken breast	58	1.65
Sirloin steak	44	3.88
Pork chop	42	2.65
Swiss cheese	37	3.75
White bread	34	2.70
Jelly	29	2.78
Margarine	16	7.21
Chocolate	13	5.18
Bacon	8	6.00
Cereals (dry)	4	2.90
Butter	0	7.17
Oils	0	8.84
Lard	0	9.00

Table 7.5 demonstrates that foods high in water content (e.g., lettuce and tomatoes) have a low caloric density (ca. 0.20 cal/g), whereas butter, oils, and lard, which have essentially no water, have the maximum caloric density of any food (ca. 9.0 cal/g). Foods with intermediate water content have intermediate caloric densities. The caloric variation between carbohydrates and lipids is seen for dry cereals, white sugar, and the lipids. These foods are all low in water content, but the caloric density of the lipid foods; i.e., butter, oils, and lard, is twice that of sugar and dry cereals, owing to the higher proportion of total hydrocarbon.

ANABOLIC PATHWAYS

Much of the ATP produced in the mitochondrion by the electron transport array of enzymes and cytochromes, the final common catabolic pathway for the oxidation of nutrients, is consumed by the anabolic pathways during biosynthesis. The major anabolic processes that consume ATP energy are the synthesis of glucose and glycogen, gluconeogenesis and glycogenesis, respectively; the synthesis of fatty acids and triglycerides; and the synthesis of the nucleic acids, deoxyribonucleic acid and ribonucleic acids, and proteins. Compounds that contain isoprene, such as cholesterol and its derivatives, also require ATP for their synthesis.

Gluconeogenesis

Of all the nutrient energy stored by the body, carbohydrate constitutes the smallest energy reserve, being found in muscle, heart, and liver. In the face of depleted carbohydrate (glycogen) stores and in the absence of carbohydrate intake, blood glucose levels will be maintained around 80 mg/dl by the synthesis of glucose from noncarbohydrate metabolites. The glycogenic amino acids, glycerol from triglycerides, and pyruvic and lactic acids, all contribute to the synthesis of glucose by gluconeogenesis (Figure 7.9).

Gluconeogenesis occurring in muscle, heart, and liver, beginning with pyruvic or lactic acids, follows nearly the same metabolic pathway as glycolysis but in reverse. It may be recalled that in glycolysis, ATP was made in a substrate-level phosphorylation during the conversion of phosphoenolpyruvate to pyruvate. During gluconeogenesis, pyruvic and lactic acids cannot be converted directly to phosphoenolypyruvate because the reaction is thermodynamically "uphill." Thus direct conversion of pyruvate (or lactate) to phosphoenolpyruvate is circumvented by reactions using carboxybiotin, ATP, and GTP. In the first reaction pyruvate is converted to oxaloacetate, which in a second reaction (oxaloacetate) is decarboxylated to phosphoenolpyruvate. Both reactions require the expenditure of high-energy phosphorylated compounds as either ATP or GTP. The conversion of pyruvate to phosphoenolpyruvate is shown in Equation 7.16.

Equation 7.16
Conversion of pyruvate to phosphoenolpyruvate.

$$\text{pyruvate + carboxybiotin + ATP} \longrightarrow \text{oxaloacetate + ADP + P}_i \text{ + biotin}$$

$$\text{oxaloacetate + GTP} \longrightarrow \text{phosphoenolpyruvate + GDP}$$

Thus two ATP equivalents (one ATP and one GTP) are expended in glyconeogenesis in converting one molecule of pyruvate (or lactate) to phosphoenolpyruvate. A second energy-requiring reaction in gluconeogenesis is the phosphorylation of fructose-6-phosphate, forming fructose-1,6-diphosphate (Equation 7.17).

Equation 7.17
Phosphorylation of fructose-6-phosphate.

$$\text{fructose-6-phosphate + ATP} \longrightarrow \text{fructose-1,6-diphosphate + ADP}$$

Fructose-1,6-diphosphate may now be converted to glucose-6-phosphate, ending the *de novo* synthesis of glucose from either pyruvate or lactate. In liver, glucose-6-phosphate may be dephosphorylated and enter the blood or be converted to glycogen. In muscle and heart, glucose-6-phosphate is converted only to glycogen. The total requirement for the conversion of either pyruvate or lactate to glucose-6-phosphate (gluconeogenesis) is equivalent to six molecules of ATP (Table 7.6) and consumes two equivalents of $NADH_2$. Comparison of the energy requirement for gluconeogenesis with the energy yield of glycolysis shows these two pathways

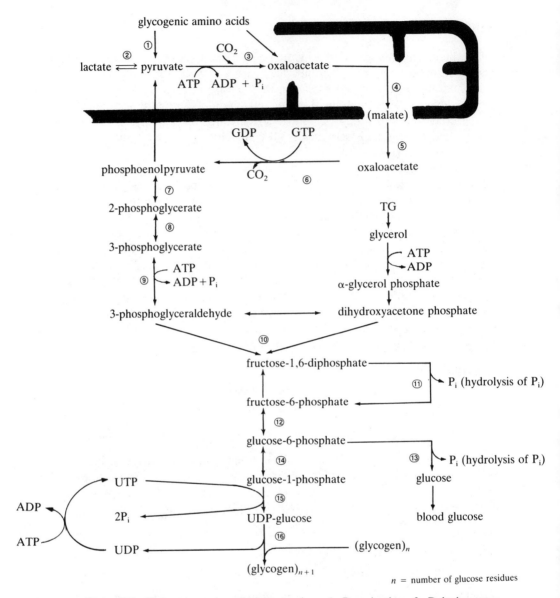

Figure 7.9 Gluconeogenesis and glycogenesis. 1. Deamination 2. Dehydrogenase
3. Pyruvate carboxylase 4. Malate dehydrogenase (mitochondrial) 5. Malate dehydrogenase (cytoplasmic) 6. Phosphoenolpyruvate carboxykinase 7. Enolase
8. Phosphoglycerolmutase 9. Phosphoglycerolkinase 10. Aldolase 11. Fructose diphos-
phatase 12. Isomerase 13. Glucose-6-phosphotase (liver, kidney enzyme)
14. Phosphoglucomutase 15. UDP-glucose pyrophosphorylase 16. Glycogen synthetase (liver,
kidney, muscle enzyme).

Table 7.6 ENERGY REQUIREMENTS FOR GLUCONEOGENESIS AND GLYCOGENESIS FROM PYRUVATE, LACTATE, OR GLYCOGENIC AMINO ACIDS

	ATP	GTP	UTP
Conversion of pyruvate (lactate) to phosphoenolpyruvate	1	1	—
Reduction of 3-phosphoglycerate to 3-phosphoglyceraldehyde	1	—	—
2 pyruvate (lactate) $\longrightarrow$ glucose	4	2	—
Conversion of glucose $\longrightarrow$ (glycogen)$_{n+1}$	1	—	1
2 pyruvate (lactate) $\longrightarrow$ (glycogen)$_{n+1}$	5	2	1

to be thermodynamically very different. The net energy yield from glycolysis is +2 ATP, whereas the net energy requirement for gluconeogenesis is +6 ATP.

Additional energy requirements are needed for the conversion of glucose to glycogen (glycogenesis). For each glucose to be transferred to a growing polysaccharide or glycogen molecule, it must first be activated by the nucleotide uridine triphosphate (UTP) shown in Equation 7.18.

Equation 7.18
Activation of glucose by uridine triphosphate.

$$\text{glucose-1-phosphate} + \text{UTP} \longrightarrow \text{UDP—glucose} + 2\ P_i$$

The product, uridine diphosphate-1-glucose, results in the activation and specific cofactor configuration for the enzymatic transfer of glucose to glycogen (Equation 7.19).

Equation 7.19
Transfer of glucose to glycogen.

$$\text{UDP—glucose} + \text{(glucose)}_n\text{glycogen} \longrightarrow \text{(glucose)}_{n+1}\text{glycogen} + \text{UDP}$$

Having transferred glucose, thereby extending the glycogen molecule by one glucose residue, the UDP must again be phosphorylated, forming UTP for activation of an additional glucose molecule. This is accomplished by ATP (see phosphorylation of nucleic acids, Figure 8.4). One ATP (as UTP) is therefore required for the incorporation of each glucose residue into glycogen.

Glycogenic Amino Acids and Glycerol

Any amino acid that can be converted to an intermediate of the citric acid cycle or pyruvate following either deamination or transamination is a glycogenic amino acid. Each amino acid may become blood glucose or glycogen via gluconeogenesis (glycogenesis). Leucine is the only amino acid that cannot be converted to glucose. Glycerol, from triglycerides, is readily converted to the glycolytic intermediate dihydroxyacetonephosphate (Equation 7.20).

Equation 7.20
Conversion of glycerol to dihydroxyacetonephosphate.

$$\text{TG} \xrightarrow[\text{3 FAS}]{} \text{glycerol} \xrightarrow[\substack{\text{ATP} \quad \text{ADP}}]{\text{NADH}_2 \quad \text{NAD}^+} \text{dihydroxyacetonephosphate}$$

Dihydroxyacetonephosphate entering the gluconeogenic pathway may then be converted to glucose-6-phosphate by combining with 3-phosphoglyceraldehyde (Figure 7.9).

Fatty Acids and Triglyceride Synthesis

Excess nutrient energy intake above and beyond energy requirements for BMR and physical exercise is converted to and stored mainly as triglyceride in depot fat. Triglycerides are formed from dietary fatty acids, fats and oils, or from dietary carbohydrates and protein via the cytoplasmic synthesis of fatty acids which are esterified with glycerol within adipose tissue. To a large degree, the synthesis and storage of triglycerides are controlled by the levels of circulating hormones, particularly insulin.

Fatty Acid Synthesis

Fatty acid synthesis begins with acetyl-CoA; which may be formed from carbohydrates (pyruvate), glycogenic or ketogenic amino acids, and fatty acids themselves (β-oxidation). Acetyl-CoA formed within the mitochondrion is transported across the mitochondrial membrane to the cell cytoplasm by carnitine. Carnitine combines with acetyl-CoA, forming mitochondrial acylcarnitine (Equation 7.21).

Equation 7.21
Transfer of mitochondrial acetyl-CoA by carnitine.

$$\underset{\text{carnitine}}{(CH_3)_3 \overset{+}{-}N-CH_2-\underset{\underset{OH}{|}}{CH}-CH_2-COOH} + \underset{\text{acetyl-CoA}}{CH_2-\overset{\overset{\displaystyle O}{\parallel}}{C}-CoA} \longrightarrow$$

$$\underset{\text{acylcarnitine}}{(CH_3)_3 \overset{+}{-}N-CH_2-\underset{\underset{\underset{\underset{CH_3}{|}}{\overset{\parallel}{C=O}}}{\overset{|}{O}}}{CH}-CH_2-COOH} + \underset{\text{coenzyme A}}{CoASH \text{ (mitochondrial)}}$$

Acylcarnitine condenses with another molecule of coenzyme A of cytoplasmic origin and forms cytoplasmic acetyl-CoA (Equation 7.22).

Equation 7.22
Condensation of mitochondrial acetyl-CoA with cytoplasmic CoASH.

$$(CH_3)_3 \overset{+}{-}N-CH_2-CH-CH_2-COOH \; + \; CoASH \text{ (cytoplasmic)} \longrightarrow$$

coenzyme A

with the chain substituent:
$$|$$
$$O$$
$$|$$
$$C{=}O$$
$$|$$
$$CH_3$$

acylcarnitine

$$(CH_3)_3 \overset{+}{-}N-CH_2-CH-CH_2-COOH \; + \; CH_2-\overset{O}{\overset{||}{C}}-CoA$$

with substituent OH on the CH.

carnitine   acetyl-CoA

The net effect of these reactions is the transfer of acetyl-CoA from the mitochondrion to the cytoplasm with the regeneration of carnitine and mitochondrial coenzyme A. In the cytoplasm, acetyl-CoA is converted to malonyl-CoA as the initiating step of fatty acid synthesis. This reaction, the synthesis of malonyl-CoA, requires the participation of carboxybiotin and the expenditure of ATP energy (Figure 7.10, Equation 7.23). Following the synthesis of malonyl-CoA, it is attached to a thiol residue of a protein (1). The protein is known as an acyl carrier protein (ACP). In a separate reaction, (2), a second ACP combines with a molecule of acetyl-CoA which provides the structural framework for the synthesis of the fatty acid. In step (3), the malonyl-ACP and the acetyl-ACP combine, forming a four-carbon unit, acetoacetyl-ACP. In this reaction, one carbon is lost as CO_2, which had originally been added in the synthesis of malonyl-CoA from acetyl-CoA (Equation 7.23).

Equation 7.23
Synthesis of malonyl-CoA from acetyl CoA.

$$CH_3-\overset{O}{\overset{||}{C}}-CoA \; + \; HO_2C\text{-biotin} \xrightarrow[\text{ATP} \quad \text{ADP + Pi}]{} HOOC-CH_2-\overset{O}{\overset{||}{C}}-SCoA \; + \; \text{biotin}$$

Acetyl-CoA   Malonyl-CoA

Acetoacetyl-ACP represents the combining of two molecules of acetyl-CoA and the formation of a four-carbon unit. The remaining steps of fatty acid synthesis

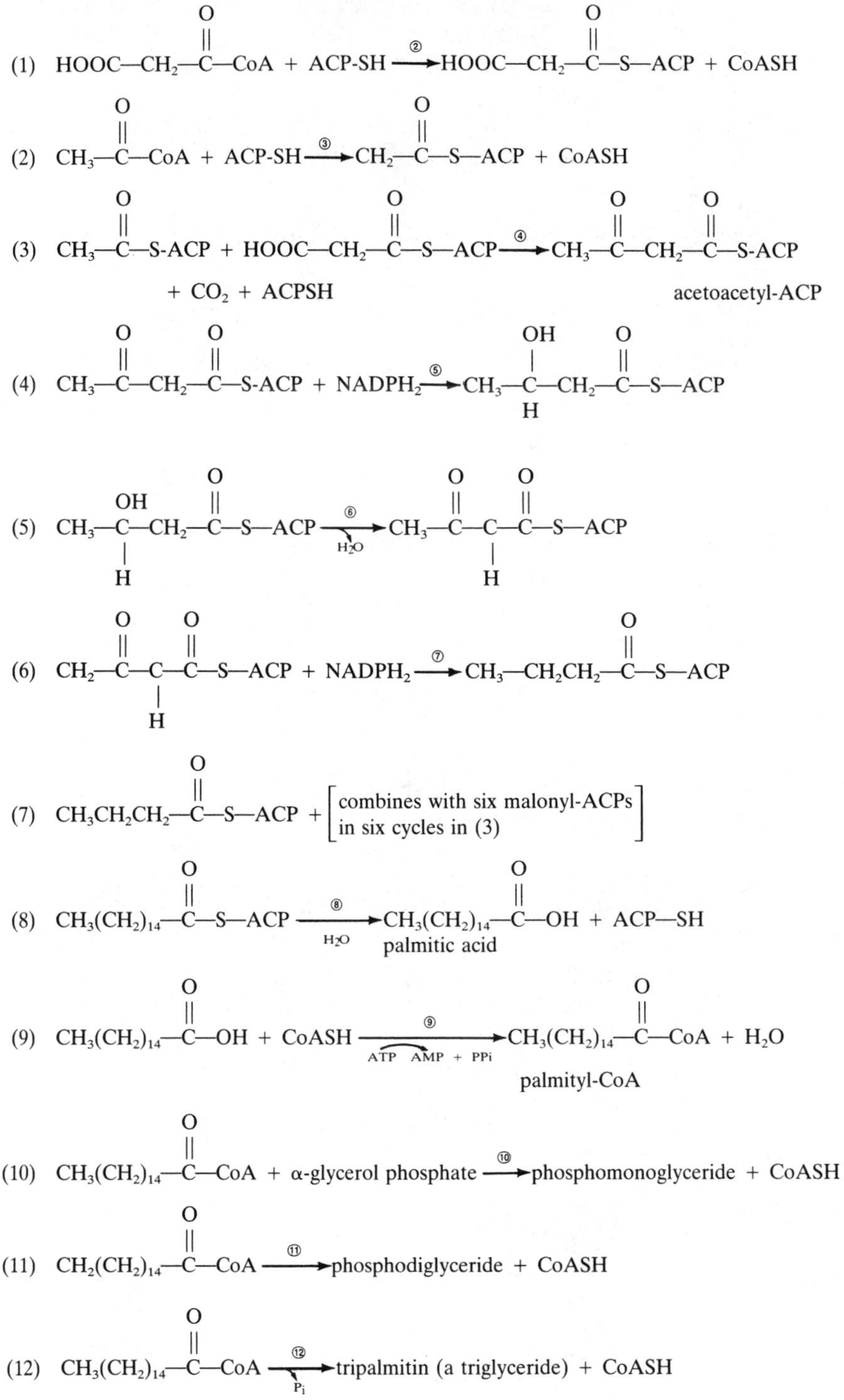

(1) $HOOC-CH_2-\overset{\overset{\displaystyle O}{\|}}{C}-CoA + ACP\text{-}SH \xrightarrow{②} HOOC-CH_2-\overset{\overset{\displaystyle O}{\|}}{C}-S-ACP + CoASH$

(2) $CH_3-\overset{\overset{\displaystyle O}{\|}}{C}-CoA + ACP\text{-}SH \xrightarrow{③} CH_2-\overset{\overset{\displaystyle O}{\|}}{C}-S-ACP + CoASH$

(3) $CH_3-\overset{\overset{\displaystyle O}{\|}}{C}-S\text{-}ACP + HOOC-CH_2-\overset{\overset{\displaystyle O}{\|}}{C}-S-ACP \xrightarrow{④} CH_3-\overset{\overset{\displaystyle O}{\|}}{C}-CH_2-\overset{\overset{\displaystyle O}{\|}}{C}-S\text{-}ACP$

$+ CO_2 + ACPSH \hspace{3cm} \text{acetoacetyl-ACP}$

(4) $CH_3-\overset{\overset{\displaystyle O}{\|}}{C}-CH_2-\overset{\overset{\displaystyle O}{\|}}{C}-S\text{-}ACP + NADPH_2 \xrightarrow{⑤} CH_3-\overset{\overset{\displaystyle OH}{|}}{\underset{\underset{\displaystyle H}{|}}{C}}-CH_2-\overset{\overset{\displaystyle O}{\|}}{C}-S-ACP$

(5) $CH_3-\overset{\overset{\displaystyle OH}{|}}{\underset{\underset{\displaystyle H}{|}}{C}}-CH_2-\overset{\overset{\displaystyle O}{\|}}{C}-S-ACP \xrightarrow[H_2O]{⑥} CH_3-\overset{\overset{\displaystyle O}{\|}}{C}-\underset{\underset{\displaystyle H}{|}}{C}-\overset{\overset{\displaystyle O}{\|}}{C}-S-ACP$

(6) $CH_2-\overset{\overset{\displaystyle O}{\|}}{C}-\underset{\underset{\displaystyle H}{|}}{C}-\overset{\overset{\displaystyle O}{\|}}{C}-S-ACP + NADPH_2 \xrightarrow{⑦} CH_3-CH_2CH_2-\overset{\overset{\displaystyle O}{\|}}{C}-S-ACP$

(7) $CH_3CH_2CH_2-\overset{\overset{\displaystyle O}{\|}}{C}-S-ACP + \left[\begin{array}{l}\text{combines with six malonyl-ACPs}\\ \text{in six cycles in (3)}\end{array}\right]$

(8) $CH_3(CH_2)_{14}-\overset{\overset{\displaystyle O}{\|}}{C}-S-ACP \xrightarrow[H_2O]{⑧} CH_3(CH_2)_{14}-\overset{\overset{\displaystyle O}{\|}}{C}-OH + ACP-SH$

$\hspace{7cm}\text{palmitic acid}$

(9) $CH_3(CH_2)_{14}-\overset{\overset{\displaystyle O}{\|}}{C}-OH + CoASH \xrightarrow[\underset{ATP \quad AMP + PPi}{}]{⑨} CH_3(CH_2)_{14}-\overset{\overset{\displaystyle O}{\|}}{C}-CoA + H_2O$

$\hspace{8cm}\text{palmityl-CoA}$

(10) $CH_3(CH_2)_{14}-\overset{\overset{\displaystyle O}{\|}}{C}-CoA + \alpha\text{-glycerol phosphate} \xrightarrow{⑩} \text{phosphomonoglyceride} + CoASH$

(11) $CH_2(CH_2)_{14}-\overset{\overset{\displaystyle O}{\|}}{C}-CoA \xrightarrow{⑪} \text{phosphodiglyceride} + CoASH$

(12) $CH_3(CH_2)_{14}-\overset{\overset{\displaystyle O}{\|}}{C}-CoA \xrightarrow[P_i]{⑫} \text{tripalmitin (a triglyceride)} + CoASH$

Figure 7.10 Fatty acid and triglyceride (tripalmitate) synthesis from acetyl-CoA, 1. Carboxylase, 2. ACP-malonyltransferase, 3. ACP-acyltransferase, 4. β-Ketoacyl-ACP-synthase, 5. β-Ketoacyl-ACP-reductase, 6. Enoyl-ACP-hydrotase, 7. Enoyl-ACP-reductase, 8. ACP-thiolesterase, 9. Acyl-CoA-synthetase, 10. Glycerolphosphate acyltransferase, 11. Glycerolphosphate acyltransferase, 12. Phosphatase and diacylglycerol acyltransferase

(Figure 7.10) consist of reduction reactions by $NADPH_2$ saturating the hydrocarbon. Elongation of the growing fatty acid in two-carbon units is made by coupling a malonyl-CoA to the ACP with simultaneous loss of CO_2 followed by further reduction of the fatty acid by $NADPH_2$. Thus each cycle in the synthesis of a fatty acid consumes one ATP in the synthesis of malonyl-CoA, uses two molecules of $NADPH_2$ for reduction of the added hydrocarbon, and results in a two-carbon extension in the *de novo* synthesis of a fatty acid. Seven cycles are completed before palmitic acid ($C_{16}H_{32}O_2$) is formed upon hydrolysis of the hydrocarbon from the acyl carrier protein (8).

Triglycerides may be formed from the fatty acids synthesized *de novo* by activation with ATP and coenzyme A. Activated fatty acids then sequentially combine [(10)–(12)] with α-glycerolphosphate or dihydroxyacetonephosphate, forming mono-, di-, and triglycerides. Addition of choline to the phosphodiglyceride would result in the synthesis of lecithin. Lecithin is not dietarily essential, but controversy exists as to whether choline is dietarily essential.

Cholesterol and Steroid Biosynthesis

A third major anabolic pathway that consumes ATP and $NADPH_2$ is the synthesis of cholesterol, principal sterol of animals and humans, and its many derivatives. Blood cholesterol levels are maintained by a combination of dietary cholesterol and endogenous *de novo* synthesis of cholesterol starting from acetyl coenzyme A. The *de novo* synthesis of cholesterol by the liver, intestinal epithelium, and skin is affected primarily by dietary cholesterol intake, but it also is affected to a lesser degree by caloric intake, fiber, exercise, and the recirculation of the bile acids via the hepatic portal system. The liver dominates the synthesis and metabolism of cholesterol. Cholesterol synthesis occurs in other tissues, however, as it is a precursor to other important compounds, 7-dehydrocholesterol (vitamin D) in the skin, adrenocortosteroids produced by the adrenal gland, and the major sex hormones, testosterone and estrogens (Figure 3.19).

Cholesterol, $C_{27}H_{46}O$, whose biosynthesis was established by Konrad Block and for which he received the Nobel Prize in 1964, has all of its 27 carbons derived from acetylcoenzyme A and may be viewed as a polymer of five isoprene units (Equation 7.24).

Equation 7.24
Acetyl-CoA or isoprene from cholesterol.

acetyl-CoA   isoprene

cholesterol carbon skeleton

$\bigcirc$, $\square$: carbons in cholesterol from acetate

The initial step in cholesterol biosynthesis (Figure 7.11) is the condensation of two molecules of acetyl-CoA to form acetoacetyl-CoA (1), which combines with a third molecule of acetyl-CoA, forming β-hydroxy-β-methylglutaryl-CoA (2). An alternative metabolic route for acetoacetyl-CoA is the formation of acetoacetic acid and the other ketones (Figure 7.12). Reduction of β-hydroxy-β-methylglutaryl-CoA by two molecules of $NADPH_2$ yields a six-carbon molecule, mevalonic acid, which is the reduced product of three combined molecules of acetylcoenzyme A. (3) Mevalonic acid is synthesized in the cytoplasm and is the immediate precursor of isoprene and ultimately cholesterol and its derivatives. In the synthesis leading to cholesterol, mevalonic acid is sequentially phosphorylated by three molecules of ATP and decarboxylated to yield the five-carbon isopentenylpyrophosphate. (4) Through a series of metabolic steps, six isopentylpyrophosphates are combined, forming squalene, a 30-carbon polymer of six isoprene units. (5) Through a series of metabolic steps, squalene is hydroxylated via formation of a 3,4-epoxide, is cyclized, demethylated, and reduced with four molecules of $NADPH_2$, all of which results in the final synthesis of cholesterol. Equation 7.25 summarized the synthesis of cholesterol from acetyl-CoA.

Equation 7.25
Chemical summary for the synthesis of cholesterol.

$$18\,\text{acetyl-CoA} + 18\text{ATP} + 5\text{NADPH}_2 + \text{H}_2\text{O} + \text{O}_2 \xrightarrow{\quad 6\text{CO}_2 \quad} \text{cholesterol}\,(\text{C}_{27})$$
$$+ 3\text{ADP} + 6\text{P}_i + 6\text{PP}_i + 5\text{NADP}^+ + (\text{R}-\text{CH}_3)_3$$

As Equation 7.25 indicates, 18 molecules of ATP and five molecules of $NADPH_2$ are required to synthesize one molecule of cholesterol *de novo*. The same energy requirement is, of course, expended in the synthesis of adrenocorticoids (C_{21}), androgens (C_{19}), and estrogens (C_{18}), all of which are metabolically derived from cholesterol (Figure 3.19).

Acetoacetic acid, β-hydroxybutyric acid, and acetone, "the ketones," which normally do not accumulate metabolically, are alternative end products to cholesterol and fatty acid synthesis. In the diabetic, these ketones accumulate, owing

(1) $2CH_3-\overset{\overset{O}{\|}}{C}-CoA \xrightarrow{①} CH_3-\overset{\overset{O}{\|}}{C}-CH_2-\overset{\overset{O}{\|}}{C}-CoA + CoASH$

acetyl CoA   acetoacetyl-CoA

(2) $CH_3-\overset{\overset{O}{\|}}{C}-CH_2-\overset{\overset{O}{\|}}{C}-CoA + CH_3-\overset{\overset{O}{\|}}{C}-CoA \xrightarrow[②]{H_2O} HOOC-CH_2-\underset{\underset{CH_3}{|}}{\overset{\overset{OH}{|}}{C}}-CH_2-\overset{\overset{O}{\|}}{C}-CoA$

β-OH, β-CH₃ glutaryl-CoA

(3) $HOOC-CH_2-\underset{\underset{CH_3}{|}}{\overset{\overset{OH}{|}}{C}}-CH_2-\overset{\overset{O}{\|}}{C}-CoA + 2\,NADPH_2 \xrightarrow{③} HOOC-CH_2-\underset{\underset{CH_3}{|}}{\overset{\overset{OH}{|}}{C}}-CH_2-CH_2OH + CoASH$

mevalonic acid

(4) $HOOC-CH_2-\underset{\underset{CH_3}{|}}{\overset{\overset{OH}{|}}{C}}-CH_2-CH_2OH + 3ATP \underset{④\,3Pi}{\overset{3CO_2}{\rightleftharpoons}} H_2C{=}\underset{\overset{|}{CH_3}}{\overset{\overset{CH_3}{|}}{C}}-CH_2-CH_2-O-℗-℗ + 3AMP$

isopentylpyrophosphate

(5) $\left(\underset{H_2C=C-CH_2-CH_2-O-℗-℗}{\overset{\overset{CH_3}{|}}{}}\right)_6 + NADPH_2 \xrightarrow{⑤} 4PP_i + NADP^+ + H^+ +$

(. . . . . indicates isoprene unit separations)

(6)

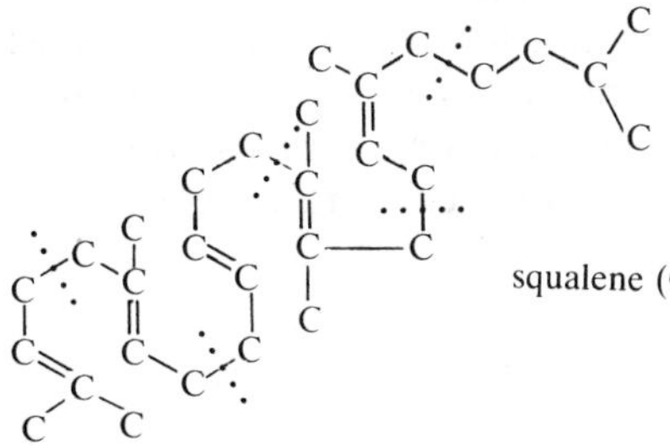

squalene (C₃₀)

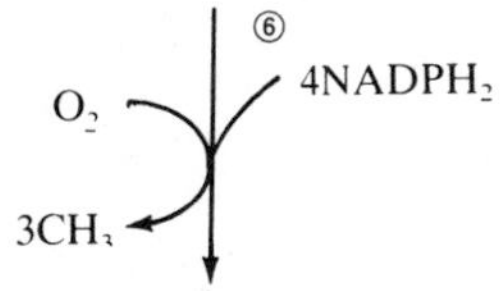

O_2 ⟍ ⟋ 4NADPH₂

3CH₃ ⟍

(steps: hydroxylation, cyclization, demethylation)

Figure 7.11 Synthesis of cholesterol from acetyl-CoA.

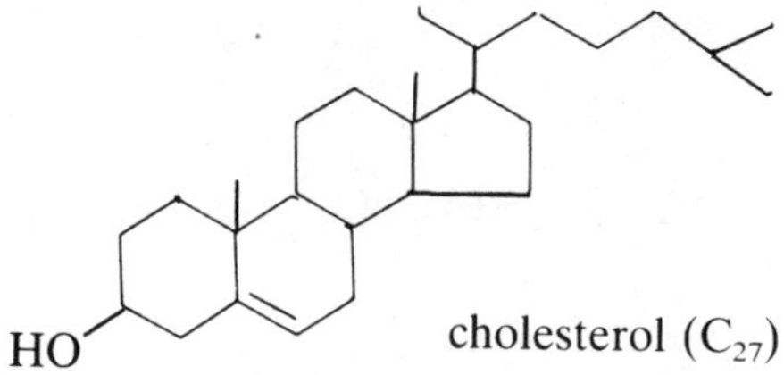

cholesterol (C_{27})

1. Condensation of 2 acetyl-CoA
2. β-Hydroxymethyl-glutaryl-CoA synthase
3. β-Hydroxymethyl glutaryl-CoA reductase
4. Mevalonic kinase
   Phosphomevalonic kinase   } combined reactions
   Phosphomevalonic decarboxylase

5. Isopentyl pyrophosphate isomerase
   Dimethylallyl transferase   } combined reactions
   Squalene synthase

6. Squalene monooxygenase
   Squalene epoxidase
   Lanosterol cyclase   } combined reactions
   7-Dehydrocholesterol reductase

Figure 7.11   (continued)

to the absence, or malfunction, of insulin and excessive β-oxidation.   If the diabetic state remains uncorrected, accumulating ketones may lead to ketoacidosis, coma, and death.   The ketones are also formed during fasting and starvation states, during gestation, and may occur postsurgically in response to ether anesthesia.   Under normal metabolic conditions, ketones, which are potential sources of caloric energy, are metabolized via the citric acid cycle.

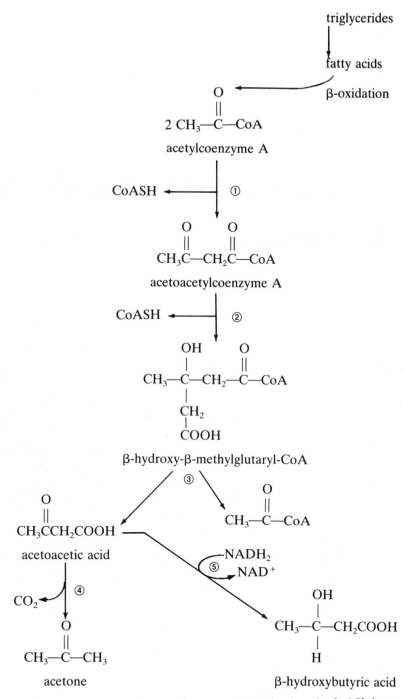

Figure 7.12 Synthesis of ketones from acetyl coenzyme A. 1. Condensation 2. β-Hydroxy-β-methylglutaryl-CoA synthetase 3. Cleavage 4. Acetoacetic decarboxylase 5. Acetoacetic reductase.

8

Nucleic Acids and Protein Synthesis

PURINES

The purines (adenine and guanine), components of the nucleic acids and hypo-xanthine, are synthesized from three amino acids, carboxybiotin, the N^{10}-formyl and N^5,N^{10}-methenyl derivatives of tetrahydrofolic acid (Figure 8.1). Six ATPs are consumed in the synthesis of the initial purine derivative, inosine monophosphate (IMP). The ATPs are expended in the incorporation of glycine, the nitrogens from aspartic acid and glutamine, and the activation of ribose-5-phosphate, forming 5-phosphoribosyl-1-pyrophosphate, which phosphorylates the mononucleotide, IMP (Figures 8.1 and 8.2). Figure 8.2 shows the pathway for the synthesis of adenosine monophosphate (AMP) and guanosine monophosphate (GMP) from IMP. Additional amounts of ATP are expended in synthesizing AMP and GMP. Two additional ATPs are consumed in converting each of the mononucleotides into

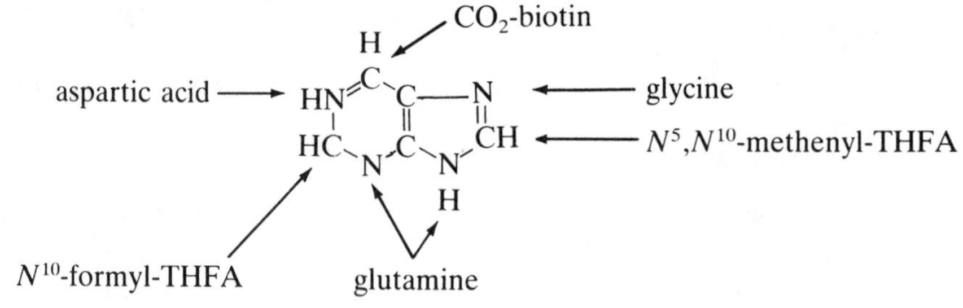

Figure 8.1 Synthesis of purines.

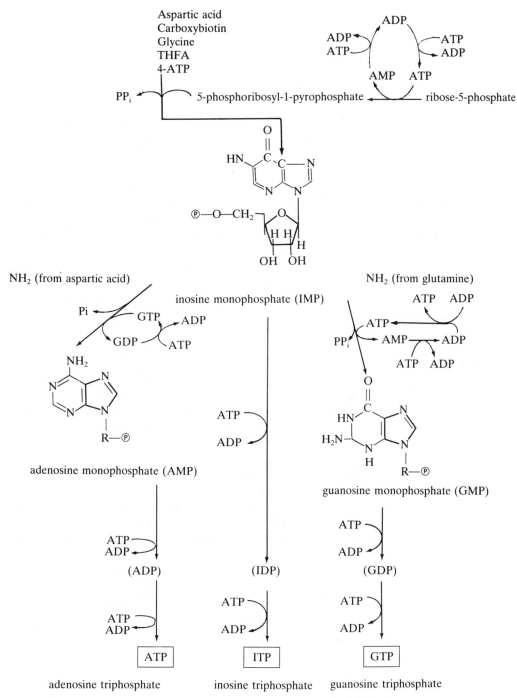

Figure 8.2 Abbreviated de novo synthesis of purines.

trinucleotides with a total of 10 ATPs expended in the synthesis of one molecule of guanine triphosphate, GTP.

PYRIMIDINES

Pyrimidines (Figure 8.3; cytosine, thymine, and uracil) components of the nucleic acids are synthesized from carbamoyl phosphate and aspartic acid (see the urea cycle, Figure 7.7). Four ATPs are consumed in the synthesis of the initial pyrimidine derivative, uridine monophosphate (UMP). Two ATPs are consumed in the cytosolic synthesis of carbamoyl phosphate and two additional ATPs are consumed in the formation of the ribotide, UMP (Figure 8.4). Cytidine triphosphate is derived from UTP with expenditure of an additional ATP for incorporating its amine being derived from glutamine. Thymidine triphosphate, through a series of metabolic steps, is derived from UMP and UTP, which yields pyrophosphate. N^5,N^{10}-Methenyltetrahydrofolic acid, probably in association with vitamin B_{12}, donates its methyl group in the synthesis of thymidine monophosphate (TMP) from UTP. TMP is then phosphorylated by two ATPs forming TTP. Nine ATP are ultimately expended in the *de novo* synthesis of one molecule of thymidine triphosphate, TPP.

NUCLEOTIDES

Nucleotides (nucleic acids) are ubiquitous in animal and human diets, but they are not dietarily essential, as they are synthesized from rather simple components. The nucleic acids, deoxyribonucleic acid (DNA) and ribonucleic acid (RNA) are carriers of cellular genetic information. The nucleic acid adenosine triphosphate (ATP) is the universal carrier of metabolic energy and adenine is also found as a component of the coenzymes NAD^+($NADP^+$), FAD, CoA, and cyclic AMP. The building blocks of the nucleic acids are the nitrogenous heterocyclic bases, derivatives of purine or pyrimidine. Addition of the carbohydrates, ribose or deoxyribose, to a nitrogen base produces a nucleoside. Nucleosides with one phosphate moiety are called nucleotides. Adenosine mononucleotide, for example, is AMP.

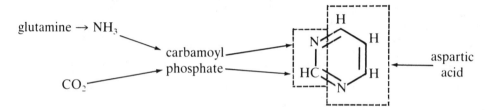

Figure 8.3 Synthesis of pyrimidines.

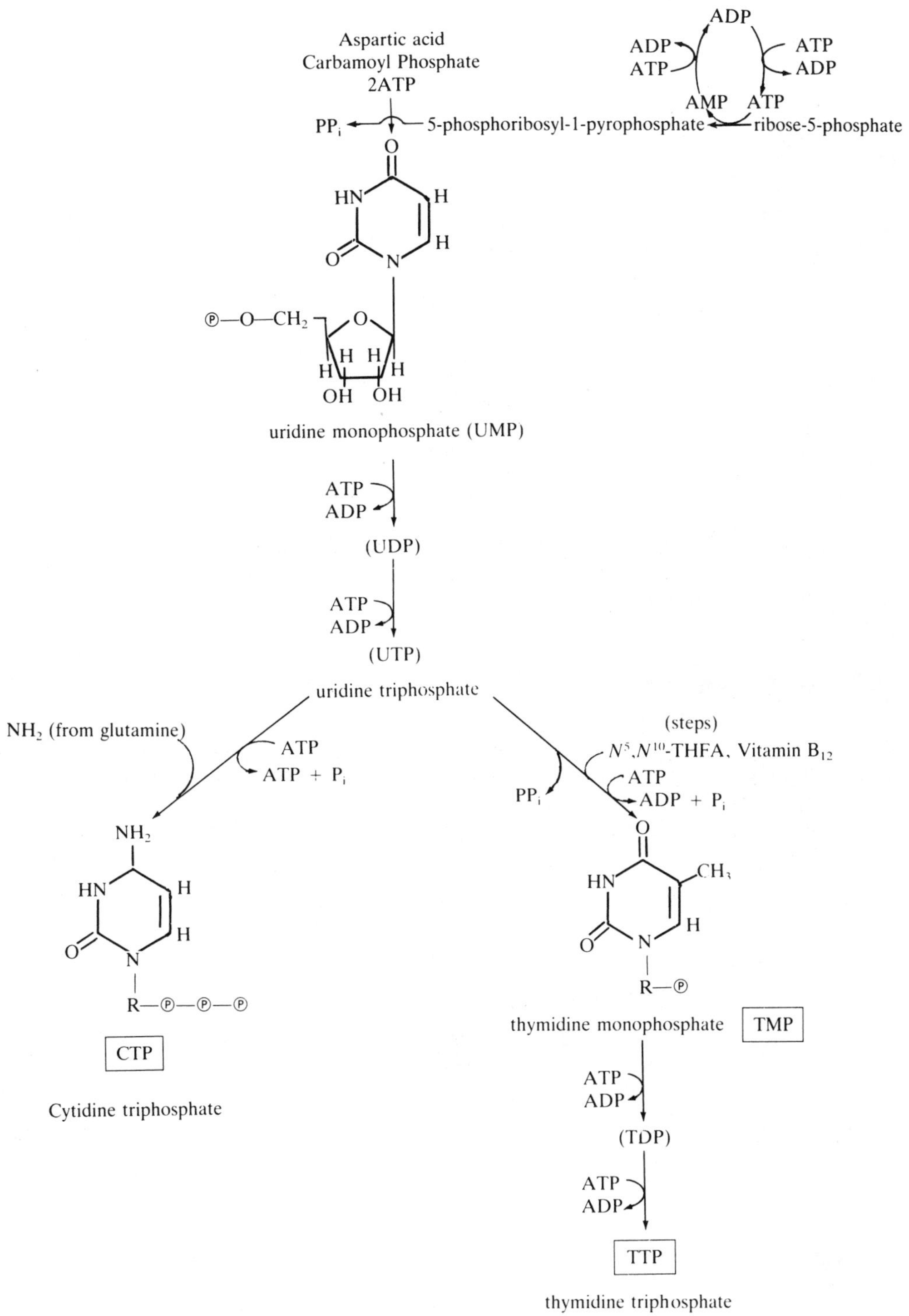

Aspartic acid
Carbamoyl Phosphate
2ATP

ADP

ADP → → ATP
ATP → → ADP

AMP   ATP

PP$_i$ ← 5-phosphoribosyl-1-pyrophosphate ← ribose-5-phosphate

uridine monophosphate (UMP)

ATP
ADP

(UDP)

ATP
ADP

(UTP)

uridine triphosphate

NH$_2$ (from glutamine)

ATP
ATP + P$_i$

(steps)
N^5,N^{10}-THFA, Vitamin B$_{12}$

PP$_i$

ATP
ADP + P$_i$

R—℗—℗—℗

CTP

Cytidine triphosphate

thymidine monophosphate   TMP

ATP
ADP

(TDP)

ATP
ADP

TTP

thymidine triphosphate

Figure 8.4   Abbreviated *de novo* synthesis of pyrimidines.

TABLE 8.1   NOMENCLATURE OF THE NUCLEIC ACIDS

Heterocyclics	Nitrogen bases	Nucleosides	Mononucleotides	Dinucleotides	Trinucleotides
Purine(s)	Adenine Guanine Hypoxanthine	Adenosine Guanosine Inosine	Adenosine monophosphate (AMP) Guanosine monophosphate (GMP) Inosine monophosphate (IMP)	(ADP) (GDP) (IDP)	(ATP) (GTP) (ITP)
Pyrimidine(s)	Cytosine Thymine Uracil	Cytidine Thymidine Uridine	Cytidine monophosphate (CMP) Thymidine monophosphate (TMP) , Uridine monophosphate (UMP)	(CDP) (TDP) (UDP)	(CTP) (TTP) (UTP)

Additional phosphates yield the nucleotides adenosine diphosphate (ADP) and adenosine triphosphate (ATP). Names of purine and pyrimidine bases, and nucleosides and nucleotides, are given in Table 8.1.

DNA AND RNA

The previous sections of this chapter have shown how energy (ATP) is used in the *de novo* synthesis of the purine and pyrimidine trinucleotides. In this section we examine how the high-energy trinucleotides are used in the synthesis of deoxyribonucleic acid (DNA) and ribonucleic acid (RNA). DNA is a polymer assembled from the trinucleotides, dATP, dGTP, dCTP, and dTTP, in which the carbohydrate ribose has been reduced by $NADPH_2$, forming 2-deoxyribose (dADP) (Equation 8.1).

Equation 8.1
Synthesis of 2-deoxyribose (dADP).

ribose (ADP)   2-deoxyribose (ADP)

RNA is a polymer assembled from the trinucleotides ATP, GTP, CTP, and UTP. RNA differs from DNA in that the base thymidine is replaced by uricil and the carbohydrate ribose is utilized in place of 2-deoxyribose. The remaining struc-

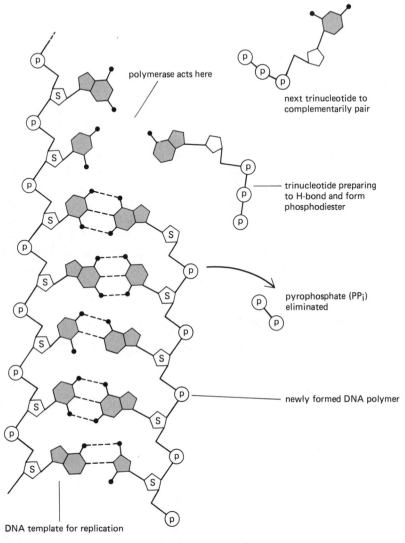

polymerase acts here

next trinucleotide to
complementarily pair

trinucleotide preparing
to H-bond and form
phosphodiester

pyrophosphate (PP$_i$)
eliminated

newly formed DNA polymer

DNA template for replication

Figure 8.5 DNA replication.

tural differences between DNA and RNA are that DNA is predominantly double stranded, while RNA exists primarily in single-stranded form. Three forms of RNA have been distinguished in nature: messenger RNA (mRNA), transfer RNA (tRNA), and ribosomal RNA (rRNA). Each form of RNA participates and functions differently in protein synthesis. RNA and DNA are structurally similar in that the phosphodiester linkage between ribose or 2-deoxyribose exists in 5′→3′ linkage. As DNA is predominantly double stranded, hydrogen bonding takes place between the complement base pairs: adenine (A) and thymine (T), and guanine (G) and cytosine (C).

DNA is complementarily copied from a DNA template in a process called replication. In this process one strand of the double-stranded DNA serves as a template and the complementary base trinucleotides hydrogen bonds to its complement with the formation of the $5' \rightarrow 3'$ phosphodiester bond being established. As the phosphodiester bond is formed, pyrophosphate (PP_i) is eliminated. DNA as well as RNA are therefore polymers of mononucleotides. The energy used to synthesize the polymer existed within the trinucleotides prior to polymerization (Figure 8.5).

RNA is also complementarily copied from a DNA template. The difference between the DNA and the RNA is that the trinucleotides forming the RNA contain ribose and not 2-deoxyribose, and the pyrimidine uracil (as UTP) replaces thymine (as TTP) by the RNA polymerase. The process of complementarily copying DNA by RNA polymers and forming messenger RNA (mRNA) is called transcription. From DNA originates also the various transfer (tRNA) RNA molecules and ribosomal (rRNA) RNA. Two molecules of ATP are therefore expended in adding one mononucleotide in establishing a $5' \rightarrow 3'$ phosphodiester bond, extending either DNA or RNA by one nucleotide. This is demonstrated for cytosine monophosphate (CMP) and DNA in Equation 8.2.

Equation 8.2
Extension of nucleic acids (DNA and RNA) by one nucleotide.

$$dCMP + ATP \longrightarrow dCDP + ADP$$

$$dCDP + ATP \longrightarrow dCTP + ADP$$

$$dCTP(CTP) + DNA(RNA) \longrightarrow DNA\text{—}dCMP \text{ or } RNA\text{—}CMP$$

$$5' \rightarrow 3' \text{ phosphodiester bond formed}$$

Codons, Anticodons, and tRNAs

The sequence of nitrogen bases along the DNA molecule ultimately determines the amino acid sequence of a specific protein. This statement is the basis of the one gene–one protein theory of genetic regulation of protein synthesis of François Jacob and Jacques Monod, who received the Nobel Prize in Medicine in 1965. The one gene–one protein theory provides not only for the coding of proteins, but for the control of protein synthesis. Our primary interest here is in the structural component of the (gene) DNA sequence. Within every gene, three nitrogen bases pair in sequence along the DNA code for one amino acid. Thus a protein of 100 amino acids would have a structural gene within a cell's nucleus of 300 sequential nitrogen bases coding for the 100 amino acids. During translation of these 300 DNA bases, complementary base pairing and mRNA synthesis would occur, resulting in the transfer of coded information to mRNA. Each of the 100 nitrogen base triplets is a codon that codes information for one amino acid. Table 8.2 gives a mRNA codon for each of the 20 amino acids commonly found in protein.

TABLE 8.2 CODONS OF THE AMINO ACIDS COMMONLY FOUND IN PROTEINS[a]

Glycine	GGU	Phenylalanine	UUU
Alanine	GCC	Proline	CCU
Valine	GUU	Histidine	CAU
Leucine	CUU	Aspartic acid	GAU
Threonine	ACU	Glutamic acid	GAA
Serine	UCU	Lysine	AAA
Methionine	AUG	Argine	AGA
Cysteine	UGU	Asparagine	AAU
Tyrosine	UGG	Glutamine	GAA

[a]Some amino acids have more than one codon; for simplicity, only one codon is shown.

Messenger mRNA is directed from the cell's nucleus to the ribosomes of the endoplasmic reticulum, where protein synthesis occurs.

Derived also from DNA is transfer RNA (tRNA). Transfer RNA of approximately 80 mononucleotides may contain several unusual nucleic acid bases and is folded back upon itself in paper-clip fashion, with three or more arms. On one arm of a tRNA molecule is a complementary base sequence to the mRNA codon: the anticodon. Attached to the tRNA through a terminal CCA sequence of bases is an amino acid. For each amino acid found in protein there is at least one specific tRNA which transfers that specified amino acid to the ribosome. The amino acids are activated by attachment to its specific tRNA, as shown in Equation 8.3.

Equation 8.3
Amino acid activation.

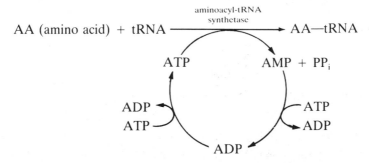

Two ATP equivalents are required to activate each amino acid, forming an aminoacyl-tRNA prior to peptide (protein) synthesis.

PROTEINS

Protein synthesis occurs in the rough endoplasmic reticulum of the cell's cytoplasm in association with ribosomes. Ribosomes, composed of rRNA and protein, are the focal point for the *de novo* synthesis of protein. It is at the ribosome that activated aminoacyl-tRNAs bearing their amino acids and mRNA come together to form a protein in the translation process. The ribosomes, moving along an mRNA, keys in the anticodon of each tRNA to the complementary base pair with each codon along the mRNA. As the translational process occurs, peptide bonds are formed between amino acids in a growing polypeptide chain. The polypeptide is synthesized from the terminal free amine and as each amino acid is added to the growing polypeptide chain, the tRNA is cleaved from the amino acid which it had carried to the ribosome. Energy is required for the synthesis of each peptide bond in the new polypeptide chain and for the movement (translocation) of the ribosome along the mRNA. The energy for these events is provided by the aminoacyl-(activated) tRNA and two molecules of GTP. These reactions, summarized in Equation 8.4, take place within the ribosome.

Equation 8.4
Energy requirements for peptide synthesis and translocation.

(1) *Binding of aminoacyl-tRNA to ribosome*

ADP ATP

GTP GDP + P$_i$

polypeptide + aminoacyl-tRNA ⟶ bound aminoacyl-tRNA

(2) *Peptide synthesis*

tRNA

bound aminoacyl-tRNA + polypeptide ⟶ polypeptide extended by one amino acid

(3) *Translocation*

ADP ATP

GTP GDP + P$_i$

New polypeptide ⟶ ribosome moved one codon awaiting next aminoacyl-tRNA

Two GTPs (two ATP equivalents) are expended in the elongation of a polypeptide chain by a single amino acid in the process of translation. Energy provided by the aminoacyl-tRNA, equivalent to two ATPs, is also expended in the synthesis of the new peptide bond, accounting for a total energy expenditure equivalent to four ATPs for the addition of each amino acid in polypeptide elongation. These reactions are summarized in Equation 8.5.

Equation 8.5
Summary of energy requirement for peptide synthesis.

polypeptide + amino acid + 4ATP ⟶ polypeptide + 1 amino acid + 4ADP + 4P$_i$

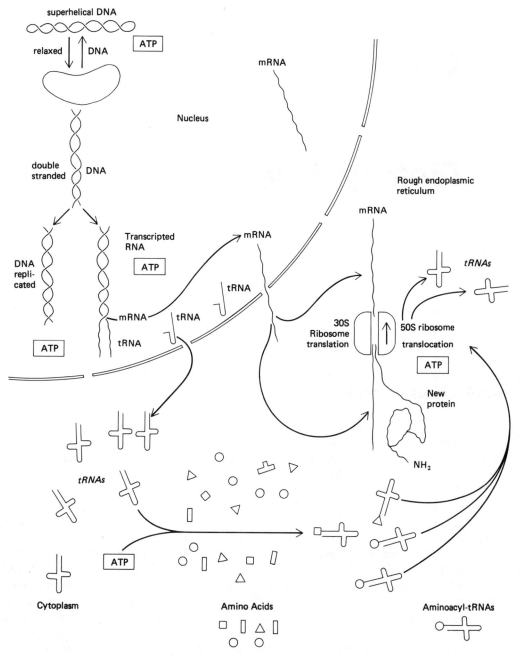

Figure 8.6 Energy use in protein synthesis.

Thus it may be appreciated that much of the ATP formed in the catabolic pathways is used in the *de novo* synthesis of nitrogen bases and nucleic acids, in the activation of amino acids, and in the formation of the new proteins (Figure 8.6).

9

Dietary Fiber

FIBER: A GENERIC TERM

Fiber is a generic term with a different meaning when used by a botanist (microfibrils), a cereal chemist (cellulose), or an animal nutritionist (indigestible feed matter). To the human nutritionist, fiber is that cell wall plant material (carbohydrates and lignin) which remains mostly undigested by the enzymes of the human gastrointestinal tract. The principal source of dietary fiber is the structural component of plant cell walls; the polymers of cellulose, hemicelluloses, and pectins; all carbohydrates. Lignin, the noncarbohydrate polymer of cell walls, is highly insoluble and is the "woody" component of plant cell walls (Table 9.1).

Also included under the generic term "fiber" are the nonstructural components of plants consisting of polysaccharides not found within the plant cell wall and other noncarbohydrate materials. Plant substances within this group include the gums, mucilages, and storage and chemically modified polysaccharides. Polysaccharides of the cell wall of seaweed and algae are distinctive in that xylans, mannans, and cellulose analogs often containing sulfates replace the normal cellulose in cell walls. Some people even argue that gums, mucilages, and so on, are not fibrous and should not be included within the definition of fiber. Such distinctions make it difficult to find a universally acceptable definition for dietary fiber.

TABLE 9.1 DIETARY FIBER COMPONENTS

Major component	Chemical composition	Colonic function	Nutritional/clinical effects
Cellulose	Homopolyglycan β-(1→4) glycosides	Nondigestible, partially fermentable, imbibes water, laxative	Dilution of colonic excretory metabolites; prevents diverticulitis
Hemicellulose	Heteropolyglycan(250 known polymers) β-(1→4) xyloside backbone; several side chains of arabinose or glucuronic acid residues	Partially fermentable, imbibes water, laxative	Dilution of colonic excretory metabolites; prevent diverticulitis; may weakly bind minerals
Pectins	Heteropolysaccharides, major component β-(1→4) linkage of galacturonic acid, uronic acid, and methyluronic side chains	Gel formation, antidiarrhetic	May reduce blood cholesterol; increased fecal steroid and lipid excretion; may have increases in Ca^{2+} and Mg^{2+} excretion proportionate to uronic acid content
Lignin	Noncarbohydrate polymers of phenylpropanes; derived from coumaryl, coniferyl, and sinapyl alcohols	Antioxidant phenols; almost chemically inert to digestion or fermentation	May bind bile acids and some cations; provides fecal bulk

235

FIBER CHEMISTRY

Cellulose

Cellulose, a β-(1→4) homoglycan (Figure 9.1), is the highly insoluble main structural component of the plant cell wall. It is the major organic hydrocarbon found
in nature and the principal fibrous component of plant cells. Because cellulose is
an unbranched linear polymer it can be densely packed into a microfibrillar structure
within the plant's cell wall. Cellulose remains mostly undigestible in monogastric
animals and humans because of the lack of synthesis of a β-(1→4) glucosidase
(cellulose). Cellulase, however, is readily digested by the microflora of polygastric
animals. Cellulose, like cooked starch, can imbibe water, increasing fecal weight.
Cellulose may also bind bile acids, increasing the excretion of these cholesterol
metabolites, thereby lowering serum cholesterol.

Hemicellulose

The hemicelluloses (unrelated to cellulose) comprise a diverse group of heteropolysaccharides. Unlike cellulose, which contains no branching, hemicelluloses
are highly branched. The main homopolymer chain consists mainly of β-(1→4)
linked xylose, mannose, and galactosides. From the primary chain are found
branches of arabinose, galactose, and 4-O-methylglucuronic acid. Hemicelluloses
are those plant cell wall polysaccharides isolated from the extraction of plant cells
with dilute base (Figure 9.1).

Pectins

Pectins are derived from intracellular and plant cell wall materials. Fruits and
vegetables contain a proportionately high dry weight content of pectins. The
pectins are chemically complete hetero- and homopolysaccharides whose principal
polymer is D-galacturonic acid (Figure 9.1). Many other carbohydrates including
arabinose, galactose, fucose, and so on, are found in the hydrolyzates of pectins,
which form the side-chain linkages from the major polymer. Some of the carbohydrates, like xylose and fucose, may be O-methylated (—OCH_3). Structurally,
the pectins within plants chelate calcium ions, which contributes to their insolubility.

Lignin

Lignin is a term referring to the noncarbohydrate aromatic polymers of the plant
cell wall. It constitutes the "woody" material usually obtained from maturing
plants. Lignin is a complex, highly variable polymer of 40 or more phenylpro-
panoids. Since lignin is variable in structure, no specific chemical structure can
be assigned. Three major aromatic alcohols—coumaryl, coniferyl, and sinapyl

(1) Cellulose

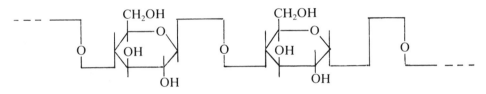

MW 50,000 to 2.5 million β-(1 → 4) glycosides

(2) Hemicellulose (xylans): β-(1 → 4) xylose

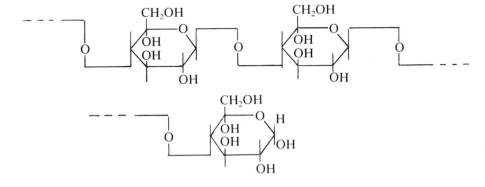

(3) Pectins: β-(1 → 4) galacturonic acid

(4) Lignin: varied aromatic noncarbohydrate polymer

phenylpropyl
monomeric
precursor

coniferyl alcohol
monomic precursor

Figure 9.1 Dietary fiber chemistry.

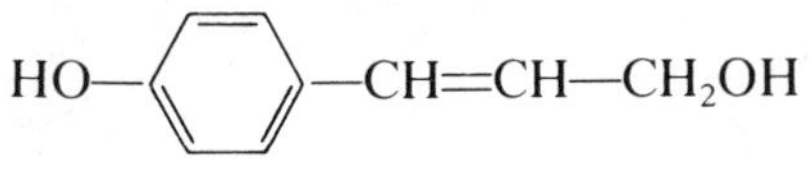

$$HO\!-\!\langle\!=\!\rangle\!-\!CH\!=\!CH\!-\!CH_2OH$$

p-courmarie oil

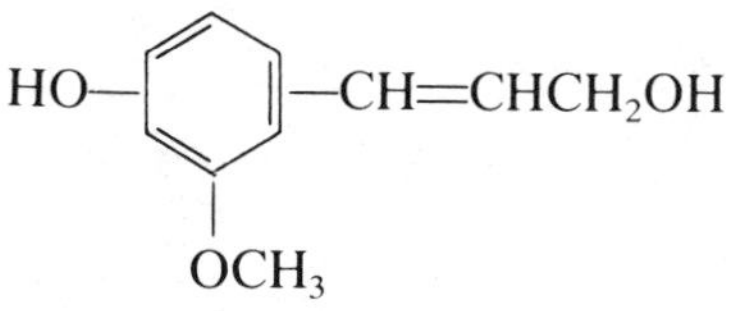

$$HO\!-\!\langle\!=\!\rangle\!-\!CH\!=\!CHCH_2OH$$
$$\overset{|}{OCH_3}$$

coniferyl alcohol

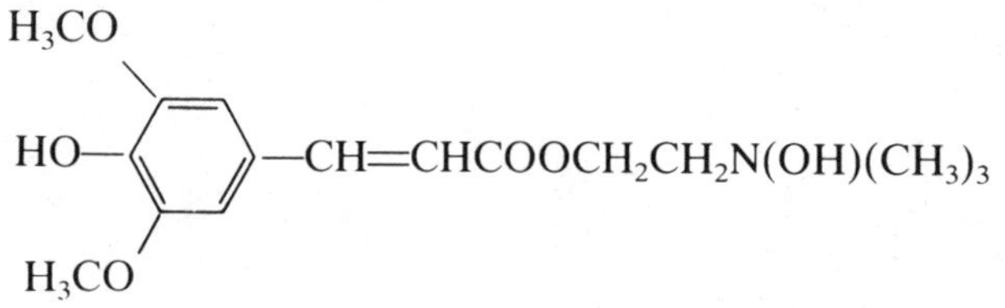

$$H_3CO$$
$$HO\!-\!\langle\!=\!\rangle\!-\!CH\!=\!CHCOOCH_2CH_2N(OH)(CH_3)_3$$
$$H_3CO$$

sinapine

Figure 9.2 Monomeric units of lignin.

alcohol—are the major monomers contributing to the final lignin polymer (Figure 9.2). Lignin is highly insoluble and resistant to digestive enzymes and fermentation reactions.

Gums, Mucilages, and Algal Polysaccharides

Gums (resins) are polysaccharides synthesized by plants in response to, and at the site of, an injury. Mucilages are polysaccharides produced by secretory cells of plants to prevent excessive transpiration. Algal polysaccharides are composed of mannans, xylose, and other carbohydrate polymers which serve functionally to replace the cellulose found in the cell walls of other plants. These carbohydrates, comprising a small proportion of the total carbohydrate portion of the diet, are often included in classifications of dietary fiber.

NUTRITIONAL PROPERTIES OF DIETARY FIBER

Dietary fiber, such as the fiber from vegetables and bran, chemically purified cellulose, gums and mucilages, and so on, each possess one or more important nutritional properties based on its inherent chemical composition. In general, the nutritional properties that various fibers possess are fermentability, contributions to the bulk density of fecal material, ability to imbibe water, and their general capacity to bind minerals. Collectively, the chemical composition of dietary fiber affects the physiology and microbiology of the gastrointestinal tract and the digestive process through fermentations, production of flatus, and changes in intraluminal pressures.

Fermentation

A major contribution to the ever-changing composition of the intestinal content of the gut is fiber. The composition of the fiber interacts with and changes the microfloral population, resulting in the fermentation of some fibrous components principally in the ascending colon of the large intestine. Here, fiber of vegetable origin, and to a lesser degree fiber from bran, are fermented by bacteria under nearly anaerobic conditions. The fermentation products are notably gases: some hydrogen, carbon dioxide, and methane. These gases are voided either through the pulmonary system or are passed as flatus. Additional fermentation products include the formation of some alcohols and volatile fatty acids: commonly acetic, proprionic, and butyric acids. Absorption of these fermentation products is a source of available calories. During fermentation, fecal weight is increased by the rapid increase in the mass of the bacterial population which can constitute as much as 40 to 50% of the fecal dry weight. Lignin is not fermented as it passes through the gastrointestinal tract.

Hydration

Fiber and polysaccharides in general have the capacity to imbibe and hold water within the fiber's structural matrix. The amount of water imbibed by fiber is dependent on its structure and solubility, which are determined in part by the number of hydrophilic moieties—hydroxyl, carboxyl, sulfoxyl, and carbonyls—which permit the hydration of fiber to occur. Generally, vegetable fibers have a greater capacity to hold water, gram for gram, than do bran or lignin. Because vegetable fibers are highly fermentable, the actual ability of dietary fiber to become hydrated and retain water, contributing to fecal bulk throughout digestion, may be quite different. Fecal bulking agents used in pharmaceutical preparations are often combinations of cellulose and vegetable fibers.

Metal Binding

Fiber, because of its carboxylic-containing carbohydrates, has the ability to bind various nutritional and toxic cations—Ca^{2+}, Zn^{2+}, (toxic) Cd^{2+}, Hg^{2+}, and so on—thereby preventing absorption. Most vegetable fibers and fiber-containing residues of uronic acids function like weak cation-exchange resins, binding these minerals. Persons with adequate mineral nutriture do not seem to be affected adversely by high-fiber diets. However, persons eating high-fiber diets and having a marginal intake of certain minerals, such as zinc, may be in jeopardy of establishing a chronic mineral deficiency.

In addition to binding cations and preventing the absorption of minerals, fiber may bind organic molecules, notably the bile acids. Although controversial, fiber, particularly pectins and lignin, appears to be hypocholesteremic by lowering the ileal reabsorption of bile acids, which have been chemically modified by the bacterial flora of the gastrointestinal tract. The effects of fiber binding the bile acids are complex and vary considerably within and between individuals as changes in dietary practices occur.

IMPORTANCE OF FIBER AS A NUTRIENT

Present-day nutritional interest in the role of dietary fiber in the prevention of disease was renewed in the early 1970s by a British surgeon, Dennis Burkett. Its importance in the diet is seen by many nutritionists and by the public at large to be so important that it could be a seventh nutrient class.

The list of diseases that fiber is claimed to prevent or ameliorate is extensive, but there is no definitive proof. Diseases of the colon—constipation, appendicitis, hemorrhoids, ulcers, precancerous polyps, and cancer—are believed by some people to be reduced or prevented by a high dietary fiber intake. Fiber's importance in reducing these diseases is thought to be derived from fiber bulk, hydration, binding of bile acids, increased fecal transit time, and dilution of fecal mutagens and carcinogens. Metabolic diseases for which fiber has been deemed preventative include obesity, diabetes, heart diseases, hypertension, vascular diseases of various types, embolisms, gallstones, and senile osteoporosis in addition to others. Endocrine diseases, hiatal hernias, Crohn's disease, and dental caries are also thought to be ameliorated by dietary fiber. The physical, chemical, and metabolic mechanisms whereby dietary fiber may affect these diseases remains largely speculative. Clearly, dietary fiber affects dietary practices and the physiology of the gastrointestinal tract by providing fecal bulk, altering fecal transit time and intestinal physiology and microbiology. In addition, dietary fiber can provide a feeling of satiety, reducing the caloric density of the diet. Whether or not dietary fiber is truly a nutrient class and significantly affects the health of people to which such claims have been attributed remains to be decided by additional research and deliberation.

Fiber and Cholesterol

In 1961, A. Keys and co-workers reported that pectins in the human diet lowered levels of serum cholesterol. *In vitro* studies of D. Kritechevsky and J. Story in 1974 provided evidence that nonnutritive fiber (cellophane and cellulose) did not bind the bile salts tarocholate or glycocholate but that some nutritive fibers did bind the bile salts. These and other studies provided evidence for the hypothesis that a lower serum cholesterol, hypocholesteremia, could be produced by increasing the amounts of dietary fiber, thereby increasing the fecal excretion of these bile salts and decreasing serum cholesterol through a reduction in bile acid reabsorption.

Not all fiber components have been shown to be effective in reducing serum cholesterol levels. Fiber components most consistent in lowering total serum cholesterol in various animal and human experiments include pectin, guar, and other gums and legumes—those fiber components that are viscous and imbibe water. Wheat bran and nonnutritive fiber apparently do not bind bile acid salts *in vivo*, as total fecal excretion in humans remains unaffected. In contrast, oat bran fed to human subjects over an 11-day period lowered total serum cholesterol approximately 25%. LDL cholesterol was reduced, whereas HDL cholesterol and VLDL cholesterol remained unchanged.

It is apparent that the bile acid binding resins, such as cholestyramine and probably lignin, are hypocholesteremic by facilitating excretion of bile acids, preventing intestinal reabsorption. Less apparent is the experimental effect of other components of fiber in reducing serum cholesterol. While fecal excretion of bile salts may be slightly enhanced by the dietary addition of pectin, guar, and other gums, legumes and oat bran (similar to the mechanism of cholestyramine), clofibrate, nicotinic acid and analogs, these fiber components also have a hypolipidemic effect by reducing hepatic lipogenesis. These and other complex physiological and metabolic factors confound the exact mechanism as to how soluble fiber is hypocholesteremic. As reduction in serum cholesterol is considered a positive factor in the overall risk reduction of atherosclerosis and heart disease, the effects of fiber and individual fiber components as hypercholesteremic agents are likely to be further investigated.

Fiber and Colon Cancer

Investigations of human colon (large bowel) cancer and fiber ingestion were rekindled in 1956 by T. L. Cleave, and later by D. P. Burkett in 1971, in epidemiological studies of Africans. Numerous epidemiological investigations (about 70%) have been able to confirm an inverse correlation between ingestion of diets high in fiber content and the incidence of colon cancer. This inverse correlation is most strongly associated with consumption of cereal fiber, is less strongly associated with the consumption of vegetable fibers, and there has been little or no correlation with consumption of legume and fruit fibers. In controlled human studies that have investigated the effects of fiber in reducing the incidence of colon cancer, with the exception of vegetable fiber, conclusive evidence for the ameliorating effect of fiber on colon cancer has not been found. The effect of vegetable fiber in protecting against colon cancer may be due to the higher consumption of certain vitamins, such as vitamins E, A, β-carotene, and other retinoids found in plants.

Highly controllable experimentation with animals and fiber suggest that fiber from wheat, corn, soybean, and oat bran may even enhance the appearance of some chemically induced colon cancer. Other animal experiments with different brans have shown either limited protection against colon cancer or no experimental effect at all. To the extent that fiber may be effective in the prevention of colon cancer, the effects observed are probably related in some manner to reduced exposure to mutagens and carcinogens by fecal dilution and increased bowel transit time, a modified intestinal microflora, binding and excretion of fecal mutagens and carcinogens, or a combination of two or more of these factors.

Bile acid and metal binding to dietary fiber may reduce the facilitation of mutagenic substances in colon cancer induction, while fermentation of fiber is known to produce additional amounts of butyric acid, an anticarcinogen, and lower intestinal pH by production of butyric and other short-chain fatty acids. The role of both nonfermentable and fermentable dietary fiber in the prevention of colon cancer, if significant at all, remains to be deciphered experimentally.

10

The Essential Fatty Acids: Precursors of the Prostaglandins

ESSENTIAL FATTY ACIDS

The requirement for fat in the diets of rats was first demonstrated in 1929 by George and Mildred Burr, who found that a rigid exclusion of dietary fat caused caudal necrosis, loss of body weight, and early death in the animals. Inclusion of three drops of fat daily or 2% fatty acids to the diet of rats prevented the deficiency disease. A year later, these authors described the effects of various oils, fats, and fatty acids in preventing the observed deficiency disease in rats fed the fat-free diets. They found that coconut oil, hydrogenated coconut oil, and methylstearate did not prevent the deficiency disease when added to the fat-free diet of rats, but that linseed, corn, and poppyseed oil, as well as methyllinolate and oleate, when added to the same diet, prevented the deficiency disease. These experiments established for the first time the quantitative need for small amounts of dietary lipid and demonstrated the qualitative dietary requirement for a specific fatty acid (i.e., linoleic acid) in the diet of rats.

The concept and recognition of the need for the essential dietary fatty acid(s) had now been firmly established. The dietary need for the essential fatty acids (EFAs) is met by ingestion of linoleic and linolenic acids. Whereas animals and humans are able to synthesize and elongate many fatty acids *de novo* (the principal product is palmitic acid) and oxidize them to mono- and biunsaturated fatty acids (dienes) up to C_9, animals and humans lack the necessary enzymes to oxidize these fatty acids further and introduce double bonds into fatty acids beyond C_9. It is for this reason that oleic acid ($C_{18}:2^{\Delta 6,9}$) can be synthesized by cells in the endoplasmic reticulum from palmitic acid, but linoleic acid ($C_{18}:2^{\Delta 9,12}$) and γ-linolenic

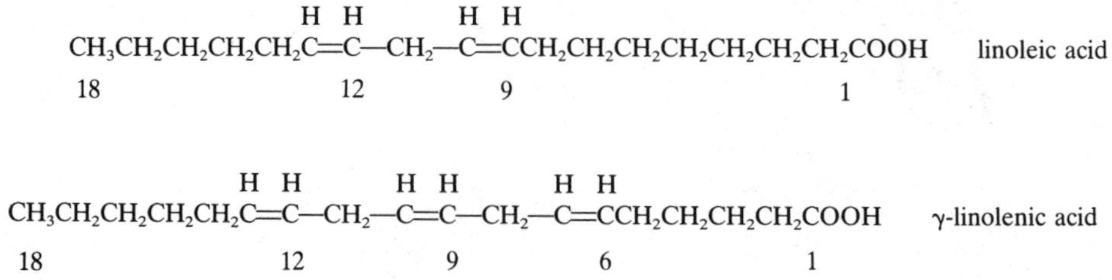

$$\underset{18}{CH_3CH_2CH_2CH_2CH_2}\overset{H}{C}\!\!=\!\!\overset{H}{C}\!\!-\!\!\underset{12}{CH_2}\!\!-\!\!\overset{H}{C}\!\!=\!\!\overset{H}{C}\underset{9}{C}CH_2CH_2CH_2CH_2CH_2CH_2\underset{1}{COOH}$$ linoleic acid

$$\underset{18}{CH_3CH_2CH_2CH_2CH_2}\overset{H}{C}\!\!=\!\!\overset{H}{C}\!\!-\!\!\underset{12}{CH_2}\!\!-\!\!\overset{H}{C}\!\!=\!\!\overset{H}{C}\!\!-\!\!\underset{9}{CH_2}\!\!-\!\!\overset{H}{C}\!\!=\!\!\overset{H}{C}\underset{6}{C}CH_2CH_2CH_2CH_2\underset{1}{COOH}$$ γ-linolenic acid

Figure 10.1 Essential fatty acids.

acid ($C_{18}:3^{\Delta6,9,12}$) with unsaturation beyond C_9 cannot be synthesized and must be obtained dietarily. These essential fatty acids are shown in Figure 10.1. Since only plants have the enzymes capable of inserting Δ^{12} and Δ^{15} double bonds into C_{18} fatty acids, plant oils containing esterified linoleic acid and linolenic acids should be components of an adequate diet.

SYNTHESIS OF EICOSATRIENOIC, EICOSATETRAENOIC, AND EICOSAPENTAENOIC ACIDS

The essential fatty acid linoleic ($C_{18}:2^{\Delta9,12}$) acid can be oxidized by enzymes of the endoplasmic reticulum of mammalian liver cells to γ-linolenic acid ($C_{18}:\Delta^{6,9,12}$). This essential fatty acid, γ-linolenic acid, is elongated by addition of two carbons (acetyl-CoA) and oxidized to form eicosatetraenoic acid, ($C_{20}:4^{\Delta5,8,11,14}$); better known as arachidonic acid. Arachidonic acid is then esterified and made a component of membrane phospholipids. In addition to its function in membrane structure, arachidonic acid serves as a pool of immediate precursor for the prostaglandins, a variety of hormone-like molecules (Figure 10.2).

Eicosatrienoic Acid

The synthesis of eicosatrienoic acid, first in a series of C_{20} polyunsaturated fatty acids, is formed by oxidation of linoleic ($C_{18}:2^{\Delta9,12}$) to γ-linolenic acid ($C_{18}:3^{\Delta6,9,12}$) by the enzymes of the endoplasmic reticulum of mammalian liver cells. This essential fatty acid, γ-linolenic (as opposed to α-linolenic acid; $C_{18}:3^{\Delta9,12,15}$), is elongated by the addition of two carbon atoms (an acetyl-CoA) to form dihomo-γ-linolenic acid ($C_{20}:3^{\Delta8,11,14}$). This PUFA, also known as eicosatrienoic acid, is stored as a phospholipid within cell membranes, where it serves as a precursor to a group of compounds within the family of prostaglandins designated E_1 (Figure 10.2).

Eicosatetraenoic Acid

Oxidation of eicosatrienoic acid ($C_{20}:3^{\Delta8,11,14}$) by the endoplasmic reticulum produces the $C_{20}:4$ PUFA, eicosatetraenoic acid ($C_{20}:4^{\Delta5,8,11,14}$), better known as ar-

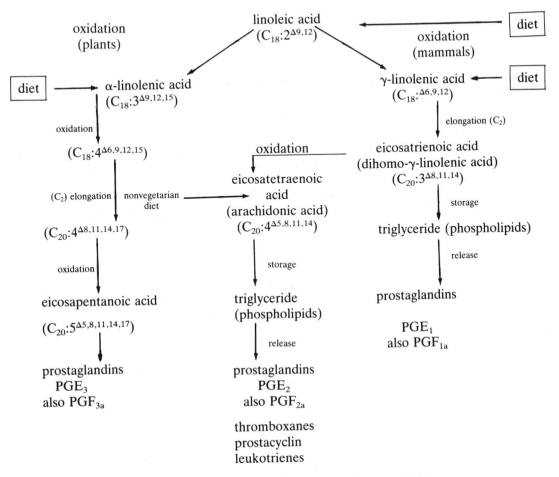

Figure 10.2 Synthesis of prostaglandin precursors from essential fatty acids.

achidonic acid. This PUFA is also stored within the phospholipid fraction of cell membranes, where it resides as a precursor to the family of prostaglandins designated E_2 (Figure 10.2).

Eicosapentaenoic Acid

The synthesis of eicosapentaenoic acid ($C_{20}:5^{\Delta5,8,11,14,17}$) is dependent on the precursor α-linolenic acid ($C_{18}:3^{\Delta9,12,15}$). α-Linolenic acid, oxidized by the same endoplasmic reticulum enzymes, is converted to a $C_{18}:4^{\Delta6,9,12,15}$ fatty acid. This fatty acid is further elongated by two carbon atoms (acetyl-CoA) and oxidized to form eicosapentaenoic acid. This longer polyene, like the other C_{20} PUFAs, is stored within the phospholipid fraction of all membranes, where it may be converted to the family of prostaglandins designated E_3 and thromboxanes.   The route of synthesis of all these fatty acids is shown in Figure 10.2.

PROSTANOIC ACID AND PROSTAGLANDINS

The prostaglandins are a diverse array of hydroxylated C_{20} fatty acids which originate from the dietary C_{18} essential fatty acids, linoleic acid and linolenic acid. The discovery of this group of C_{20} fatty acids was initiated in 1930 by R. Kurzrok and C. Lieb, whose observations of smooth muscle contractions following application of semen prompted a search for the cause of the physiological action.   U. S. von Euler, having observed similar effects of glandular extracts on smooth muscle in 1935, named the affective compounds prostaglandins, after the prostate gland. Subsequently, these first fatty acid compounds, some quite unstable, were isolated

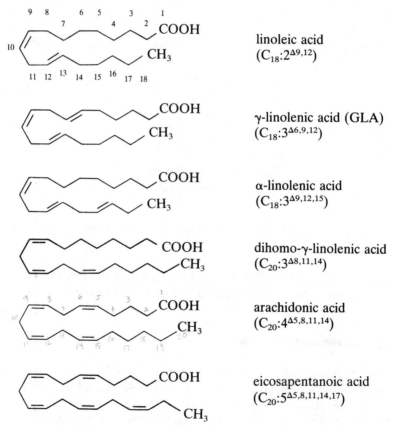

linoleic acid
$(C_{18}:2^{\Delta9,12})$

γ-linolenic acid (GLA)
$(C_{18}:3^{\Delta6,9,12})$

α-linolenic acid
$(C_{18}:3^{\Delta9,12,15})$

dihomo-γ-linolenic acid
$(C_{20}:3^{\Delta8,11,14})$

arachidonic acid
$(C_{20}:4^{\Delta5,8,11,14})$

eicosapentanoic acid
$(C_{20}:5^{\Delta5,8,11,14,17})$

Figure 10.3 Structural chemistry of the essential fatty acids, prostanoic acid, prostaglandins, and derivatives.

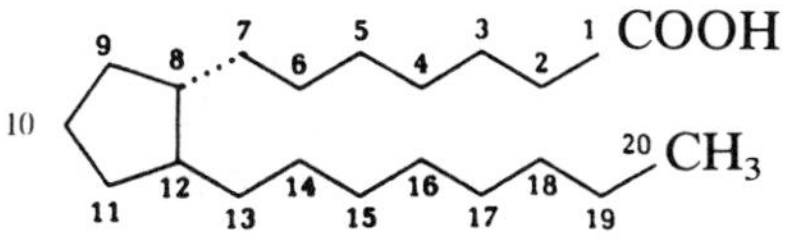

prostanoic acid
$(C_{20}:0)$

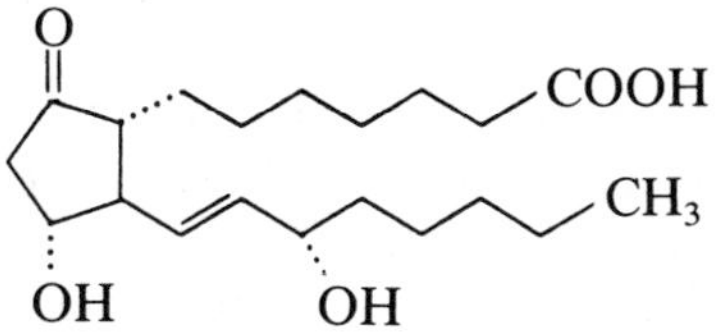

prostaglandin E_1
(PGE_1)

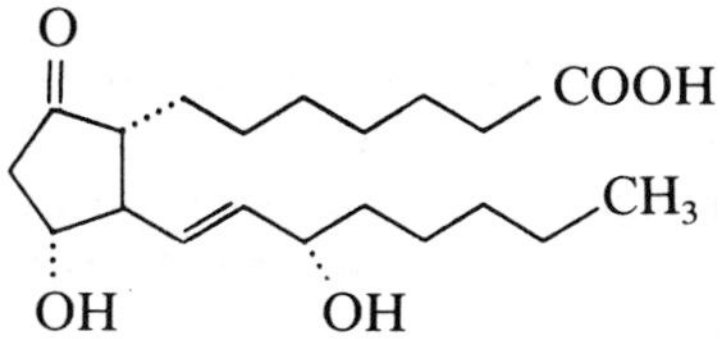

prostaglandin E_2
(PGE_2)

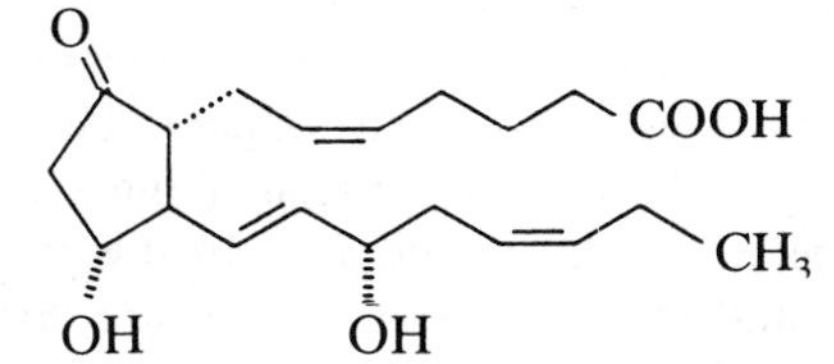

prostaglandin E_3
(PGE_3)

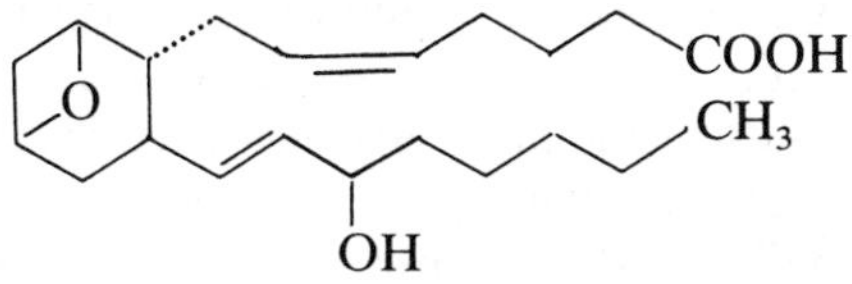

thromboxane A_2
(TXA_2)

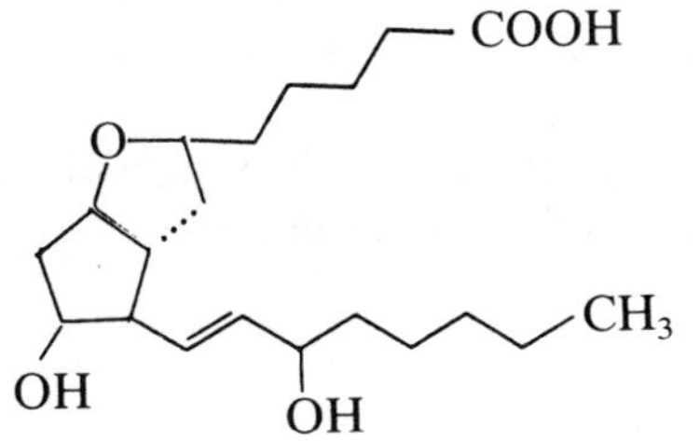

prostacyclin
(PGI_2)

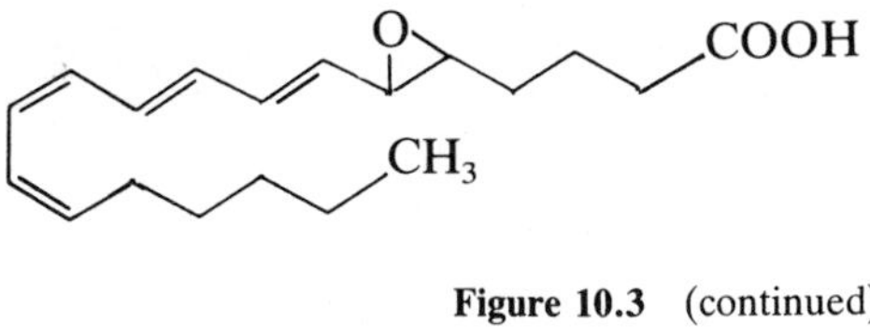

leukotriene A
(LTA)

Figure 10.3 (continued)

and structurally identified in 1962 by S. Bergström and colleagues.   Recognition that the prostaglandins were derived from the essential fatty acids came in 1964, the association having been made by Bergström.   These remarkable intuitive discoveries have led researchers to discover an array of C_{20}-derived fatty acids, almost all of which are hydroxylated and include the prostaglandins, thromboxanes, and prostacyclins (Figure 10.3).

Prostaglandins, synthesized by most cells, are made in response to mechanical, chemical, immunological, or inflammatory insults.   They may not be hormones per se, but certainly they appear to modulate hormonal responses.   As molecules with specific and potent pharmacologic effects, they are under intensive investigation by pharmaceutical companies and independent researchers for physiologic application in the treatment of diseases.

Among the noted biochemical and physiological responses to prostaglandins are induction of cyclic AMP and subsequent effects; vasoconstriction and vasodilation and their consequences for maintenance of blood pressure; inhibition of platelet cell aggregation; induction of erythema; increased vascular permeability; edema; and inflammatory responses.

While a detailed description of the entire chemistry of the prostaglandins would exceed the intent of this introductory chapter, we should note that the parent molecule of the prostaglandins is prostanoic acid (C_{20}:O; Figure 10.3), formed upon oxidation of C_8 and C_{12} by the enzyme prostaglandin synthase, forming a five-membered ring of carbons 8, 9, 10, 11, and 12.   In this manner the prostaglandins of the PGE_1, PGE_2, and PGE_3 and other series are derived from eicosanoids: eicosatrienoic, eicosatetraenoic (archidonic), and eicosapentaenoic acids. Further chemical modifications to either the mono-, di-, or triene fatty acid side chains (hydroxylations or ketal formation) or to the C_{8-12} ring (hydroxylations and/or ketal formations) results in the synthesis of a chemically different prostaglandin.   Insertion of an oxygen into the C_{8-12} ring produces the family of thromboxanes; addition of a second oxygen ring produces the family of prostacyclins, and side-chain epioxidation of arachidonic acid leads to the leukotrienes.   Representative structures of all these families of prostaglandins are given in Figure 10.3.

Presently, there are more than 100 known prostaglandins, isomers, and derivatives, with more likely to be discovered in the future.

11

Lipid Peroxidation

TOXIC OXYGEN SPECIES

On earth, most life exists in a toxic atmosphere of oxygen. Oxygen is so toxic that an anaerobic organism can exist only in its absence. Aerobic organisms, including humans, require oxygen for cellular respiration and have concurrently evolved chemical and enzymatic systems to resist the toxicity of oxygen and its metabolites.

Oxygen (really dioxygen) is an oxidant with an affinity for electrons and hydrogen. This fact is apparent in the mitochondrion, where oxygen accepts electrons and protons, forming metabolic water at the terminal end of the electron transport chain. This oxidative process is both desirable and normal. It is when dioxygen or one of its active reduced products uncontrollably and randomly oxidizes other biological molecules, such as a lipid component of a membrane, that biological damage is done. It is the oxidation of lipids, nucleic acids, and other molecules by oxygen and the reactive species of oxygen that is believed by many, but not all scientists, to be the molecular basis of aging. Such reactive oxygen species are produced by single electron reductions (Equation 11.1).

Equation 11.1
Pathways for the synthesis of reactive oxygen species.

$$O_2^+ \xleftarrow{-e^-} O_2 \xrightarrow{e^-} O_2^- \xrightarrow{e^-} O_2^{2-} + 2H^+ \longrightarrow H_2O_2 \xrightarrow[M^{2+}]{-e^-} \cdot OH \xrightarrow{RH} H_2O$$
$$\downarrow{hv} \qquad\qquad\qquad\qquad\qquad\qquad\qquad\qquad OH^-$$
$$^1O_2$$

TABLE 11.1   REACTIVE OXYGEN SPECIES

Oxygen species	Name
O_2	Oxygen (dioxygen)
O_2^-	Superoxide
$^1O_2$	Single oxygen
H_2O_2	Hydrogen peroxide
$\cdot OH$	Hydroxyl radical
O_3	Ozone (environmental pollutant)
RO_2H	Organic peroxide
NO_2	Nitrogen dioxide

The most important species of reactive oxygen in biological systems are given in Table 11.1. Oxygen, superoxide anion, singlet oxygen, hydrogen peroxide, and the hydroxyl radical are all potentially reactive and capable of oxidizing organic molecules (RH), particularly unsaturated hydrocarbons. Peroxidation of mono- or polyunsaturated fatty acids (oxidation) is the cause of fats and oils becoming rancid, the cause of damage to cell membranes, and is perhaps a component of aging itself. Lipid peroxidation is caused by an initiator, an environmental component that induces formation of an organic free radical $(R\cdot)$, or one of the reactive species of oxygen (Table 11.1) which may react with an organic molecule, also initiating an organic free radical. The environmental initiators of lipid peroxidation *in vitro* include the presence of oxygen and trace metals (M^{2+}), the absence of antioxidants, and moderate to high temperatures. Lipid peroxidation of cells *in vivo* is initiated by a variety of natural and environmental initiators. Since body temperature of most vertebrates is regulated, lipid peroxidation is initiated and controlled at essentially constant temperature. Table 11.2 lists some *in vitro* and *in vivo* initiators of lipid peroxidation. Whereas lipid peroxidation is initiated by a number of species of oxygen derivatives, many endogenous metals and enzymes can either initiate directly, or be produced from organic substrates of these highly reactive and toxic oxygen derivatives, which cause lipid peroxidation. Many environmental factors, such as cigarette smoke, polluted air containing ozone, oxides of nitrogen, chlorinated hydrocarbons, and heavy metals when inhaled, cause lipid peroxidation and damage living tissues. Either intensive or extensive exposure to ultraviolet light and x-irradiation can cause cellular peroxidation and when extreme, even cell death. Clearly, endogenous and environmental initiators of lipid peroxidation are diverse and extensive.

The result of lipid peroxidation by these initiators is membrane and genetic damage (i.e., aging), with the formation of degradative lipid products. The products of lipid peroxidation (Figure 11.1) are ethane, pentane, malondialdehyde, and lipofusion pigments. Ethane (C_2H_6) and pentane (C_5H_{12}) are gases formed as a result of lipid peroxidation and sission, and are exhaled.

TABLE 11.2   INITIATORS OF LIPID PEROXIDATION

In vitro (fats and oils)	*In vivo* (living cells)
Oxygen	Oxygen
Metals	Ultraviolet radiation
High temperatures	X-irradiation
Ultraviolet light (?)	Metals: Fe, Cu; heavy metals: Pd, Cd, Hg, Ag
	Superoxide anion
	Singlet oxygen
	Hydrogen peroxide
	Hydroxyl radical
	Organic peroxide
	Ozone
	Nitrogen dioxide
	Alcohol
	Smoke (from cigarettes and other combustibles)
	Organic halogens
	Enzymes (e.g., glucose oxidase)
	Some drugs

CHAIN REACTIONS: ETHANE, MALONDIALDEHYDE, AND LIPOFUSION SYNTHESIS

Malondialdehyde is one of several aldehydes and ketones that may be synthesized from unsaturated fatty acids by sission of lipid hydroperoxides. Malondialdehyde is capable of acting as a cross-linking agent of protein and DNA, which contributes to cellular damage and the formation of lipofusion. Lipofusion pigments are fluorescent protein-derived molecules not found in young cells, but which accumulate in cells roughly proportionate with time. Such pigment formation and cellular deposition is thought to be associated with aging. Malondialdehyde, because it can cross-link protein to DNA, is at least mutagenic and may be carcinogenic.

In addition to lipid peroxidation, resulting in the formation of gases, malondialdehyde, and lipofusion, it may also result (if undetected) in the synthesis of other free radicals, as shown in Equation 11.2. Once lipid peroxidation is initiated, a single free radical can lead to the formation of many other free radicals and more ethane and pentane, more malondialdehyde, more lipofusion pigments, and so on. Such uncontrolled free-radical events are called chain reactions, and these reactions may continue until the reaction is quenched. A chain reaction is given schematically in Equation 11.2.

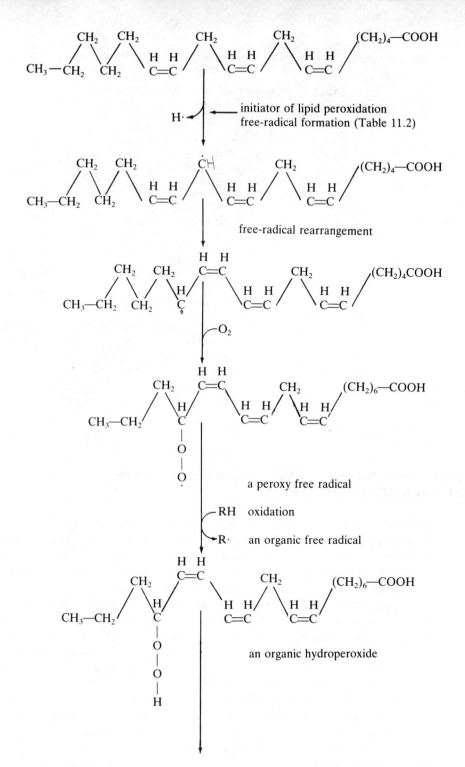

Figure 11.1 Formation of ethane (pentane), malondialdehyde and lipofusion from peroxidation of linolenic acid.

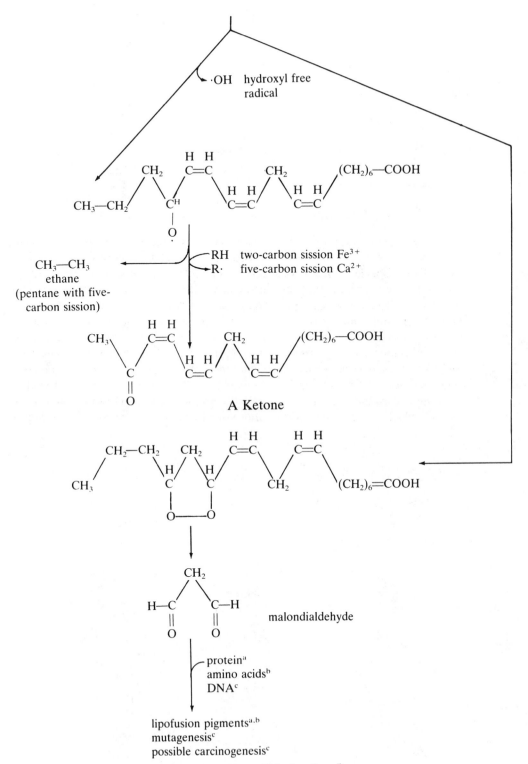

Figure 11.1 (continued)

Equation 11.2
Chain reaction of lipid peroxidation.

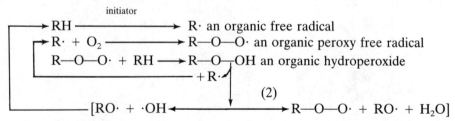

Following initiation of lipid peroxidation, the formation of an organic peroxy free radical (ROO·) and an organic hydroperoxide (ROOH) can rapidly lead to a variety of new species of free radicals (R·, RO·, and ·OH) which in chain reactions result in the oxidation of still other molecules.   These free-radical events are kept as low as possible by cells not allowing a lot of "free" oxygen to be available in tissues to promote uncontrolled oxidations.   In addition, diet provides a variety of antioxidants to cells which prevent free-radical reactions from being sustained. *In vivo*, additions to the dietary antioxidant armament are formed as cells synthesize molecules and enzymes which eliminate the cellular presence of most reactive oxygen species that initiate lipid peroxidation.   These dietary factors and endogenous molecules and enzymes are the cell's defenses against peroxidation and cell damage, which are collectively the antioxidant defense system of cells (Chapter 12).

12

The Antioxidants

ANTIOXIDANTS: INTRODUCTION

All cells contain endogenous initiators of lipid peroxidation and are also subject to a variety of environmental insults (Chapter 11), which upon generating organic or inorganic free radicals, can lead to membrane damage and mutations that may contribute to aging and even produce cell death. These same cells contain antioxidants, a variety of small and macromolecules whose purpose is to prevent lipid peroxidation by either breaking free-radical chain reactions or preventing the cellular accumulation of the toxic molecular species of oxygen. The cellular antioxidant armamentarium can be divided into four classes of molecules. Group 1 molecules include the natural dietary antioxidants; group 2, the antioxidants found in foods as additives; group 3, the small-molecular-weight antioxidants synthesized by cells; and group 4, the antioxidant enzymes synthesized by cells. Table 12.1 lists these antioxidants.

Molecules found naturally in foods—vitamins A, C, E, and β-carotene—are the cell's first line of defense against free-radical reactions, peroxidation, and cellular damage. These molecules protect the cell against peroxidation by becoming oxidized themselves, reacting with the toxic species of oxygen when they are found in the cell's cytoplasm, organelles, or membrane. They are free-radical traps. Each vitamin generally protects a certain part of the cell and some antioxidants are found predominantly in certain types of cells. Vitamins A, E, and β-carotene, because they are lipid soluble, seem to protect cell membranes. They are the free-radical traps in membranes. Vitamin A and β-carotene are particularly effective

TABLE 12.1   ANTIOXIDANTS FOUND IN FOODS AND SYNTHESIZED *DE NOVO* BY CELLS

Natural antioxidants in foods	Antioxidant food additives
Vitamin A	BHT (butylated hydroxytoluene)
β-Carotene	BHA (butylated hydroxyanisole)
Vitamin C	Sodium benzoate
Vitamin E	Ethoxyquin
	Propyl galate
Minerals contributing to antioxidant enzymes	
Selenium	
Manganese	
Copper	
Zinc	
Iron	
Antioxidants synthesized by cells	Antioxidant enzymes synthesized by cells
Glutathione	Glutathione peroxidase
Cysteine	Glutathione transferase
Uric acid	Catalase
Hydroquinones	CuZn-superoxide dismutase
	Mn-superoxide dismutase
	Fe-superoxide dismutase (bacterial)

in protecting ectodermal tissue: skin and the tissues lining the oral cavity and gastrointestinal tract.   Vitamin C, being water soluble, complements the lipid-soluble antioxidants by trapping free radicals in the aqueous portion of cells, the cytoplasm.   Vitamin C is so easily oxidized that it may even help to protect vitamins A and E and even β-carotene from oxidation.

Figure 12.1 shows the proposed pathways for free-radical chain reactions following initiation, formation of hydrogen and lipid peroxides, and the points of prevention of cellular oxidation by the major antioxidants.   The small dietary food additives and cellularly synthesized antioxidants are shown to block initiation and break closed-loop free-radical-chain reactions.   The enzymes present in the cytoplasm and organelles of cells serve to protect the cells by catalytic elimination of superoxide, hydrogen, and organic hyperoxides.

As examples of the action of antioxidants, free-radical trapping by vitamin E (α-tocopherol) is shown in Figure 12.2.   One vitamin E molecule readily accepts two free radicals, either from superoxide or the organic peroxy radical.   One electron oxidation of vitamin E results in the formation of an intermediate methyl-tocophenyl radical.   Two electron reduction of vitamin E results in the formation of the tocophenyl quinone.   The one-electron methyltocophenyl radical may be reduced by cellular glutathione.   Vitamin E is normally present in cell membranes in a 1:1000 ratio with polyunsaturated fatty acids.   Its absence from the diet leads to increased cellular production of ethane and pentane, malondialdehyde, and lipofusion pigments.

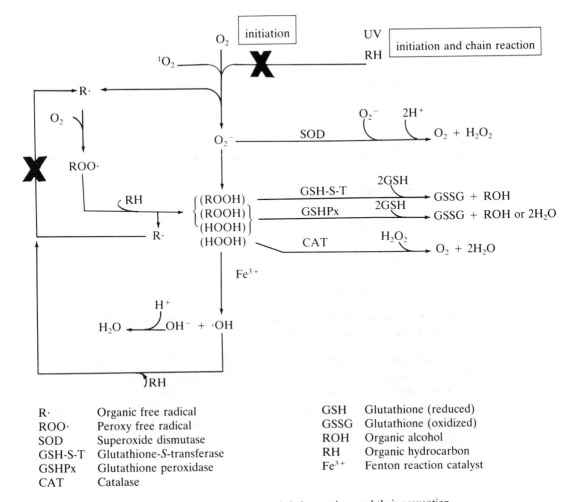

Figure 12.1 Free-radical chain reactions and their prevention.

R·	Organic free radical	GSH	Glutathione (reduced)
ROO·	Peroxy free radical	GSSG	Glutathione (oxidized)
SOD	Superoxide dismutase	ROH	Organic alcohol
GSH-S-T	Glutathione-S-transferase	RH	Organic hydrocarbon
GSHPx	Glutathione peroxidase	Fe^{3+}	Fenton reaction catalyst
CAT	Catalase		

Vitamin C, ascorbic acid, may be both an intracellular quencher of free radicals and an extracellular quencher of free radicals for the epithelial cellular lining of the lung. Intracellular ascorbate quenches the superoxide free radical, the organic peroxy free radical and possibly the hydroxyl free radical. In the lung, ascorbate protects against free radicals generated from smoke, oxygen, and ozone. Ascorbate also protects organs from the peroxidative damage of drugs, chlorinated hydrocarbons, and peroxides.

Like vitamin E, ascorbic acid readily oxidizes and quenches free radicals in a two-electron process (Figure 12.3). Carotenoids and β-carotene in particular, like vitamins C and E are an effective quencher of free-radical reactions *in vivo* in

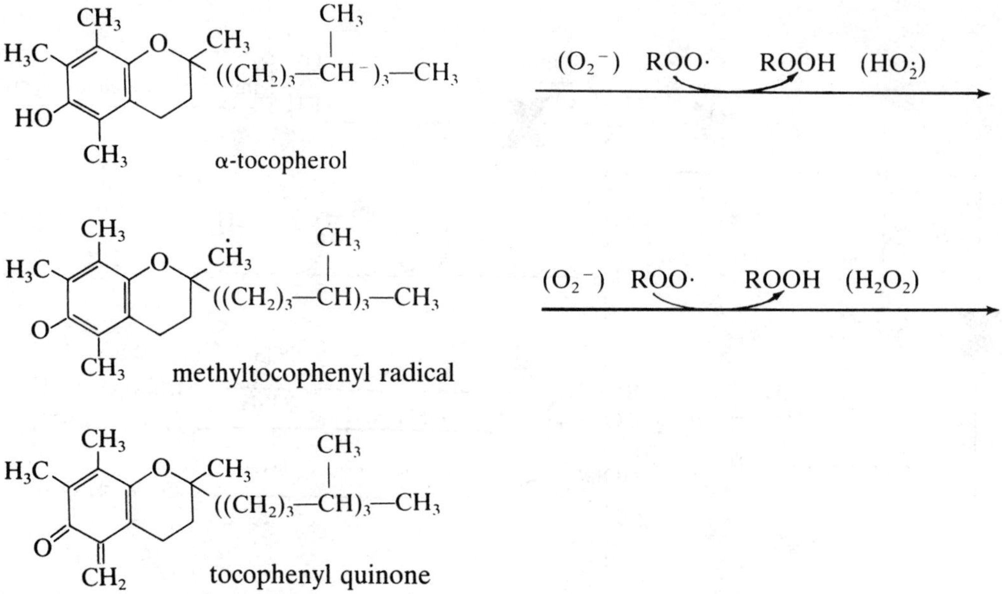

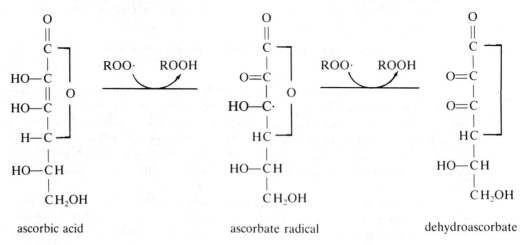

Figure 12.2 Antioxidant function of vitamin E. (Reproduced from *Nutrition of the Chicken*, with permission of M. Scott, Publishers, Ithaca, N.Y., 1977.)

which π (double) bonding electrons are oxidized. More important, β-carotene quenches induction of free radicals by ultraviolet light, a property not shared by any of the other antioxidants. β-Carotene in skin blocks these free-radical chain reactions from occurring by quenching singlet oxygen. This reaction, unique to β-carotene is shown in Figure 12.4. In this reaction, UV light interacting with oxygen produces excited singlet ($^1O_2$) oxygen. Singlet oxygen, instead of producing

ascorbic acid ascorbate radical dehydroascorbate

Figure 12.3 Antioxidant function of ascorbic acid.

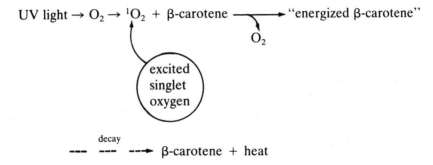

Figure 12.4 Quenching singlet oxygen by β-carotene.

free radicals, interacts with β-carotene, transferring its energy to form "energized β-carotene." The UV energy now present in β-carotene is dissipated from the molecule as heat.

Vitamin A, like β-carotene, vitamin C, and vitamin E, can also act as an antioxidant and quench free-radical reactions, but unlike β-carotene, it does not quench singlet-oxygen reactions. Other antioxidant molecules, BHA, BHT, benzoate, and so on, function similarly to the examples given for vitamins E and C in protecting cells from free-radical damage.

ANTIOXIDANT ENZYMES

There exists in aerobic cells enzymes that act catalytically on free-radical substrates, and peroxides that generate free radicals, protecting cells from oxidative damage. These enzymes, which are present in the cytoplasm, are the superoxide dismutases and peroxidases. Four of these enzymes contain at least one mineral which participates in the dismutation of the superoxide anion or the reduction of peroxides. Table 12.2 provides data on each of these enzymes and shows the catalytic reaction in which it participates.

TABLE 12.2 ANTIOXIDANT ENZYMES FOUND IN AEROBIC CELLS

Enzyme	Mineral	Reaction
Superoxide dismutase (EC 1.15.1.1) MW 32,500	CuZn Mn Fe (bacterial)	$2O_2^- + 2H^+ \rightarrow O_2 + H_2O_2$
Glutathione peroxidase (EC 1.11.1.9) MW 84,000	Se	$H_2O_2 + 2GSH \rightarrow GSSG + 2H_2O$ $ROOH + 2GSH \rightarrow GSSG + ROH + H_2O$
Catalase (EC 1.11.1.6) MW 250,000	Fe	$2H_2O_2 \rightarrow 2H_2O + O_2$
Glutathione-S-transferases (EC 2.5.1.18) MW various	—	$ROOH + 2GSH \rightarrow GSSG + ROH + H_2O$

Superoxide dismutase

Superoxide dismutase (SOD) catalyzes the dismutation of the superoxide anion into oxygen and hydrogen peroxide. This enzyme is ubiquitous in nature in aerobic cells, providing them with protection from the superoxide free radical. Two SOD enzymes are known in mammals, a CuZn-SOD, blue-green in color, and a Mn-SOD, reddish in color. A pale yellow Fe-SOD has been isolated from *E. coli*.

Glutathione Peroxidase

Glutathione peroxidase (GSHPx) catalyzes the reduction of H_2O_2, which is produced by SOD via the dismutation of superoxide. The reduction of H_2O_2 and ROOH by GSHPx requires the reduced tripeptide, glutathione (GSH), as a cofactor. GSHPx is a major protein containing selenium. In mammals, including humans, this enzyme is found in many tissues and is especially concentrated in erythrocytes and liver, both tissues being highly exposed to oxygen.

Catalase

Catalase (CAT) catalyzes the oxidation of hydrogen peroxide without need for a cofactor. The enzyme contains heme-iron and is widely found in nearly all aerobic cells.

Glutathione-S-Transferase

The glutathione-*S*-transferases are a family of enzymes catalyzing conjugation of glutathione to xenobiotics (Chapter 13). In addition, some enzymes of this family catalyze the reduction of organic hydroperoxides (ROOH) to alcohols. The GSH-*S*-transferases help to protect cells from the damage that can occur from organic hydroperoxides. Cellular levels of these enzymes can be found elevated in some tissues when GSHPx is absent.

13

Digestive and Metabolic Interactions between Drugs and Nutrients

DRUG–NUTRIENT INTERACTIONS

It is well know that many drugs, particularly when used in chronic long-term drug therapy, can affect the nutritional status of individuals for certain nutrients. Effects on appetite, digestion of food, absorption, metabolism, and excretion of nutrients are consequences of some chronic drug therapies. Conversely, foods and the specific nutrient composition of certain foods can adversely affect the desired pharmacologic action of some drugs. Clinical practitioners of medicine and dietetics should be aware of both drug–nutrient and nutrient–drug interactions. Drug–nutrient interactions can be the consequence of chronic over-the-counter (OTC) or prescription drug therapy, particularly among the elderly, who are the principal consumers of drugs. Adverse nutrient-drug interactions can have short-term effects, usually reducing drug effectiveness without serious long-term nutritional consequences.

Drugs and nutrients are both chemical entities and their interaction occurs because of (1) direct chemical reactivity, (2) competitive or noncompetitive inhibition of vitamins or coenzymes with enzymes, or (3) by alteration of membrane permeability or receptor sites.

Drugs are chemical substances used as medicines or as an ingredient in medicines. They may or may not be toxic, and when they are toxic, toxicity is often dose related. Nutrients are chemical substances that are ingested to support growth, maintenance, and repair of tissues. When some nutrients are ingested in excess of 150% of the RDA for that nutrient, they may have a pharmacologic action, be toxic, and are considered drugs. In such cases when nutrients can have pharmacologic activity, nutrient–nutrient metabolic interactions are possible.   Interest in drug–nutrient, nutrient–drug, and nutrient–nutrient interactions is the branch of science called pharmacology.   Pharmacologists study, describe, and try to understand how chemicals (i.e., drugs) interact with living organisms.   These goals are not much different from that of a nutritionist—only the molecules are different. The present status of understanding the many individual drug interactions with nutrients is often extensive, and such individual details exist well beyond the author's imposed limitations of this chapter.   Table 13.1 lists many specific drug–nutrient interactions by chemical reactivity, interference with enzymatic activity, or alteration of membrane permeability or receptive sites.   Three commonly used examples of drug–nutrient interactions are described for each category of pharmacologic effect.

Direct Chemical Reactivity: Chelation of Calcium by Tetracycline

Several drugs and nutrients react directly with minerals by chelation, a process whereby organic molecules directly bind minerals usually through coordinate covalent bonding.   The chelation of calcium (Ca^{2+}) and other divalent cations by the antibiotic tetracycline (Figure 13.1) in the gastrointestinal tract may reduce absorption of both the drug and the calcium by forming the chelate.   Although short-term medicinal use of tetracycline would probably have little impact on the calcium status of an individual, the effect of calcium on reducing absorption of tetracycline would restrict the antibiotic's therapeutic effectiveness.

Other drugs acting on minerals by chelation include penicillamine and EDTA (ethylenediaminetetraacetic acid) affecting calcium, copper, iron, and zinc absorption.   In the treatment of some forms of arthritis, gold (gold-thioglucose) used in therapy may affect selenium metabolism.

Competitive Inhibition of Dihydrofolate by Methotrexate

Tetrahydrofolic acid (THFA) (Chapter 3) is an important coenzyme in the synthesis of purines and pyrimidines (Chapter 8) and in one carbon metabolism.   Reduction of dihydrofolic acid (DHFA) to the active form of folic acid, THFA, is inhibited

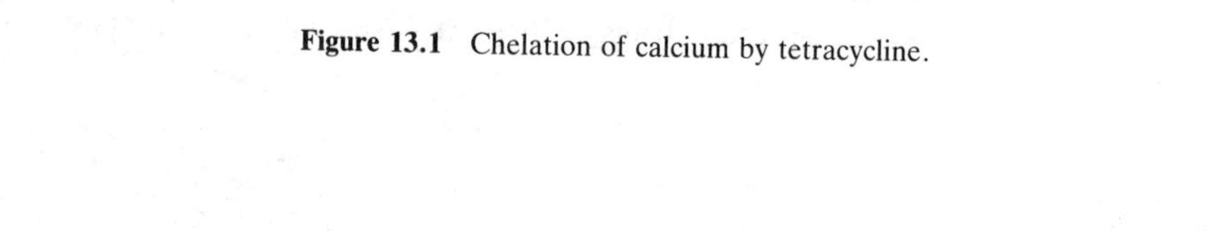

Figure 13.1   Chelation of calcium by tetracycline.

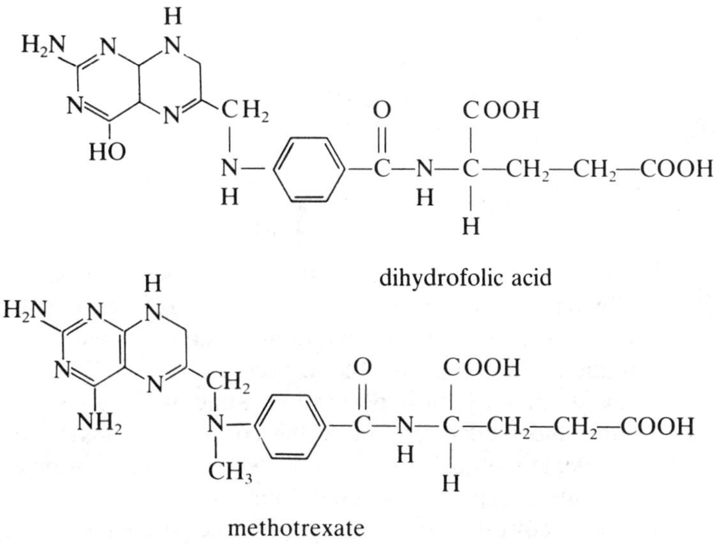

dihydrofolic acid

methotrexate

Figure 13.2 Structural similarity of dihydrofolic acid and methotrexate.

by the anticancer drug methotrexate (aminopterin), resulting in a blockage of nucleic acid synthesis. This inhibition adversely affects replication and subsequently, cellular division. The reason that methotrexate blocks THFA synthesis is that it effectively competes with and blocks the binding site of DHFA on the enzyme dihydofolate reductase because of its structural similarity to DHFA (Figure 13.2).

Many other drugs effectively compete to displace normal coenzymes and vitamins from their enzymes and block enzymatic catalysis because the drugs are structurally very similar to the coenzyme. This is particularly true of many of the vitamins for which there are known antimetabolites (i.e., drugs and poisons). Examples of drugs (poisons) that are competitive inhibitors of vitamins include isoniazid (vitamin B_6) used in the treatment of tuberculosis and dicoumerol, and its derivatives, such as warfarin, which are antagonistic to vitamin K (see Chapter 3). Consumption of folic acid, vitamin B_6, and vitamin K supplements would help to reduce the effectiveness of these drugs during therapy and should probably be avoided. Many other drugs function similarly as metabolic inhibitors.

Drug Action on Membrane Receptor Sites

Receptor sites on membranes are similar conceptually to the binding sites of coenzymes or substrates on enzymes. In the latter case, drugs may block catalysis. On membranes, blocking of receptor sites (which are probably proteins in many cases), may alter the membrane permeability affecting molecular or ion transport. Furosemide is the generic name of a very commonly prescribed drug used as an antihypertensive to lower blood pressure. Furosemide pharmacologically is a di-

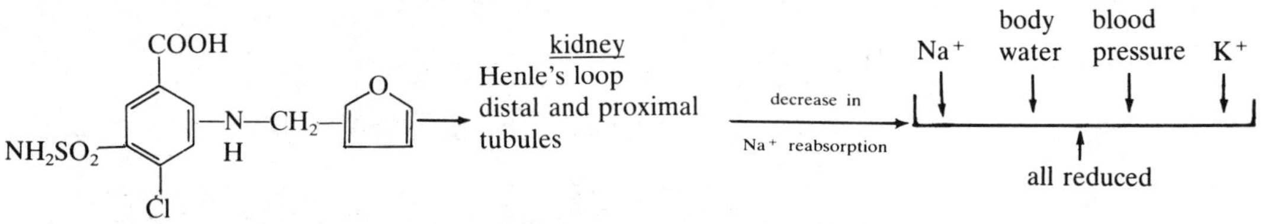

Figure 13.3 Alteration of Na^+ reabsorption by furosemide.

uretic drug which acts upon the receptor sites for Na^+ in the proximal, distal, and Henle's loop nephrotic tubules. The drug's action alters the ability of the tubules to reabsorb Na^+ ions, facilitating excretion, which effectively reduces water retention and may lower blood pressure (Figure 13.3). The consequence of furosemide therapy for hypertension, in addition to loss of Na^+, reduced blood pressure, and fluid retention, is the concomitant loss of potassium, K^+. Potassium supplementation is therefore a frequent dietary supplement taken by furosemide patients to replace lost renal potassium.

Many other drugs alter membrane permeability or affect membrane receptors. In addition, the diuretics and psychotropic drugs act on membranes and may affect utilization of nutrients. Phenytoin, an anticonvulsant used in the control of epilepsy, alters the metabolism and may increase the need for folic acid and vitamins D and K.

Table 13.1 provides a list of some drugs and their interaction with some

TABLE 13.1 COMMONLY PRESCRIBED AND OTC DRUGS: INTERACTION WITH NUTRIENTS

Drug (compound)	Use	Indicated nutrient interaction
Acetaminophen	Analgesic	Absorption reduced or delayed by pectins
Adrenal corticosteroids	Water balance; sodium, potassium balance	Inhibits Ca^{2+} absorption by inhibition of vitamin B_1
Alcohol	Abusive	Increased excretion of Mg^{2+} and zinc, vitamin B_6 displacement of calories and other nutrients
Aluminum hydroxide	Antacid	Inhibits PO_4^{2-} absorption, may inhibit fluoride absorption, may reduce vitamin A absorption, may destroy vitamin B
Aspirin	Analgesic	Causes or aggravates ulcers affecting nutrient absorption, increased vitamin C and potassium excretion, reduces iron absorption.
Barbiturates	Sedatives	Decreased absorption of vitamin B_{12} and D
Bisacodyl	Laxative	Loss of fluids, Na^+, K^+, Cl^-
Chlorpromazine	Sedative	Decreased absorption of vitamin B_2
Chlortetracyline	Antibiotic	Decreased absorption of vitamins C and B_2, Ca^{2+}

TABLE 13.1 (cont.)

Drug (compound)	Use	Indicated nutrient interaction
Cholestyramine	Resin, anticholesteremic and lipemic	Malabsorption of lipids, fat-soluble vitamins, β-carotene, reduced Fe^{2+}, Ca^{2+} absorption
Clofibrate	Anticholesteremic	Vitamins B_6 and B_{12}, folic acid; decrease absorption of Fe^{2+}, glucose
Cloridine	Antihypertensive	Retention of Na^+, edema
Colchicine	Antigout	Decreased absorption of Na^+, K^+, lipids, β-carotene
Contraceptives (oral)	Contraception	Decreased absorption of vitamins C, B_2, B_6, and folic acid
Coumarin	Anticoagulant	No vitamin K supplements
Cycloserine	Antibiotic	Vitamins B_6, B_{12}, folate, Ca^{2+}, Mg^{2+} affected
Digitalis	Cardiotonin	Decreased absorption of vitamin Ca^{2+}
Estrogens	Estrogen replacement	Vitamin D-induced hypercalcemia, edema, retention of Na^+, water
Furosemide	Diuretic	Depletion of K^+, Ca^{2+}, Mg^{2+}, Na^+, Cl^-, and fluid
Glutethmide	Sedative	Interference with vitamin D, loss of Ca^{2+} from bone
Guanethidine	Antihypertensive	Na^+ retention, edema
Hydralazine	Hypotensive	Supplement vitamin B_6; B_6 excreted with drug
Indomethacin	Anti-inflammatory	Supplement Fe^{2+}
Isoniazid	Antitubercular	Supplement with vitamins B_6, D, and niacin, competitive inhibitor
Isotretinoin	Acne	No vitamin A supplementation
L-dopa	Parkinsonism	Competitive with phenylalanine
Lithium	Antidepressant	Competitive with Mg^{2+}, Na^+
Methotrexate	Chemotherapeutic	Competitive with dihydrofolic acid
Mineral oil	Laxative	Malabsorption of lipid-soluble vitamins, β-carotene
Neomycin	Antibiotic	Malabsorption of vitamins A and B_{12}
Penicillamine	Chelate	Chelation of Cu^{2+}, Fe^{2+}, Zn^{2+}
Phenolphthalein	Laxative	Malabsorption of vitamin D and some minerals
Phenytoin	Anticonvulsant	Inactivation of vitamin D
Primidone	Anticonvulsant	Supplement with vitamins D, B_6, B_{12}, K, and folic acid
Pyrimethamine	Antimalarial	Competitive against dihydrofolic acid
Sulfasalazine	Anti-inflammatory	Malabsorption of folic acid
Tetracycline	Antibiotic	Chelates Ca^{2+}, increased vitamin C excretion
Thioridazine	Sedative	Supplement with riboflavin
Triamterene	Diuretic	Competitive with dihydrofolic acid

Note: This table should not be used for self-medication or ascertaining requirements for supplementation. Consult your physician or clinical nutritionist if you have a personal concern.

Adapted by permission from V. F. Thiele, *Clinical Nutrition*, St. Louis, 1980, The C. V. Mosby Co.

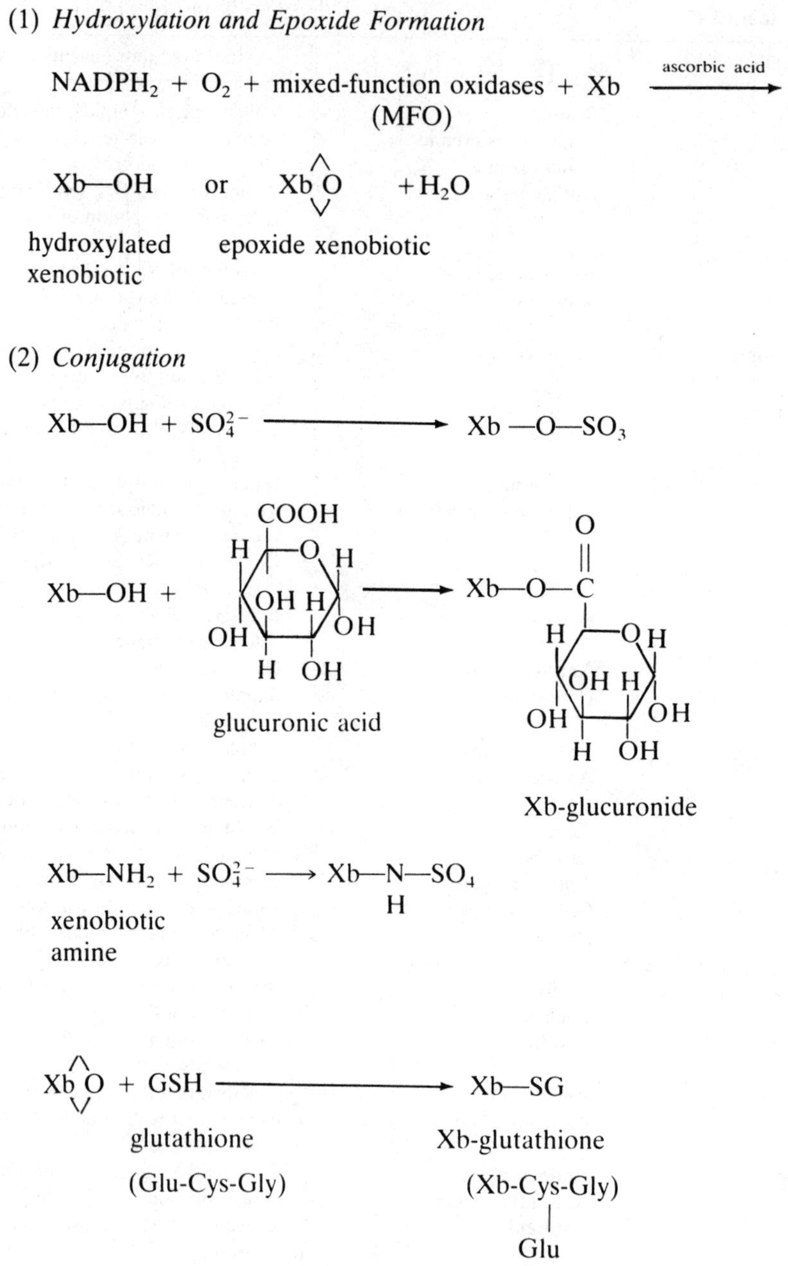

(1) *Hydroxylation and Epoxide Formation*

$$NADPH_2 + O_2 + \text{mixed-function oxidases} + Xb \xrightarrow{\text{ascorbic acid}}$$
$$(MFO)$$

$$Xb—OH \quad \text{or} \quad Xb\overset{\wedge}{\underset{\vee}{O}} \quad +H_2O$$

hydroxylated   epoxide xenobiotic
xenobiotic

(2) *Conjugation*

$$Xb—OH + SO_4^{2-} \longrightarrow Xb—O—SO_3$$

$$Xb—OH + \text{glucuronic acid} \longrightarrow Xb\text{-glucuronide}$$

$$Xb—NH_2 + SO_4^{2-} \longrightarrow Xb—\underset{H}{N}—SO_4$$

xenobiotic
amine

$$Xb\overset{\wedge}{\underset{\vee}{O}} + GSH \longrightarrow Xb—SG$$

glutathione   Xb-glutathione

(Glu-Cys-Gly)   (Xb-Cys-Gly)
                             |
                            Glu

Figure 13.4 Two-step metabolism and conjugation of xenobiotics (Xb) and non-nutritive food chemicals.

nutrients. In addition to direct drug–nutrient interaction, foods and fiber in the diet often affect drug absorption by altering gastrointestinal pH, diluting drugs, and causing nonspecific binding. These effects may alter the efficacy of medication by reducing drug absorption. Thus the timing of medications with or without food is important, as foods may decrease drug effectiveness or the drug(s) may affect nutrient absorption and metabolism.

DRUG METABOLISM: EFFECT OF NUTRITIONAL STATUS

In addition to consuming drugs, we also consume food dyes, agricultural chemicals, and other unnatural compounds. Such manufactured compounds are called xenobiotics, from the Greek word, *xenor*, meaning "strange," "foreign," or "extraneous." We also consume naturally, in many foods, chemical compounds which are not nutrients, which if homogeneously isolated and consumed in sufficient quantity would possibly be mutagenic, carcinogenic, or at the least, toxic. All such molecules have to be metabolized, conjugated, and excreted.

A good nutritional status influences the metabolisms of xenobiotics and natural toxins. Most of these molecules are metabolized by the liver in a two-step process (Figure 13.4). In the first step, (1) mixed-function oxidases (MFOs) make nonpolar hydrocarbons more polar, usually by inserting a hydroxyl moiety or epoxide. Two cytochrome enzymes in the endoplasmic reticulum complete the polarization process. $NADPH_2$ and O_2 are enzymatically combined for either the hydroxylation or epoxide reactions. These reactions make the compounds more water soluble. In a second set of reactions, (2) a conjugating enzyme adds to a xenobiotic phenol, alcohol, or amine, either sulfate, glucuronic acid, or glutathione to the hydroxyl amine, or epoxide moiety. The conjugated hydrocarbon is then excreted in the urine.

Adequate protein intake (for methionine), vitamins (niacin for $NADPH_2$), vitamins A, C, and E (antioxidants), and minerals are all important for the metabolism of xenobiotics and nonnutritive food chemicals.

Appendix

Recommended Dietary Allowances*

ESTIMATED SAFE AND ADEQUATE DAILY DIETARY INTAKES OF SELECTED VITAMINS AND MINERALS[a]

	Age (years)	Vitamins		
		Vitamin K (μg)	Biotin (μg)	Pantothenic acid (mg)
Infants	0–0.5	12	35	2
	0.5–1	10–20	50	3
Children and	1–3	15–30	65	3
Adolescents	4–6	20–40	85	3–4
	7–10	30–60	120	4–5
	11+	50–100	100–200	4–7
Adults		70–140	100–200	4–7

	Age (years)	Trace elements[b]					
		Copper (mg)	Man- ganese (mg)	√Fluoride (mg)	√Chromium (mg)	√Selenium (mg)	Molyb- √denum (mg)
Infants	0–0.5	0.5–0.7	0.5–0.7	0.1–0.5	0.01–0.04	0.01–0.04	0.03–0.06
	0.5–1	0.7–1.0	0.7–1.0	0.2–1.0	0.02–0.06	0.02–0.06	0.04–0.08
Children and	1–3	1.0–1.5	1.0–1.5	0.5–1.5	0.02–0.08	0.02–0.08	0.05–0.1
Adolescents	4–6	1.5–2.0	1.5–2.0	1.0–2.5	0.03–0.12	0.03–0.12	0.06–0.15
	7–10	2.0–2.5	2.0–3.0	1.5–2.5	0.05–0.2	0.05–0.2	0.10–0.3
	11+	2.0–3.0	2.5–5.0	1.5–2.5	0.05–0.2	0.05–0.2	0.15–0.5
Adults		2.0–3.0	2.5–5.0	1.5–4.0	0.05–0.2	0.05–0.2	0.15–0.5

*Ninth Revised Edition, *Committee on Dietary Allowances Food and Nutrition Board*, Division of Biological Sciences Assembly of Life Sciences National Research Council (National Academy of Sciences: Washington, D.C., 1980).

RECOMMENDED DAILY DIETARY ALLOWANCES,[a] REVISED 1980

	Age (years)	Weight (kg)	Weight (lb)	Height (cm)	Height (in)	Protein (g)	Fat-soluble vitamins Vita-min A (µg RE)[b]	Vita-min D (µg)[c]	Vita-min E (mg α-TE)[d]
Infants	0.0–0.5	6	13	60	24	kg × 2.2	420	10	3
	0.5–1.0	9	20	71	28	kg × 2.0	400	10	4
Children	1–3	13	29	90	35	23	400	10	5
	4–6	20	44	112	44	30	500	10	6
	7–10	28	62	132	52	34	700	10	7
Males	11–14	45	99	157	62	45	1000	10	8
	15–18	66	145	176	69	56	1000	10	10
	19–22	70	154	177	70	56	1000	7.5	10
	23–50	70	154	178	70	56	1000	5	10
	51+	70	154	178	70	56	1000	5	10
Females	11–14	46	101	157	62	46	800	10	8
	15–18	55	120	163	64	46	800	10	8
	19–22	55	120	163	64	44	800	7.5	8
	23–50	55	120	163	64	44	800	5	8
	51+	55	120	163	64	44	800	5	8
Pregnant						+30	+200	+5	+2
Lactating						+20	+400	+5	+3

	Water-soluble vitamins							Minerals					
	Vitamin C (mg)	Thiamin (mg)	Riboflavin (mg)	Niacin (mg NE)[c]	Vitamin B-6 (mg)	Folacin[f] (μg)	Vitamin B-12 (μg)	Calcium (mg)	Phosphorus (mg)	Magnesium (mg)	Iron (mg)	Zinc (mg)	Iodine (μg)
	35	0.3	0.4	6	0.3	30	0.5[g]	360	240	50	10	3	40
	35	0.5	0.6	8	0.6	45	1.5	540	360	70	15	5	50
	45	0.7	0.8	9	0.9	100	2.0	800	800	150	15	10	70
	45	0.9	1.0	11	1.3	200	2.5	800	800	200	10	10	90
	45	1.2	1.4	16	1.6	300	3.0	800	800	250	10	10	120
	50	1.4	1.6	18	1.8	400	3.0	1200	1200	350	18	15	150
	60	1.4	1.7	18	2.0	400	3.0	1200	1200	400	18	15	150
	60	1.5	1.7	19	2.2	400	3.0	800	800	350	10	15	150
	60	1.4	1.6	18	2.2	400	3.0	800	800	350	10	15	150
	60	1.2	1.4	16	2.2	400	3.0	800	800	350	10	15	150
	50	1.1	1.3	15	1.8	400	3.0	1200	1200	300	18	15	150
	60	1.1	1.3	14	2.0	400	3.0	1200	1200	300	18	15	150
	60	1.1	1.3	14	2.0	400	3.0	800	800	300	18	15	150
	60	1.0	1.2	13	2.0	400	3.0	800	800	300	18	15	150
→	60	1.0	1.2	13	2.0	400	3.0	800	800	300	10	15	150
	+20	+0.4	+0.3	+2	+0.6	+400	+1.0	+400	+400	+150	—[h]	+5	+25
	+40	+0.5	+0.5	+5	+0.5	+100	+1.0	+400	+400	+150	—[h]	+10	+50

DESIGNED FOR THE MAINTENANCE OF GOOD NUTRITION OF PRACTICALLY ALL HEALTHY PEOPLE IN THE U.S.A.

[a] Allowances are intended to provide for individual variations among most normal persons as they live in the United States under usual environmental stresses. Diets should be based on a variety of common foods in order to provide other nutrients for which human requirements have been less well defined.

[b] Retinol equivalents. 1 retinol equivalent = 1 μg of retinol or 6 μg of β-carotene.

[c] As Cholecalciferol. 10 μg of cholecalciferol = 400 IU of vitamin D.

[d] α Tocopherol equivalents. 1 mg of d-α tocopherol = 1 α-TE. See text for variation in allowances in calculation of vitamin E activity of the diet as α-tocopherol equivalents.

[e] 1 NE (niacin equivalent) is equal to 1 mg of niacin or 60 mg of dietary tryptophan.

[f] The folacin allowances refer to dietary sources as determined by *Lactobacillus casei* assay after treatment with enzymes (conjugases) to make polyglutamyl forms of the vitamin available to the test organism.

[g] The recommended dietary allowance for vitamin B$_{12}$ in infants is based on average concentration of the vitamin in human milk. The allowances after weaning are based on energy intake (as recommended by the American Academy of Pediatrics) and consideration of other factors, such as intestinal absorption; see text.

[h] The increased requirement during pregnancy cannot be met by the iron content of habitual American diets nor by the existing iron stores of many women; therefore, the use of 30–60 mg of supplemental iron is recommended. Iron needs during lactation are not substantially different from those of nonpregnant women, but continued supplementation of the mother for 2–3 months after parturition is advisable in order to replenish stores depleted by pregnancy.

ESTIMATED SAFE AND ADEQUATE DAILY DIETARY INTAKES OF SELECTED VITAMINS
AND MINERALS[a] (cont.)

	Age (years)	Electrolytes		
		Sodium (mg)	Potassium (mg)	Chloride (mg)
Infants	0–0.5	115–350	350–925	275–700
	0.5–1	250–750	425–1275	400–1200
Children and	1–3	325–975	550–1650	500–1500
Adolescents	4–6	450–1350	775–2325	700–2100
	7–10	600–1800	1000–3000	925–2775
	11+	900–2700	1525–4575	1400–4200
Adults		1100–3300	1875–5625	1700–5100

[a]Because there is less information on which to base allowances, these figures are not given in the main table of RDA and are provided here in the form of ranges or recommended intakes.

[b]Since the toxic levels for many trace elements may be only several times usual intakes, the upper levels for the trace elements given in this table should not be habitually exceeded.

Selected References

BOOKS

AIKAWA, J. K. *Magnesium: Its Biological Significance*. CRC Press, Inc., Boca Raton, Fla. (1981).

ALFIN-SLATER, R. B., AND KRITCHEVSKY, D. *Human Nutrition: Nutrition and the Adult*, Vol. 3A, *Macronutrients*, and *Micronutrients*. Vol. 3B, Plenum Press, New York (1980).

ANGHILERI, L. J., AND TUFFET-ANGHILERI, A. M. *The Role of Calcium in Biological Systems*, Vol. III. CRC Press, Inc., Boca Raton, Fla. (1982).

ARMS, K., AND CAMP, P. *Origin of Life*, in *Biology*, 2nd ed., Chapter 19. CBS College Publishing, New York (1982).

BANNISTER, J. V., AND BANNISTER, W. H. *The Biology and Chemistry of Active Oxygen*, Vol. 26. Elsevier Science Publishers, New York (1984).

BECKER, W. M. *Energy and the Living Cell*. J. B. Lippincott Company, Philadelphia. (1977).

BELL, G. H., DAVIDSON, J. N., AND SCARBOROUGH, H. *Textbook of Physiology and Biochemistry*, 5th ed. The Williams & Wilkins Company, Baltimore, Md. (1961).

BENDER, D. A., AND BARKER, B. M. *Vitamins in Medicine*, 4th ed. William Heinemann Medical Books Ltd., London (1980).

BOWEN, H. J. M. *Trace Elements in Biochemistry*. Academic Press, Inc., New York (1966).

BRISSON, G. J. *Lipids in Human Nutrition*. Jack K. Burgess, Inc., Englewood, N.J. (1981).

CHRISTIE, W. W. *Lipid Analysis*, 2nd ed. Pergamon Press Inc., Elmsford, N.Y. (1982).

CIBA FOUNDATION SYMPOSIUM 101. *Biology of Vitamin E*. Pitman Books Ltd., London (1983).

CIBA FOUNDATION SYMPOSIUM 65. Biosynthesis of Prostaglandins, in *Oxygen Free Radicals and Tissue Damage*, R. J. Flower, ed., pp. 123–142. Excerpta Medica, Amsterdam (1979).

COMBS, JR. G. F., SPALLHOLZ, J. E., LEVANDER, O., AND OLDFIELD, J., EDS. *Proceedings, 3rd International Symposium on Selenium in Biology and Medicine, Beijing.* An AVI book by Van Nostrand Reinhold Company, Inc., New York (1987).

COMBS, JR. G. F., AND COMBS, S. B. *The Role of Selenium in Nutrition.* Academic Press, Inc., New York (1986).

FRIEDEN, E., ED. *Biochemistry of the Essential Ultratrace Elements.* Vol. 3. Plenum Press, New York (1984).

GURR, M. I. *Role of Fats in Food and Nutrition.* Elsevier Applied Science Publishers, New York (1984).

HAMILTON, E. I. *The Chemical Elements and Man.* Charles C Thomas, Publisher, Springfield, Ill. (1979).

HARRISON, P. M., AND HOARE, R. J. *Metals in Biochemistry.* Chapman & Hall Ltd., London (1980).

HENKIN, R. I., CHAIRMAN. *Zinc.* National Research Council, University Park Press, Baltimore, Md. (1979).

HOEKSTRA, W. G., ET AL., EDS. *Trace Elements in Man and Animals (TEMA-2).* University Park Press, Baltimore, Md. (1974).

HOWELL, J. M., HAWTHORNE, J. M., AND WHITE, C. L., EDS. *Trace Elements in Man and Animals (TEMA-4). Australian Academy of Science,* Canberra (1981).

IRWIN, M. I. *Nutritional Requirements of Man.* The Nutrition Foundation, Inc., Washington, D.C. (1980).

JACOBS, A. *Iron in Biochemistry and Medicine.* Academic Press, Inc., New York (1980).

KIRCHGESSNER, M., ED., *Trace Elements in Man and Animals (TEMA-3).* Technische Universitat, Munich, West Germany (1978).

KRATZER, F. H., AND VOHRA, P. N. *Chelates in Nutrition.* CRC Press, Inc., Boca Raton, Fla. (1986).

LEHNINGER, A. I. *Biochemistry,* 2nd ed. Worth Publishers, Inc., New York (1970).

LEHNINGER, A. I. *Bioengenetics: The Molecular Basis of Biological Energy Transformations,* W. A. Benjamin, Inc. New York (1965).

LEVANDER, O. A., AND CHENG, L., EDS. *Micronutrient Interactions: Vitamins, Minerals and Hazardous Elements,* Vol. 355. New York Academy of Sciences, New York (1980).

MACHLIN, L. *Handbook of Vitamins.* Marcel Dekker, Inc., New York (1984).

MEAD, J. F., ALFIN-SLATER, HAWTON, D. R., AND POPJAK, G. *Lipids: Chemistry, Biochemistry and Nutrition.* Plenum Press, New York (1986).

MERTZ, W., AND CORNATZER, W. E. *Newer Trace Elements in Nutrition (TEMA-2).* Marcel Dekker, Inc., New York (1971).

METCALFE, H. C., WILLIAMS, J., CASTKA, J., AND DULL, C. *Modern Chemistry,* Holt, Reinhart and Winston, New York (1974).

MILLS, C. F., ED. *Trace Elements in Man and Animals (TEMA-1).* E. & S. Livingstone, London (1970).

MILLS, C. F., BRENNER, I., AND CHESTERS, J. K., EDS. *Trace Elements in Man and Animals (TEMA-5).* Churchill, Edinburgh (1970).

MORTVEDT, J. S., ET AL. EDS. *Proceedings, Microelements in Agriculture.* Soil Science Society of America, Inc., Madison, Wis. (1972).

PRASAD, A. S. *Current Topics in Nutrition and Disease*, Vol. 6. Alan R. Liss, Inc. New York (1982).

RENNERT, O. M., ED. *Metabolism of Trace Elements in Man*. CRC Press, Inc., Boca Raton, Fla. (1984).

ROBINSON, M. T. *Proceedings, New Zealand Workshop on Trace Elements in New Zealand*. University of Otago, Dunedin, New Zealand (1981).

ROE, D. A. *Handbook: Interactions of Selected Drugs and Nutrients in Patients*. 3rd ed. The American Dietetic Association, Chicago (1982).

ROTH, H. P., CHAIRMAN. *Symposium on Role of Dietary Fiber in Health*. American Journal of Clinical Nutrition, Supplement 20477, Vol. 3 (1978).

SEBRELL, W. H., JR., AND HARRIS R. S., EDS. *The Vitamins: Chemistry, Physiology, Pathology, Methods*. 2nd ed. Vol. 5. Academic Press, Inc., New York (1972).

Selenium in Nutrition. National Academy of Sciences, Washington, D.C. (1976).

SIROTNAK, R. M., ED. *Folate Antagonists as Therapeutic Agents*. Academic Press, Inc., New York (1984).

SPALLHOLZ, J. E., MARTIN, J. L., AND GANTHER, H. E. *Proceedings, 2nd International Symposium on Selenium in Biology and Medicine, Lubbock, Texas*. AVI Publishing Company, Westport, Conn. (1981).

SPILLER, G. A., ED. *CRC Handbook of Dietary Fiber in Human Nutrition*. CRC Press, Inc., Boca Raton, Fla. (1987).

SPILLER, G. A., AND AMEN, R. J. *Fiber in Human Nutrition*. Plenum Press, New York (1976).

STARE, F. J., ED. *Atherosclerosis*. MedCom, Inc. New York (1974).

THIELE, V. F. Drugs, in *Clinical Nutrition*, 2nd ed. Chapter 12. The C. V. Mosby Company, St. Louis, Mo. (1980).

UNDERWOOD, E. J. *Trace Elements in Human and Animal Nutrition*, 4th ed. Academic Press, New York (1977).

VOKAL-BOREK, H. *Selenium (USIP Report 79-16)*. Institute of Theoretical Physics, University of Stockholm, Stockholm, Sweden (1979).

WHITE, A., HANDLER, P., AND SMITH, E. *Principles of Biochemistry*. 3rd ed. McGraw-Hill Book Company, New York (1964).

WINDHOLZ, M. W. *The Merck Index*, 9th ed. Merck and Co., Rahway, N.J. (1976).

WILLIS, A. L. Essential Fatty Acids, Prostaglandins and Related Eicosanoids; in *Present Knowledge in Nutrition*, 5th ed., pp. 90–1115. The Nutrition Foundation, Washington, D.C. (1984).

ZAPSALIS, C., AND BECK, R. A. *Food Chemistry and Nutritional Biochemistry*. John Wiley & Sons, Inc., New York (1985).

ARTICLES

ANDERSON, J. W. Physiological and Metabolic Effects of Dietary Fiber. *Fed. Proc. 44*, 2902–2906 (1985).

BIDLOCK, W. R., AND SMITH, C. H. The Effect of Nutritional Factors on Hepatic Drug and Toxicant Metabolism. *J. Am. Diet. Assoc. 84*, 892–898 (1984).

CARAFOLI, E., AND PENNISTON, J. T. The Calcium Signal. *Sci. Am.* (Nov. 1985).

CHANCE, B., SIES, H., AND BOVERIS, A. Hydroperoxide Metabolism in Mammalian Organs. *Phys. Rev. 59*, 527–605 (1979).

EGAMI, F. Minor Elements and Evolution. *J. Mol. Evol. 4*, 113–120 (1974).

EGAMI, F. Origin and Evolution of Transition Element Enzymes. *J. Biochem. 77*, 1165–1169 (1975).

FOLKERS, K. Perspectives from Research on Vitamins and Hormones. *J. Chem. Ed. 61*, 747–756 (1984).

FRIEDEN, E. The Chemical Elements of Life, Chapter 16, Scientific American Press, New York (1972).

HALFISCH, J., PRATHER, E. S., POWELL, A., CARAFELLI, C., AND REISER, S. Mineral Balances of Men and Women Consuming High Fiber Diets with Complex or Simple Carbohydrates. *J. Nutr. 117*, 48–55 (1987).

HARMON, D. The Aging Process. *Proc. Nat. Acad. Sci. 78*, 7124–7128 (1981).

HOPPS, H. C., AND O'DELL, B., EDS. Research Needed to Improve Data on Mineral Content of Human Tissue. *Fed. Proc. 40*, 2111–2158 (1981).

JACOBS, L. R. Relationship between Dietary Fiber and Cancer: Metabolic, Physiologic and Cellular Mechanisms. *Proc. Soc. Exp. Biol. Med. 183*, 299–310 (1986).

KEINHOLZ, E. Why Water Is So Important to Animals. *Feedstuffs 50* (3), 17–118 (1978).

KINSELLA, J. E., BRUCKNER, G., MAI, J., AND SHRIMP, J. Metabolism of Trans Fatty Acids with Emphasis on the Effects of Trans, Trans-Octadecondienoate on Lipid Composition, Essential Fatty Acid and Prostaglandin: An Overview. *Am. J. Clin. Nutr. 34*, 2307–2316 (1981).

MCCAY, P. B. Physiological Significance of Lipid Peroxidation. A Symposium. *Fed. Proc. 40*, 173–200 (1981).

MEISTER, A., AND ANDERSON, M. E. Glutathione. *Am. Rev. Biochem. 52*, 711–760 (1983).

MILLER, S. M. New Perspectives on Vitamin D. *Am. J. Med. Tech. 49*, 27–36 (1983).

MORRIS, E. R. An Overview of Current Information on Bioavailability of Dietary Iron to Humans. *Fed. Proc. 42*, 1716–1720 (1983).

NIELSEN, F. H. Ultratrace Elements: Current Status. *Nutr. Update 2*, 107–126 (1985).

POLLACK, J. B., AND YUNG, Y. L. Origin and Evolution of Planetary Atmospheres. *Ann. Rev. Earth Planet Sci. 8*, 425–487 (1980).

SCHWARZ, K. Recent Dietary Trace Element Research Exemplified by Tin, Fluorine and Silicon. *Fed. Proc. 33*, 1748–1757 (1974).

SCHWARZ, K. Trace Elements Newly Identified as Essential. *Proc. 9th Int. Congr. Nutr. Mexico 1*, 96–109 (1972).

SHAW, W. H. R. Studies in Biogeochemistry. I. A Biogeochemical Periodic Table. The Data. *Geochim. Cosmochim. Acta 19*, 196–207 (1960).

SHAW, W. H. R. Studies in Biogeochemistry. II. Discussion and References. *Geochim. Cosmochim. Acta 19*, 207–215 (1960).

SMITH, C. H., AND BIDLACK, W. R. Dietary Concerns Associated with the Use of Medications. *J. Am. Diet. Assoc. 84*, 901–914 (1984).

SMITH, J. C., AND SCHWARZ, K. A Controlled Environment System for New Trace Element Deficiencies. *J. Nutr. 93*, 182–188 (1967).

HISTORICAL

GUGGENHEIM, K. Y. *Nutrition and Nutritional Diseases*. The Collamore Press, D. C. Health and Company, Lexington, Mass. (1981).

McCOLLUM, E. V. *A History of Nutrition*. Houghton Miffin Company, Boston (1957).

MENDEL, L. B. *Nutrition: The Chemistry of Life*. Yale University Press, New Haven, Conn. (1923).

Index